Operative Techniques for Severe Liver Injury

Rao R. Ivatury

Editor

Operative Techniques for Severe Liver Injury

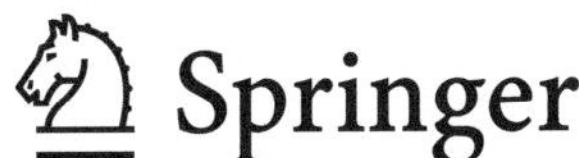 Springer

Editor
Rao R. Ivatury, MD, MS, FACS
Department of Surgery
Virginia Commonwealth University
Richmond, VA
USA

Videos to this book can be accessed at http://www.springerimages.com/
videos/978-1-4939-1199-8

ISBN 978-1-4939-5377-6   ISBN 978-1-4939-1200-1   (eBook)
DOI 10.1007/978-1-4939-1200-1
Springer New York Heidelberg Dordrecht London

Foreword

This is a unique book with chapters written by a unique grouping of surgeons about a unique organ. Although this organ – the liver – is often not the only organ injured, it is frequently the injury to the liver and its integrated vascular structures that determine the ultimate outcome of the patient. Therefore, this book is a valuable resource for anyone, whether surgeon, emergency physician, radiologist, vascular interventionalist, anesthesiologist, or others, interacting in the management of the patient with a liver injury. It will be a valuable, in-depth source document, as well as a ready reference.

The selected authors of the chapters in this book are internationally recognized, skilled technicians, teachers, and writers. Each has written other chapters and journal articles relating to liver injuries, and each has ruminated publicly and privately about never having enough time or space to give justice to this extensive subject. This comprehensive work allows adequate space to thoroughly and completely cover all aspects of the injured liver. The chapters are organized logically, with an orderly flow.

As all authors are experienced and extremely capable surgeons and writers, differing but equally acceptable approaches and opinions may be expressed. And differences will continue to occur, to include even, perhaps, new surgeon-directed endovascular therapy in the operating room for liver injuries. These accepted variations are what allow for, and, indeed, encourage academic scientific comparisons, which form the basis of large prospective clinical studies (and future editions).

This book focuses on technique – the technical aspects of exposure of hepatic and juxta-hepatic injuries, control of bleeding, and management of the injuries. Each chapter contains some history, some technique, and some data to support the author's conclusions, along with journal references, but it remains a book on technique. Surgeons like and are attracted to books on technical process, for that is what we do. It is our genomic craft. The life and function of our patients depend on the surgeon's ability to know the anatomy, understand the injury, have an ability to control hemorrhage, and expose the injury, and, of course, reconstruct the anatomy as well as possible.

Analysis of the chapter titles of this book reveals several that have not been traditionally part of past texts relating to liver injury. Several chapters at the end of the book underscore the benefit of linking the advances in trauma surgery to advances in simulation, transplantation, and non-trauma hepatobiliary surgery.

Finally, this is an ideal technical textbook to be recommended to acute care/trauma/emergency surgeons who want to continue on the cutting edge of being a "top knife surgeon."

Kenneth L. Mattox, MD, FACS
Distinguished Service Professor
Baylor College of Medicine
Chief of Staff/Chief of Surgery
Ben Taub General Hospital
Houston, TX, USA

Preface

In the present era of non-operative management of solid organ injuries, operative control of hemorrhage from liver injury has become an increasingly rare phenomenon. Damage control operations with liver packing and subsequent angio-embolization, even in situations when they may not be the most optimal approach, have become the popular methods of care. Consequently, the younger trauma surgeon has minimal experience in advanced surgical techniques of controlling hemorrhage. This surgical immaturity and inexperience are a tremendous handicap when faced with an unstable patient exsanguinating from a complex liver injury. The critical surgical skills in treating a crushed liver are now a lost art. Other factors also seem to contribute to this loss of surgical expertise. Several studies have now established that the operative experience of the surgical residents has declined due to restriction of duty hours. For instance, Lucas reported that recent graduating chief surgical residents performed a mean of 1.2 operations for hemostasis with liver injuries with most having no experience with complex techniques of liver injury management such as tractotomy or hepatic resection [1]. This becomes a serious issue when the inexperienced surgeon is faced with high grade solid organ injury in the hemodynamically unstable patient. Perihepatic packing, damage-control laparotomy, and angio-embolization are valuable ancillary techniques in such situations but are only ancillary to skillful operative techniques of bleeding control.

It is apparent, therefore, that the students and practitioners of trauma surgery must be prepared for the intra-operative challenge of uncontrollable hemorrhage from a ruptured liver or a torn retrohepatic vein. Unfortunately, our current training programs are more complete in the education of pre- and post-operative affairs rather than intra-operative techniques themselves.

Several options are currently under way to remedy this situation. Simulators, animal laboratories, and cadaveric dissections are being incorporated into the curriculum of the trainee in an attempt to give the students of trauma the necessary skills and confidence. What is perhaps equally important is the prelude for these hands-on exercises by "how-I-do-it" tutorials from seasoned "master surgeons" who gained their expertise from their everyday experience on the battle field of civilian trauma.

This book on the surgical approaches to the severely injured liver is a collection of these tutorials narrated by the masters themselves. It aims to bring all available techniques of hemostasis of a complex liver injury into one detailed volume. Their text is supplemented with line drawings, operative pictures, cadaveric dissections, and even images of simulation. Videos of important techniques bring to life the static text of descriptions. It is hoped that the reader will find these helpful to consult, even in the middle of a difficult operation. The final chapters of the book discuss the future of training in operative trauma surgery: animal lab, simulators, and time on hepato-biliary and/or transplantation services to correct a critical deficiency in our surgical training.

The distinguished authors of this volume were asked to describe their approach to liver injury as a personal account ("this is all about you in the O.R.") and they contributed their time and expertise very generously. The readers will note that some steps in liver injury management are repeated in multiple chapters. This is deliberately allowed so that the authors can set the stage for their step-wise, escalating maneuvers for the control of complex injuries. The personalized individual "tricks" of these brilliant surgeons are worth noting carefully by reading between the lines of what appears to be a repetitive description. I owe much credit and many thanks to my young and brilliant colleague Francisco Collet M.D. for his crisp videos of operating techniques. I have admired his skill for a long time and his real-time videos of life-threatening situations in the operating room are an inspiration. Gautam Ivatury lent his time and voice very graciously for the videos. My thanks also to Joni Fraser at Springer for her immense help in seeing this work to completion. First and last, this book would not have been completed without the encouragement and patience of Leela, my spouse and partner.

The painful memories of lost battles with severe liver injury in the operating room are the inspiration behind this work. This labor of love would be entirely worth it, if *one* life can be saved by timely and appropriate surgical intervention.

Reference

1. Lucas CE, Ledgerwood AM. The academic challenge of teaching psychomotor skills for hemostasis of solid organ injury. J Trauma. 2009;66:636–40.

Richmond, VA, USA   Rao R. Ivatury MD, MS, FACS

Contents

Contributors

Juan A. Asensio, MD, FACS, FCCM, FRCS (England) Department of Surgery, New York Medical College, Valhalla, NY, USA

Division of Trauma Surgery and Acute Care Surgery, Joel A. Halpern Trauma Center, International Medicine Institute, Research Institute, Westchester Medical Center, Valhalla, NY, USA

Mark W. Bowyer, MD The Norman M. Rich Department of Surgery, Uniformed Services University, Bethesda, MD, USA

L.D. Britt, MD, MPH Department of Surgery, Eastern Virginia Medical School, Norfolk, VA, USA

Brandon Bruns, MD Surgery, R Adams Cowley Shock Trauma Center, University of Maryland, Baltimore, MD, USA

Robert F. Buckman Jr., MD, FACS Operative Experience Inc., North East, MD, USA

Vicente Cortes, MD, FACS Department of Surgery, Reading Hospital, West Reading, PA, USA

Timothy C. Fabian, MD Department of Surgery, University of Tennessee Health Science Center, Memphis, TN, USA

David V. Feliciano, MD Division of General Surgery, Department of Surgery, Indiana University Medical Center, Indianapolis, IN, USA

Salvatore Gruttadauria, MD, PhD, FACS Department of Abdominal Surgery, IsMeTT/UPMC Italy, Mediterranean Institute for Transplantation and Advanced Specialized Therapies (IsMeTT), University of Pittsburgh Medical Center, Palermo, Italy

Brian G. Harbrecht, MD Department of Surgery, University of Louisville Hospital, Louisville, KY, USA

Rao R. Ivatury, MD, MS, FACS Department of Surgery, Virginia Commonwealth University, Richmond, VA, USA

Anna M. Ledgerwood, MD Department of Surgery, Detroit Receiving Hospital, Detroit, MI, USA

Mauricio Millán Division of Trauma and Acute Care Surgery, Department of Surgery, Universidad del Valle, Cali, Colombia

Charles E. Lucas, MD Department of Surgery, Wayne State University, Detroit, MI, USA

Corrado Marini, MD, FACS New York Medical College/Westchester Medical Center, Valhalla, NY, USA

James Wallis Marsh, MD, MBA Department of Surgery, University of Pittsburgh School of Medicine, Pittsburgh, PA, USA

Adrian W. Ong, MD Department of Surgery, Reading Hospital, West Reading, PA, USA

Carlos A. Ordoñez, MD Division of Trauma and Acute Care Surgery, Hospital Universitario del Valle, Fundación Valle del Lili, Cali, Colombia

Department of Surgery, Universidad del Valle, Cali, Colombia

H. Leon Pachter, MD Department of Surgery, New York University School of Medicine, New York, NY, USA

Duilio Pagano, MD, PhD Division of Abdominal Surgery and Transplantation, Department of Surgery, Istituto Mediterraneo per i Trapianti e Terapie ad Alta Specializzazione (IsMeTT), Palermo, Italy

Michael W. Parra, MD Division of Trauma Critical Care, Broward General Level I Trauma Center, Fort Lauderdale, FL, USA

Andrew B. Peitzman, MD Department of Surgery, University of Pittsburgh, Pittsburgh, PA, USA

Alejandro J. Pérez-Alonso, MD Westchester Medical Center, Valhalla, NY, USA

Patrizio Petrone, MD, MPH New York Medical College/Westchester Medical Center, Valhalla, NY, USA

K. Shad Pharaon, MD Division of Trauma, Critical Care, and Acute Care Surgery, Department of Surgery, Oregon Health and Science University, Portland, OR, USA

Department of Trauma and Acute Care Surgery, Surgery Critical Care, PeaceHealth Southwest Medical Center, Vancouver, WA, USA

Anthony Policastro, MD Westchester Medical Center, Valhalla, NY, USA

J. David Richardson, MD Department of Surgery, University of Louisville Hospital, Louisville, KY, USA

Aurelio Rodriguez, MD Division of Trauma/Critical Care, Department of Surgery, Conemaugh Memorial Hospital, Johnstown, PA, USA

Thomas M. Scalea, MD R Adams Cowley Shock Trauma Center at, University of Maryland, Baltimore, MD, USA

Marco Spada, MD, PhD Division of Abdominal Surgery and Transplantation, Department of Surgery, Istituto Mediterraneo per i Trapianti e Terapie ad Alta Specializzazione (ISMETT), Palermo, Italy

Department of Surgery, School of Medicine, University of Pittsburgh, Pittsburgh, PA, USA

S. Rob Todd, MD, FACS Trauma and Emergency Surgery, Bellevue Hospital Center, New York, NY, USA

Department of Surgery and Anesthesiology, New York University School of Medicine, New York, NY, USA

Donald D. Trunkey, MD Section of Trauma and Critical Care, Department of Surgery, Oregon Health and Science University, Portland, OR, USA

Juan Manuel Verde, MD Westchester Medical Center, Valhalla, NY, USA

Jordan A. Weinberg, MD Department of Surgery, University of Tennessee Health Science Center, Memphis, TN, USA

Surgical Anatomy of the Liver

1

Thomas M. Scalea and Brandon R. Bruns

Surgical Anatomy

Throughout medical history, the anatomy of the liver has perplexed anatomists and surgeons alike. The complex vascular anatomy of the liver produces the capacity for rapid and life-threatening hemorrhage from the injured liver. Major liver injuries requiring operation are relatively rare. Thus, the injured liver can be a challenge even to the most-skilled surgeon. The anatomic relationships within the peritoneal cavity make the liver relatively inaccessible. Complete mobilization is necessary to deliver the liver to a position where operative repair is possible. To rapidly and adequately manage the bleeding liver, the surgeon must understand the three-dimensional anatomic relationships within the liver parenchyma.

Gross Anatomy

The liver is the largest solid organ in the human body and lies in the right upper quadrant of the peritoneal cavity. It is shielded anteriorly by the confines of the thoracic cage and bordered in an anterosuperior direction by the peritoneal surface of the diaphragm. Inferiorly, the liver is in contact with intra-abdominal viscera including the right kidney (Fig. 1.1), forming the potential space of the hepatorenal recess, or Morrison's pouch. Other inferior visceral relationships include the lesser curvature of the stomach, the second and third portions of the duodenum, the gallbladder,

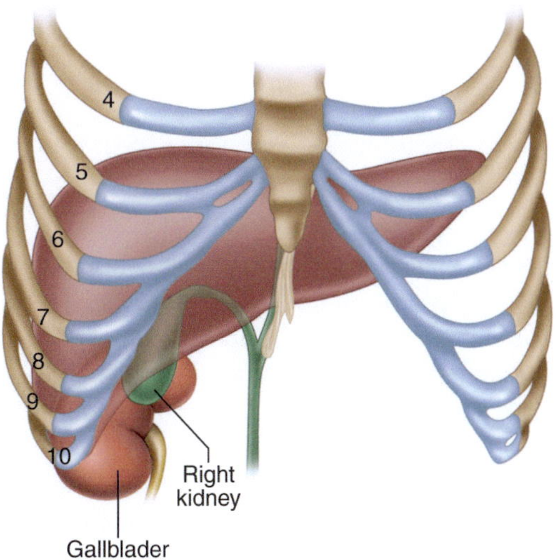

Fig. 1.1 The intrathoracic location of the liver and the inferior location of the right kidney. *4–10* indicate rib numbers

T.M. Scalea, MD (✉) • B.R. Bruns, MD
Department of Surgery,
R Adams Cowley Shock Trauma Center,
University of Maryland, 22 S. Greene Street,
Baltimore, MD 21201, USA
e-mail: tscalea@umm.edu; bbruns@umm.edu

R.R. Ivatury (ed.), *Operative Techniques for Severe Liver Injury*,
DOI 10.1007/978-1-4939-1200-1_1, © Springer Science+Business Media New York 2015

1

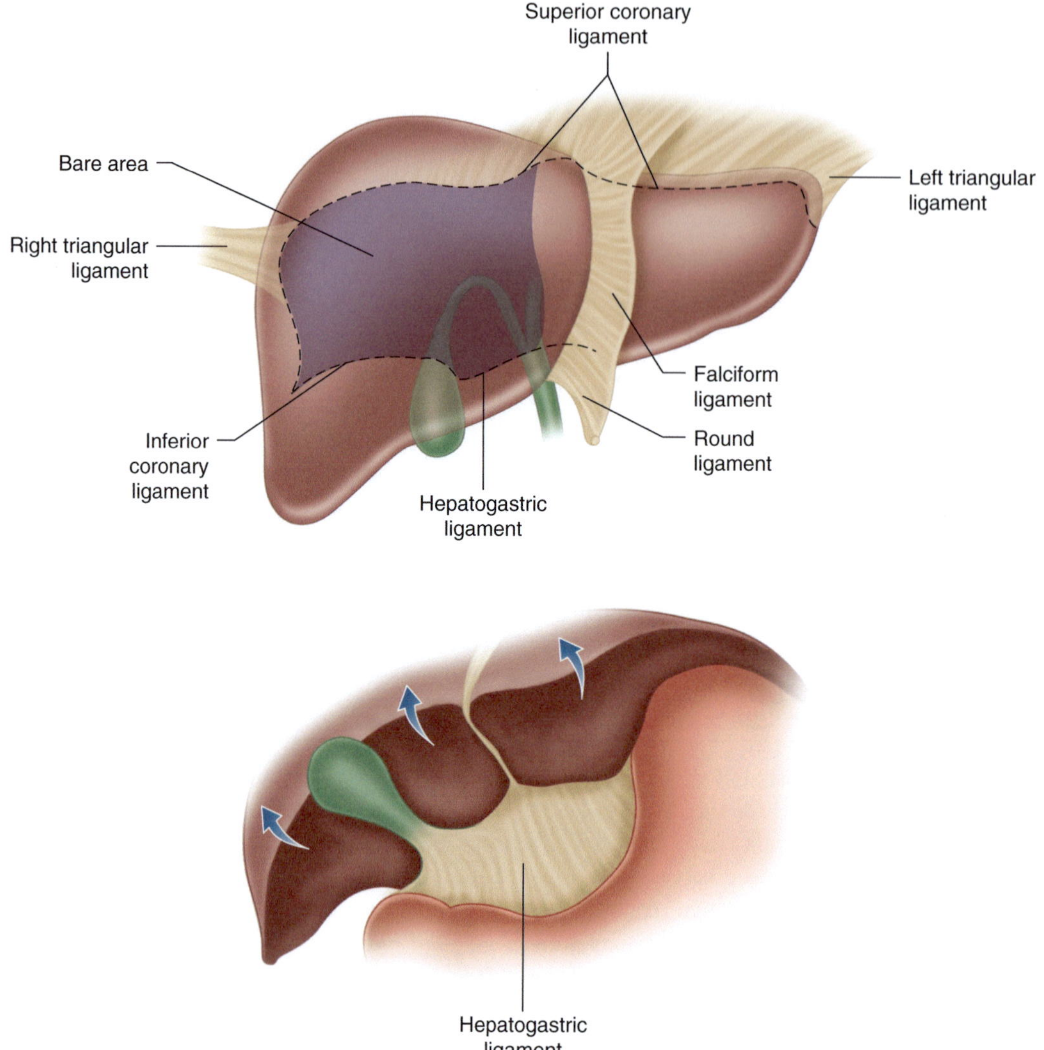

Fig. 1.2 The ligamentous attachments of the liver and the enclosed bare area. *Arrow* shows direction of mobilization, would leave un-labeled.

the porta hepatis, and the vasculature of the right kidney. Posteriorly, the surface projections of the liver lie in close approximation with the vertical diaphragm, superior pole of the right kidney, right adrenal gland, and the retrohepatic portion of the inferior vena cava.

The protected position of the liver in the recesses of the right upper quadrant mandates complete liberation of the liver from its peritoneal attachments for adequate exposure and visualization of hepatic injuries. The peritoneal attachments include the falciform ligament, coronary liga-

ment, triangular ligaments, and the hepatogastric ligament. The coronary and triangular ligaments essentially suspend the liver from the parietal peritoneum superiorly and enclose the bare area of the liver, which lies at the apex of the organ (Fig. 1.2).

The Glissonian capsule surrounds the liver parenchyma and extends to envelope the portal triad as it enters the liver consisting of the portal vein, the hepatic artery, and the bile duct. The portal vein lies deepest in the triad, with the hepatic duct normally occupying the superficial lateral position and the artery the superficial medial

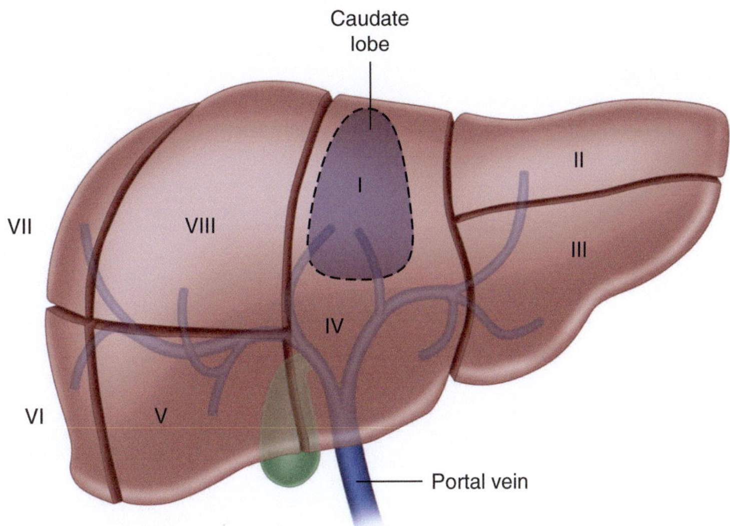

Fig. 1.3 The segmental nature of the liver and relationship to the portal vein

position. A fibrous sheath of connective tissues envelopes the triad at the hepatic hilum and is referred to as the hilar plate, which lies in continuity with the cystic and umbilical plates and acts as a protective barrier for the extrahepatic triad.

Segmental Anatomy

Many have contributed to our current understanding of hepatic anatomy, though most credit Claude Couinaud's 1954 work, *Lobes et segments hepatiques*, with the definitive documentation of hepatic segmental anatomy and the standardization of segmental terminology. Couinaud's descriptions were unique as they were based on anatomic relationships to the main portal vein and its branches, as the variability of portal vein anatomy is much less than that of the hepatic artery or duct.

Couinaud described three levels of the liver: the right and left hemi-livers, the sectors, and the segments. The portal vein bifurcation into right and left branches divides the liver into its right and left hemi-livers, as based on portal venous blood supply.

Further division of the right and left portal veins divides the right and left lobes of the livers into sectors; two are present on the right and two on the left. The right hemi-liver is divided into anterior and posterior sectors. The posterior sector consists of segments VI and VII, and the right anterior sector consists of segments V and VIII.

The left portal vein divides into two branches, one to segment II and one to segments III and IV. Thus, the left hemi-liver consists of a lateral sector (segment II) and a paramedian sector (segments III and IV), which are separated by the falciform and round ligaments. Segment I, or the caudate lobe, lies posterior to the right hemi-liver and between the portal vein bifurcation and vena cava with its own hepatic venous drainage and portal venous tributary (Fig. 1.3).

Couinaud further described the suprahepatic sectoral anatomy and its relationships to the right, middle, and left hepatic venous drainage. The course of the portal venous division overlaps with the hepatic venous drainage and thus helps define the eight portal segments and their drainage pattern.

Hepatic Arterial Anatomy

Hepatic arterial anatomy is well recognized for its multiple variations and their surgical implications in hepatic surgery. Recognition of these anatomic variations is critical when pursuing operative intervention for traumatic liver injury, as indiscriminate ligation can lead to hepatic ischemia and necrosis.

Fig. 1.4 (**a**) The most common variant of hepatic arterial supply, (**b**) replaced right hepatic artery, and (**c**) replaced left hepatic arterial variants

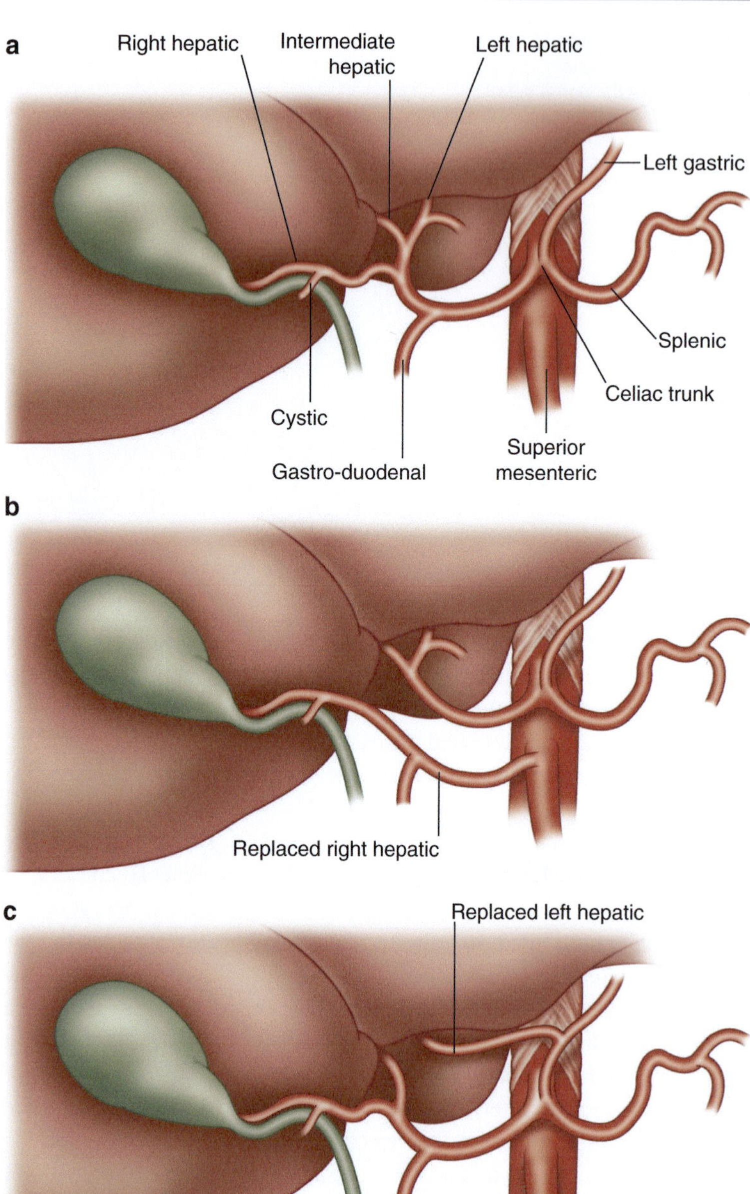

The most common variant involves the common hepatic artery originating from the celiac trunk prior to its division into hepatic artery proper and gastroduodenal artery. The proper hepatic artery then continues its course toward the hilum of the liver before bifurcating into the right and left hepatic arteries within the hilar plate.

The next two most common variants consist of the replaced or accessory origins of the right and left hepatic arteries. Replaced arteries act as the sole blood supply to its equivalent hemi-liver and accessory arteries act as an additional source of arterial blood. Replaced or accessory right hepatic arteries originate from the superior mesenteric artery and can be found intraoperatively by the presence of an arterial pulse along the lateral border of the hepatoduodenal ligament. Replaced or accessory left hepatic arteries originate from the left gastric artery and manifest as an arterial pulse in the lesser omentum (Fig. 1.4). Less common anomalies include double-replaced patterns, common hepatic arterial derivation from the superior mesenteric artery, and common hepatic artery origin directly from the aorta, among others.

Hepatic Vein Anatomy

Venous drainage is accomplished by a series of three major hepatic veins, along with a series of 10–50 smaller veins. Hepatic veins lack the Glissonian sheath surrounding the portal triad and its structures, thus contributing to their fragility. The majority of the course of these veins lies within the parenchyma of the liver, with only short segments of each lying extrahepatic before their junction with the inferior vena cava. The extrahepatic portions typically measure from 0.5 to 1.5 cm, making surgical control difficult. Additionally, a series of exceedingly fragile and short retro-hepatic veins drain directly into the inferior vena cava from the liver parenchyma.

The middle hepatic vein lies in the median fissure of the liver and joins with the left hepatic vein, to emerge from the liver as a single vein in greater than 50 % of humans. The middle and left hepatic veins serve to drain primarily segments II, III, and IV. The right hepatic vein is the largest of the three veins and lies in the right fissure on its course to the inferior vena cava. This large right hepatic vein drains segments V, VI, VII, and a portion of segment VIII. Segments V and VIII are also drained by tributaries of the middle hepatic vein. Segment I has its own drainage directly into the inferior vena cava. The hepatic venous drainage of the liver lies deep within the peritoneal cavity and complete hepatic mobilization is required for visualization and repair.

Biliary Tract Anatomy

The bile duct acts as one third of the portal triad accompanying the portal vein and hepatic artery into the hepatic hilum and subsequently branching in concert with the other two. The left and right hepatic ducts join to form the common hepatic duct at the hilum and exit the liver on its course to the duodenum. Extrahepatic bile duct variation is fairly common and must be identified during the course of operation to avoid ductal injury.

Segments V, VI, VII, and VIII (the right hemi-liver) are drained of bile by the right hepatic ductal system. Segment VI and VII bile ducts converge to form the posterior right hepatic duct and segments V and VIII converge to form the anterior right hepatic duct. These ducts then converge, with many anatomic variations, to form the right hepatic duct, which is most commonly vertical and approximately 1 cm in length.

Segments II, III, and IV (the left hemi-liver) are drained by the left bile duct with segments II and III draining in tandem, joined by the duct from segment IV. Segment I has its own biliary drainage going to both hepatic ducts 80 % of the time, solely to the left hepatic duct 15 % of the time, and solely to the right hepatic duct in approximately 5 % of cases.

The confluence of the right and left hepatic ducts occurs outside the hepatic parenchyma running anterior to the origin of the right branch of the portal vein. At the hilar level, the bile duct is joined by the hepatic artery and portal vein in the thickened and dense connective tissue of Glisson's capsule, the hilar plate. The hepatic duct continues on its course toward the duodenum with the portal vein deep and the hepatic artery immediately to the left of the duct.

The blood supply to the supraduodenal bile duct typically arises from the gastroduodenal artery, right branch of the hepatic artery, retroduodenal artery, and cystic arteries, among others. The arteries run along the lateral borders of the bile ducts in a segmental fashion with blood supply coursing from superior and inferior vessels. At the hilar plate, the bile duct enjoys a rich supply of arterial blood from the confluence of the right and left arterial systems. Venous drainage of the duct typically parallels the arterial supply.

Portal Venous Anatomy

The portal vein originates behind the neck of the pancreas and is formed by the combination of the superior mesenteric and splenic veins. Along its extrahepatic course, the portal vein measures approximately 8 cm in length and approximately 1–1.5 cm in diameter. The vein is unique in that it does not possess valves and does not return blood directly to the heart, instead filtering blood through the hepatic sinusoidal capillary network prior to return to the right heart. Surgical access to the portal vein is accomplished by performing a full Kocher maneuver of the duodenum to the level of the superior mesenteric vein, thus enabling visualization of the triad.

The extrahepatic portal vein bifurcates at the porta hepatis and continues as the right and left portal venous branches. On the left, the course of the portal vein is long and tangential, with an initial branch to segment I as it continues to its umbilical portion where it is joins the round ligament. The left portal vein differs from the left hepatic artery and duct by nature of the fact that it divides into medial and lateral segmental branches and further subdivides into superior and inferior subsegmental branches. The right branch of the portal vein is short in comparison to the left and also contributes a branch to segment I. Unlike the left, the right portal vein follows the course of the right hepatic artery and duct as it proceeds into the right hemi-liver.

Implications for Surgical Care

By virtue of its size, the liver is the most injured organ within the abdomen. Blunt force trauma often injures the liver, particularly if applied to the epigastrium or right upper quadrant. Penetrating injury to the right thoracoabdominal area virtually always injures the liver. In the past, operative therapy was used for diagnosis of abdominal injury and operating on the injured liver was relatively common. Newer diagnostic modalities have made liver operations for injury relatively rare. Thus, many surgeons have limited experience in the techniques of hepatic mobilization and repair. However, knowledge of hepatic anatomy is essential for safe operative therapy of the liver.

As the liver is located high up in the right side of the abdominal cavity, it is protected by the ribcage. The ligamentous attachments fix the liver in position posteriorly. Thus, visualizing the areas of hepatic injury can be problematic, particularly when located posteriorly on the right lobe or in the bare area of the liver. Full mobilization is essential in order to clearly identify stage and treat liver injuries. The liver must be delivered onto the anterior abdominal wall. Operating on the liver when it remains in the right upper quadrant is dangerous and fraught with difficulty.

Mobilizing the liver begins by taking down and completely dividing the falciform ligament, all the way to the level of the vena cava. The posterior ligamentous attachments must also be taken completely down in order to deliver the injured lobe, or lobes, into the surgeon's visual field. Phrenic veins can run within the substance of the posterior ligaments and care must be taken to avoid injuring them. As one approaches the vena cava, it is necessary to take the last portion of the ligaments down carefully, as iatrogenic injury to the hepatic veins will produce torrential hemorrhage.

Some liver injuries may spontaneously tamponade. Full mobilization of the liver may disturb this hemostatic clot and injuries that have spontaneously stopped bleeding may bleed again. This is particularly problematic in the area of hepatic veins. The surgeon must balance these issues when making decisions about the therapy of liver injuries.

Injury to the liver rarely follows the anatomic lines. Multiple segments are often involved. As the liver is fixed posteriorly, it is freely mobile anteriorly. Thus, long linear lacerations can occur in the liver. Examination of the external surface of the liver often underestimates the damage within the substance of the liver. Direct force injury often creates large stellate lacerations that extend deep into the central portion of the liver. The surgeon must keep this in mind and be prepared to deal with these complex injuries deep in the substance of the liver.

The liver parenchyma itself is spongy. The vascular and biliary structures that run within the parenchyma have far more substance and are obviously the structures that must be controlled. Therefore, it is often necessary to divide normal liver in order to identify and control injuries. A number of techniques exist. "Finger fracturing" the liver allows the surgeon to divide the substance of the liver, identifying biliary and vascular structures. This "fracturing" can be done between the thumb and the index finger. Alternatively, the back end of a scalpel handle is very effective at dissecting the liver parenchyma off of the vascular and biliary radicals, which can be tied or clipped as they are encountered. This often is relatively time consuming. Use of a universal stapling device makes the dissection much quicker. It is important not to force the stapler into the liver, as that will almost certainly injure vascular structures, making bleeding worse. Gentle pressure allows the stapler jaws to enter the liver parenchyma, which can then be safely divided.

It is mandatory to use meticulous technique when both mobilizing and handling the liver. Injured blood vessels often retract deep into the substance of the liver. Controlling these retracted blood vessels may be a significant problem and create a real challenge.

As the hepatic arterial, portal, venous, and biliary branches run immediately adjacent to one another, all three are virtually always injured. Techniques such as finger fracturing allows the surgeon to divide the liver, hopefully providing good visualization of the injured liver relatively deep in the parenchyma. Large liver sutures can be utilized to simply coapt the injured hepatic edges. However, this technique risks simply closing a bridge of liver over injured liver deep in the parenchyma. If there are hepatic arterial branches of any substance that have not been ligated, the bleeding will simply continue until the liver ruptures and free hemorrhage into the peritoneal cavity ensues.

The initial hemostatic maneuver often used is the Pringle maneuver. Placing a vascular clamp across the porta occludes the hepatic artery and portal vein. This should provide good hemostasis via inflow control. Of course, the Pringle maneuver does nothing to control hepatic venous bleeding. The Pringle maneuver can be used as both a diagnostic tool and for temporary hemostasis. If bleeding is not markedly reduced when the clamp is applied, there must be significant hepatic venous component to the area of injury.

Hepatic arterial and portal venous structures enter the liver via the porta and then branch to supply the left and right lobes. Hepatic injury

rarely completely divides either lobe of the liver. Thus, the vascular structures remain intact in the uninjured portion of the liver. The injured liver thus bleeds on both sides of the injury. This makes resectional debridement extremely attractive as a technique. If the surgeon simply removes the liver laterally to the injury, there is only one surface left that can bleed. Vascular structures should easily be able to be identified and ligated.

The hepatic veins enter the liver via the inferior vena cava, just below the area of the diaphragm. These large, very short vessels are thin walled and bleed impressively. Their location makes them extraordinarily difficult to control. If excessive force is applied to the liver during mobilization, iatrogenic hepatic venous injury can occur. These are difficult to visualize, even with full mobilization of the liver. Retrohepatic vena caval injuries are among the most deadly. A number of techniques exist to try to reduce hemorrhage from either the hepatic veins or the vena cava immediately adjacent to them. Inserting an atrio-caval shunt is an attractive technique as it should provide proximal and distal control of the vena cava yet allow venous return to the heart. Unfortunately, there are many small veins between the liver substance and the retrohepatic cava. Thus, the hemorrhage control with an atrio-caval shunt is less than ideal. Other techniques such as venovenous bypass also allow shunting of the blood away from the injured cava. Many techniques exist, none however, are ideal.

Conclusion

Knowledge of the surgical anatomy of the liver is imperative for safe and efficient operative management of hepatic trauma. In the current era of increasing nonoperative management of hepatic injury, fewer surgeons have the requisite operative experience necessary to confidently manage complex liver trauma. Therefore, it becomes incumbent upon the practicing trauma surgeon to approach these injuries with a full knowledge of the liver's surgical anatomy and a well-rehearsed operative plan in an effort to achieve optimal outcomes.

Treatment of Liver Injuries: An Overview

Charles E. Lucas and Anna M. Ledgerwood

Introduction

The liver is the largest organ in the body and the organ most frequently injured. This is true for both blunt and penetrating wounds [1, 2]. The morbidity and mortality associated with liver injury vary with the associated hemorrhagic shock insult, the severity of liver injury as judged by the Abbreviated Injury Score (AIS), and the presence or absence of bleeding at the time of operative intervention [3–5]. The severity of injury related to missile wounds correlates directly with the amount of energy that is dissipated as the missile traverses the liver, with the energy being calculated by the classic formula of $energy = mass \times volume^2 \div 2$. Thus, high velocity missiles have the greatest potential for creating the worst injuries. When a patient with a liver injury presents with severe hemorrhagic shock that is not rapidly reversible with preoperative resuscitation, the mortality is very high; when the hemorrhagic shock insult is corrected while in transit to the operating room, the mortality is low; when there is no associated hemorrhagic shock, the mortality is negligible [3, 5]. The presence or absence of bleeding at the time of operative intervention correlates closely with the AIS. Patients with major AIS (4, 5) have a 70 % chance of active bleeding at the time of operation compared to only a 30 % chance of active bleeding in patients with a minor liver injury (AIS 1, 2, 3) [3, 5]. Active bleeding in these patients appears to be the primary cause of death. In a prospective study of 637 patients treated over 5 years, 46 of the 68 patients who died in association with active intraoperative bleeding died within the first 24 h, whereas when bleeding from the liver was controlled with a temporary pack, only six of the 26 deaths occurred within the first 24 h [1, 2]. The mortality following liver injury is also related to the number of associated injuries, particularly those involving named intra-abdominal vessels. Mortality with isolated liver injury is less than 5 %, whereas mortality in patients with five or more associated injuries exceeds 75 % [1, 6].

C.E. Lucas, MD (✉)
Department of Surgery, Wayne State University,
4201 St. Antoine Street, Room 2V,
Detroit, MI 48201, USA
e-mail: clucas@med.wayne.edu

A.M. Ledgerwood, MD
Department of Surgery, Detroit Receiving Hospital,
4201 St. Antoine Street, Room 2V,
Detroit, MI 48201, USA
e-mail: aledgerw@med.wayne.edu

Surgical Incision

Patients about to undergo operation for suspected liver injury should have full prep of the chest and abdomen in anticipation that the thoracic

Electronic supplementary material Supplementary material is available in the online version of this chapter at 10.1007/978-1-4939-1200-1_2. Videos can also be accessed at http://www.springerimages.com/videos/978-1-4939-1199-8.

R.R. Ivatury (ed.), *Operative Techniques for Severe Liver Injury*,
DOI 10.1007/978-1-4939-1200-1_2, © Springer Science+Business Media New York 2015

Fig. 2.1 Patients presenting with a large truncal defect in the right upper quadrant/right lower chest from a close-range shotgun blast or rifle wound (**a**) should be explored by an oblique incision which extends through the large defect and, if needed, can be extended inferiorly along the midline of the abdomen (**b**)

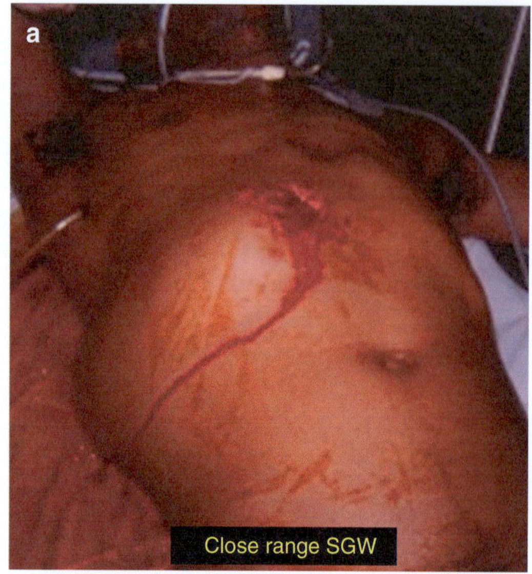

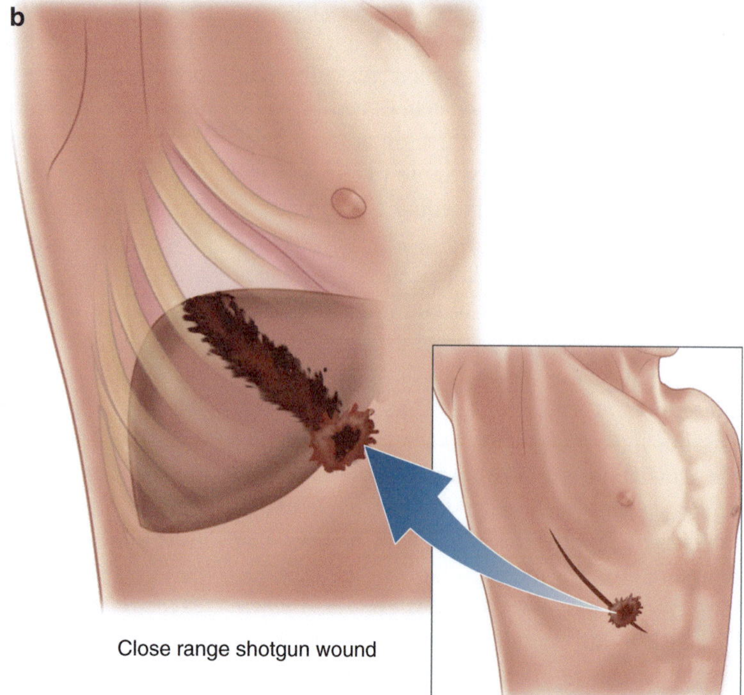

extension of an abdominal incision might be necessary [7–9]. The most efficient initial incision is the midline laparotomy extending from xiphoid to umbilicus or below depending upon intraoperative findings. Exceptions to this policy occur when a patient presents with a large truncal defect due to a high velocity rifle wound or a close-range shotgun wound. In this setting, the laparotomy or combined thoracoabdominal approach should incorporate the large truncal defect as part of the incision (Fig. 2.1) [2]. Although the thoracoabdominal incision provides excellent exposure to patients with major liver injuries, they tend to be associated with greater morbidity in comparison to the median sternotomy, which can be used to provide

Fig. 2.2 The midline laparotomy provides the most practical approach to patients with both blunt and penetrating wounds involving the liver (**a**). This incision can then be extended superiorly as a median sternotomy in order to get control of bleeding from dome of the liver or from the hepatic veins (**a**). The diaphragm can be divided in the posterior midline to facilitate this control(**b**)

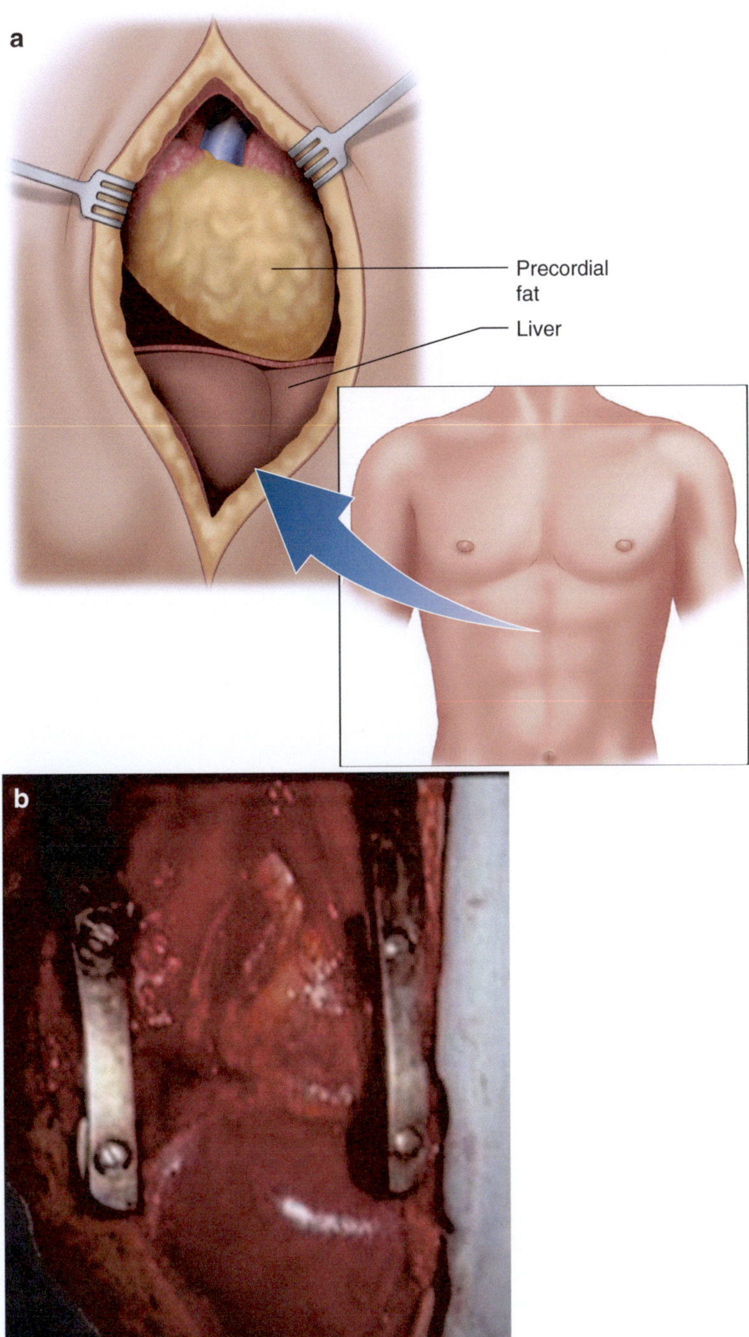

complete liver mobilization (Fig. 2.2) [2, 8]. Division of the diaphragm and the median plane from the crura anteriorly also allows for access to the IVC in patients in whom a retrohepatic IVC shunt is anticipated [2, 8].

Temporary Packs

Upon entering the abdomen, rapid packing of all four quadrants allows the anesthesia team to catch up so that sequential life-saving treatment

Fig. 2.3 Actively bleeding injuries from the right lobe can usually be temporarily contained by placing packs superiorly and inferiorly to the right lobe and then providing compression either digitally (**a**) or by way of the large right-angled retractor (**b**)

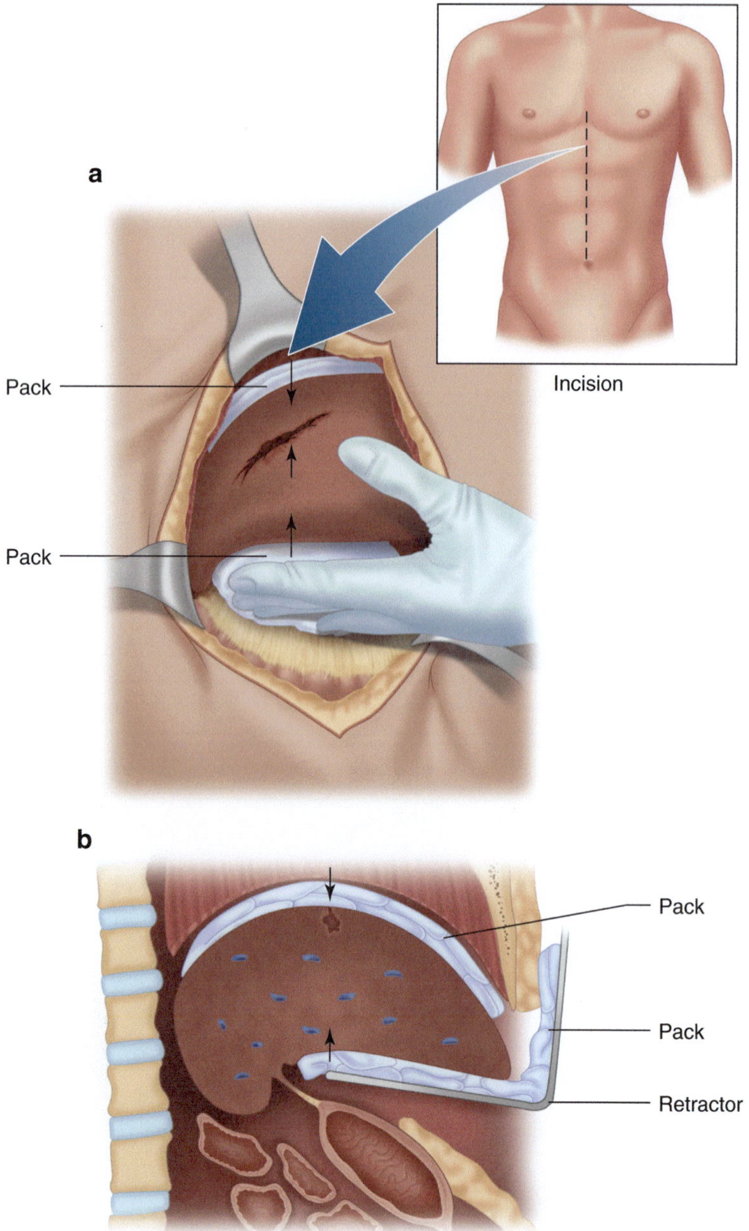

can be implemented on a priority basis [2, 10, 11]. When a major liver injury with active bleeding is identified, successful packing can usually be achieved by placing lap sponges above and below the liver and then using a large straight retractor to pull the liver up toward the diaphragm (Fig. 2.3). A penetrating wound adjacent to the gallbladder floss often can be controlled by a gauze pack but stressed by a Harrington retractor (Fig. 2.4) [2, 10]. The pack technique usually controls major hepatic bleeding; pressure should be maintained while bleeding from other sources is controlled and while a first-layer closure of hollow-viscus injuries is accomplished. When these latter objectives have been completed, the liver pack can be carefully removed. Often a major liver injury is no longer bleeding after pack removal. When this occurs, the injury should be

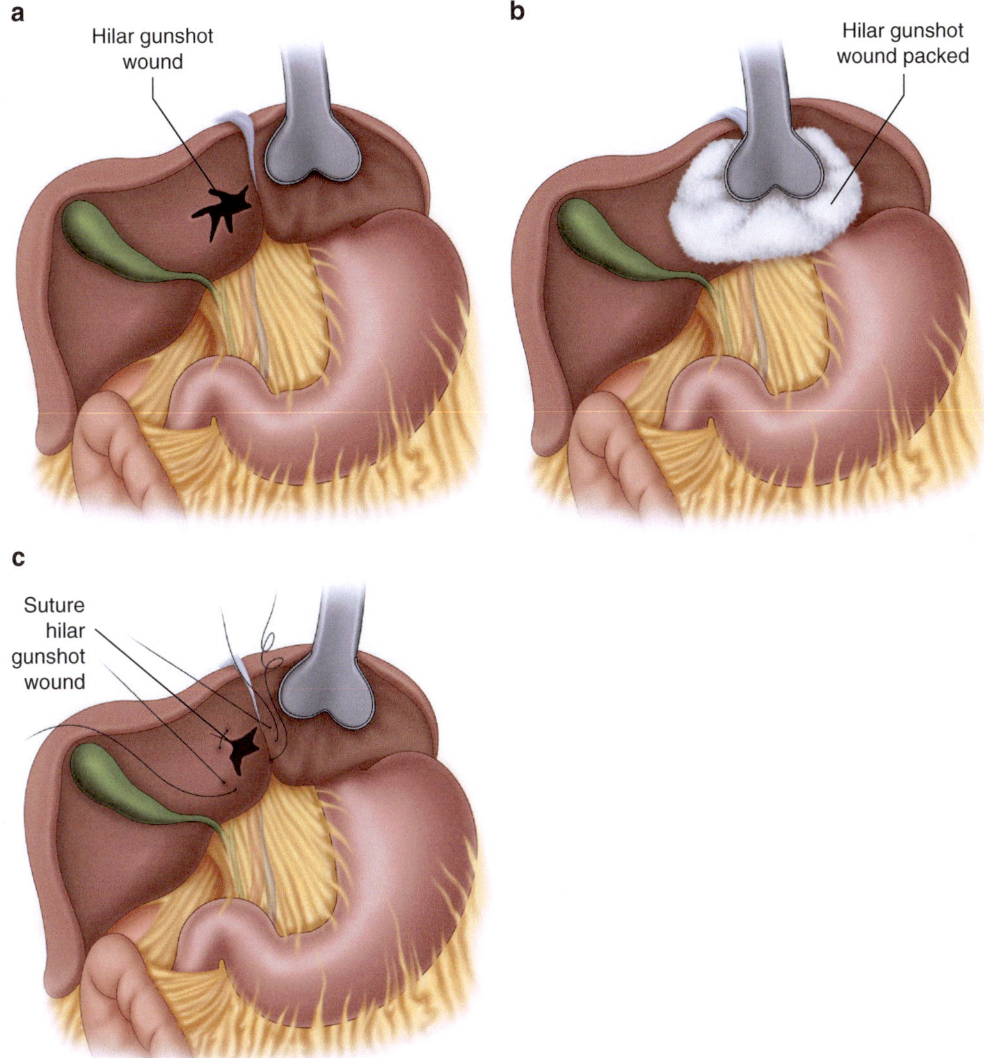

Fig. 2.4 Bleeding wounds near or at the hilum (**a**) can usually be contained by placing a pack and a Harrington retractor over the injury (**b**) until temporary hemostasis is obtained or slowed, at which time liver sutures placed on each side of the defect will provide hemostasis (**c**). Cholecystectomy is usually indicated in patients with these injuries

left alone; aggressive palpation manipulation, especially probing "to see if there is any mushiness" within the liver, may lead to recurrent hemorrhage that is lethal. When the liver rebleeds after pack removal, they should be reapplied and pressure retraction reinstituted. This will provide an opportunity to achieve proper mobilization of the portion of the liver that needs to be approached surgically [2, 12, 13].

Hepatic Mobilization (Right Lobe)

The approach to hepatic mobilization varies according to the site and extent of liver injury. Mobilization of the right hepatic lobe in patients with major injuries near the right hepatic vein, or "bare" area of the liver, is most challenging [2, 13]. The right triangular ligament extends along the dome of the right lobe and can be divided in

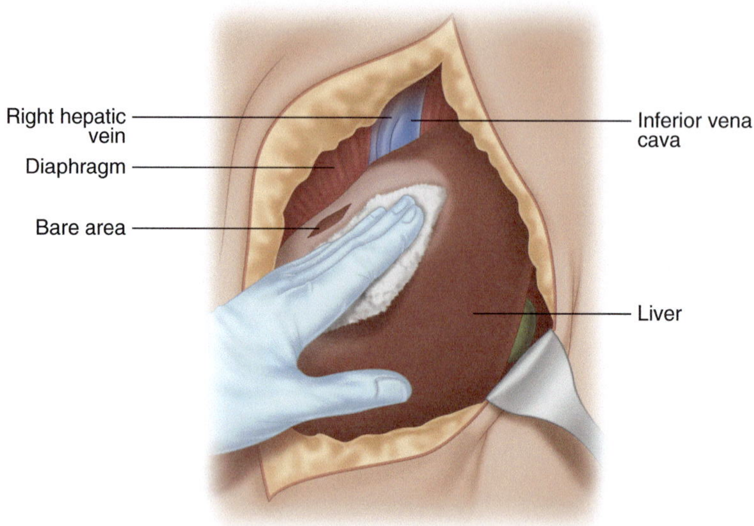

Fig. 2.5 Access to the right hepatic dome and right hepatic vein is achieved by mobilizing anteriorly and medially the right lobe beyond the bare area of the liver until the right hepatic vein is identified as it courses superiorly and posteriorly for about 2 cm to the IVC

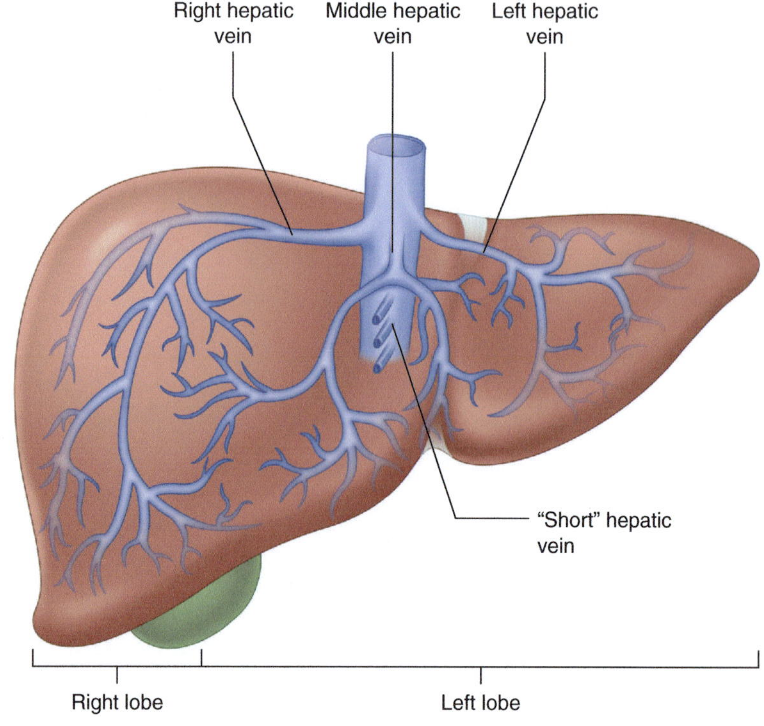

Fig. 2.6 The "short" hepatic veins run from the caudate lobe to the anterior portion of the IVC. The authors prefer that, when divided, these veins be controlled by suture ligature or ties rather than with clips which can be pulled off the vein when they get attached to a sponge being removed. The classic hepatic venous system has separate entrance of the right, middle, and left hepatic veins into the IVC. Sometimes the middle hepatic vein and left hepatic vein join before entrance into the IVC

its 1–2 cm width between the dome of the liver and the right hemidiaphragm (Fig. 2.5). When suprahepatic packs must be left in place to contain bleeding, this ligament can be divided throughout most of its length by Braille dissection. The bulk of the right lobe can then be mobilized inferiorly as the so-called "bare" area between the liver and diaphragm is reached (Fig. 2.6). The liver is mobilized anteriorly and medially as the "bare" area is dissected, being careful not to inadvertently perforate the diaphragm superiorly or dissect into the liver substance inferiorly

[7, 13]. Further mobilization in the same direction provides access to the right hepatic vein, which rises on a superior portion of the liver and extends about 2 cm superiorly into the inferior vena cava (IVC, Fig. 2.5) [2, 12]. Careful dissection of the tissues medial to the right hepatic vein along with division of the diaphragmatic crura anteriorly permits access to the right hepatic vein/IVC junction.

When further mobilization on the right lobe is needed in order to achieve anatomic resection, the right lobe can be retracted anteriorly, being careful to avoid injury to the right adrenal gland with its numerous vessels and, more medially, the short hepatic veins, which run between the caudate lobe and the inferior vena cava [2]. These veins need to be divided; the authors prefer suture ligature rather than clips, which sometimes catch onto sponges and yank off the divided veins (Fig. 2.6).

Hepatic Mobilization (Left Lobe)

Mobilization of the left hepatic lobe is much less challenging. The left triangular ligament between the left lobe and the left hemidiaphragm is more accessible and, therefore, more safely divided beyond the left lateral segment; this ligament is divided to the left medial segment where the left hepatic vein will be seen exiting on it and passing superiorly toward the left side of the IVC (Fig. 2.7) [2, 13]. The left hepatic vein usually flows directly into the IVC but, on occasion, may join with the mid-hepatic vein, in which case the entrance into the cava will be more medial. The short hepatic veins between the caudate lobe and IVC are usually not identified while mobilizing the left lobe. The entrance of the short hepatic veins is about 2–3 cm distal to the entrance of the middle and left hepatic veins into the IVC (Fig. 2.6) [2]. With full mobilization on the left lobe, however, these veins may be divided.

Hepatic Inflow

Control of arterial inflow is an important adjunct to hepatic mobilization. Temporary control can be achieved by the Pringle maneuver whereby one digitally compresses the portal triad just distal to the insertion of the cystic duct into the common bile duct (Fig. 2.8) [2, 12]. Temporary digital control can be achieved by Braille technique; vascular non-crushing clamps are used for longer term control. Long-term occlusion should not extend beyond 20 min at one time [13]. The individual branches of the hepatic artery and portal vein can then be dissected as one mobilizes the injured portion of the liver.

Vascular Anomalies

Although there are several anomalies of the hepatic arterial inflow, the most common occurs when the right hepatic artery arises as the first branch of the superior mesenteric artery; when this occurs, the right hepatic artery courses posterior to the pancreas and duodenum before curving superiorly toward the liver as the most lateral structure of the portal triad (Fig. 2.9) [2, 13]. Other less common anomalies of the hepatic arterial system include a common hepatic artery that rises from the superior mesenteric artery, a very proximal bifurcation of the common hepatic artery into the right and left hepatic arteries, and an accessory left hepatic artery that originates from the left gastric artery and perfuses the left lateral segment. The anomalous right hepatic artery provides oxygenation to all of the right lobe and the left medial segment. When this anomaly occurs, the left hepatic artery typically arises from the left gastric artery, passes through the lesser omentum, and provides oxygenation to only the left lateral segment. Portal venous anomalies are much less common.

The Non-bleeding Wound

Often, when the packs that are used to obtain temporary control of the bleeding liver are removed, no rebleeding occurs. This wound should be observed and the surgeon should be certain that the patient is fully resuscitated and has stable vital signs. The non-bleeding, thus observed wound, should be left alone. Digital or instrument probing of the wound, as noted above,

Fig. 2.7 The left hepatic vein usually flows superiorly and medially into the IVC and is accessed by dividing the left triangular ligament (**a**). After obtaining temporary control of the cava and left hepatic vein, the patient shown herein had rapid left hepatic lobectomy and oversewing of the left hepatic vein – IVC junction after placement of a Satinsky clamp (**b**). This type of patient salvage only occurs when God is not ready to receive the patient

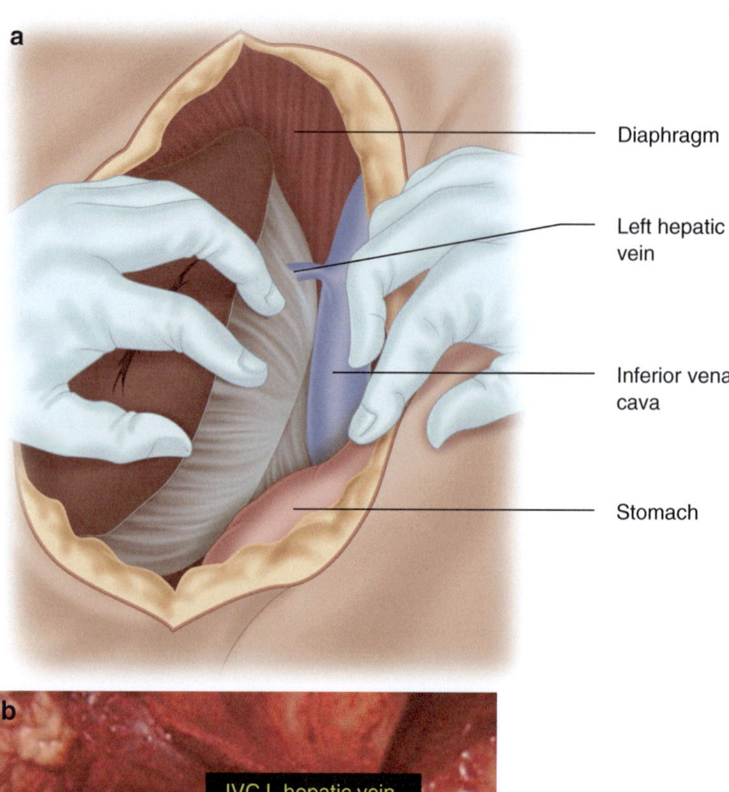

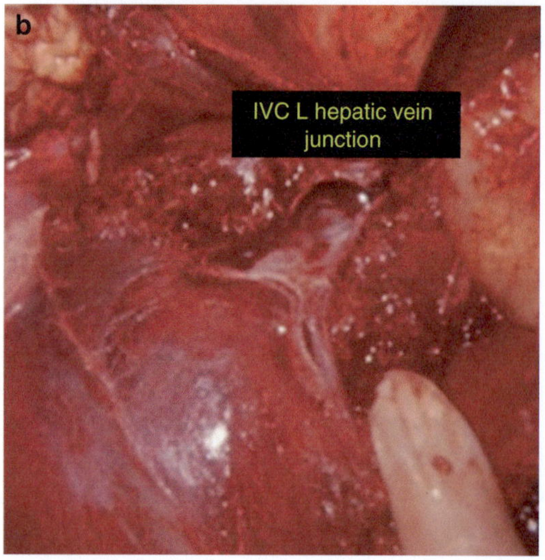

may lead to recurrent and sometimes lethal bleeding. Likewise, when a bullet has passed through the liver parenchyma into the hepatic vein and inferior vena cava with embolization to the right heart, the tract should be left alone and the known perforation of the retrohepatic IVC should not be explored (Fig. 2.10) [2]. No hemostatic techniques should be employed in a stable patient with a non-bleeding wound.

During a prospective study of 637 patients who were operated upon for liver injury during a 5-year period, there were 280 patients in whom there was no bleeding after the liver packs were removed and the vital signs were stable [1, 2, 8]. These wounds were left alone, and not one patient had postoperative bleeding from the non-bleeding liver wound. Likewise, the isolated subcapsular hematoma should be left alone (see Fig. 2.13).

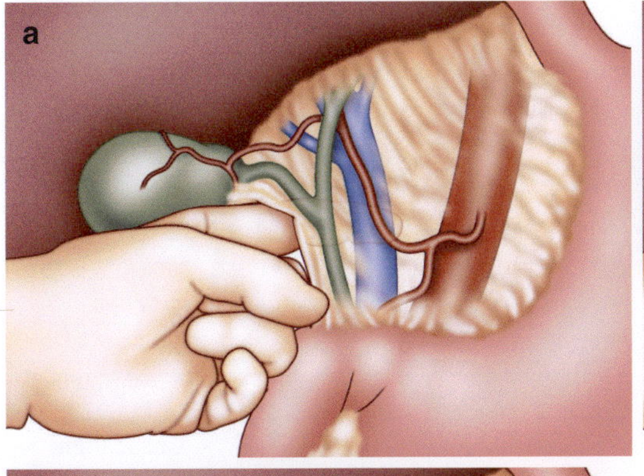
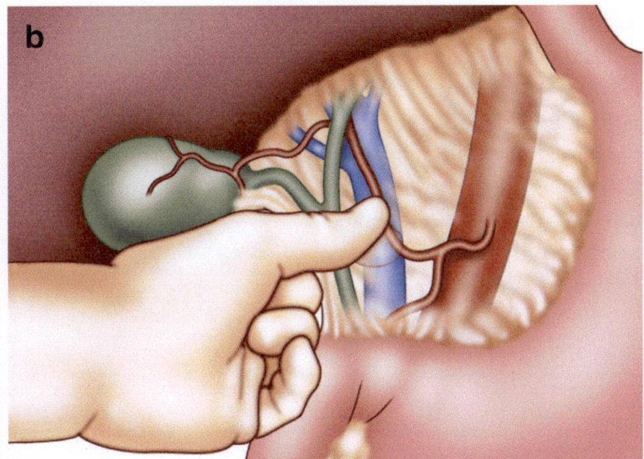
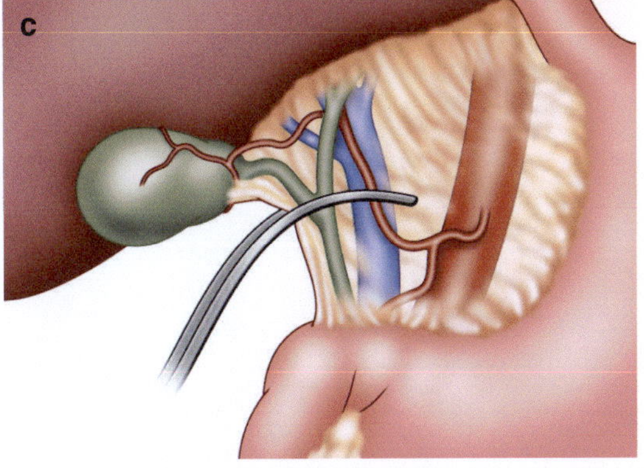

Fig. 2.8 The Pringle maneuver achieved with digital compression of the porta hepatis (**a**) not only provides good temporary inflow control of bleeding (**b**) but also is a predictor of the likelihood that hepatic dearterialization will contain active bleeding from a branch of the hepatic artery (**c**)

Patients treated nonoperatively for intrahepatic hematomas usually have normal resolution of the hematoma; some patients, particularly intravenous drug addicts, will have bacterial seeding of the hematoma leading to an abscess, which can usually be drained percutaneously.

Hemostatic Techniques/Liver Suture

The simplest and most successful technique for obtaining hemostasis from bleeding liver wounds is hepatorrhaphy using liver sutures [2, 12]. These sutures are blunt tipped, two inches in length, and swedged on to a 2-O chromic suture (Fig. 2.11) [2, 14]. The blunt-tipped needle minimizes parenchyma damage while passing through the liver and can be easily grasped by the surgeons without fear of a needle injury. The suture should be passed through the full depth of the two-inch needle, well away from the bleeding margins with large deep bites (Fig. 2.11) [2]. The sutures are then approximated in order to bring the liver substance together without strangling it and hence creating liver necrosis (Fig. 2.12) [2]. This can often be best achieved by having the first assistant hold one of the strategically placed sutures so that the liver is compressed but not strangled while the surgeon ties a second suture in order to achieve the exact degree of compression without tearing or strangulation.

One of the controversies regarding hepatorrhaphy concerns the patient with active bleeding through both the entrance and the exit sites of a liver gunshot wound. The fear of closing both the entrance and exit wounds is that there will be continued intrahepatic bleeding, which may cause a need for reoperation or become contaminated

Fig. 2.9 Normal hepatic arterial inflow is shown (**a**) along with the two common anomalies, namely, the right hepatic artery originating from the superior mesenteric artery (**b**) and the left hepatic artery originating from the left gastric artery (**c**)

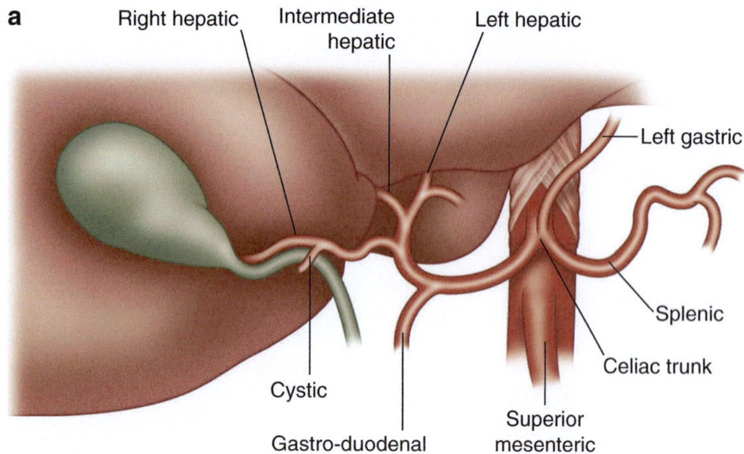

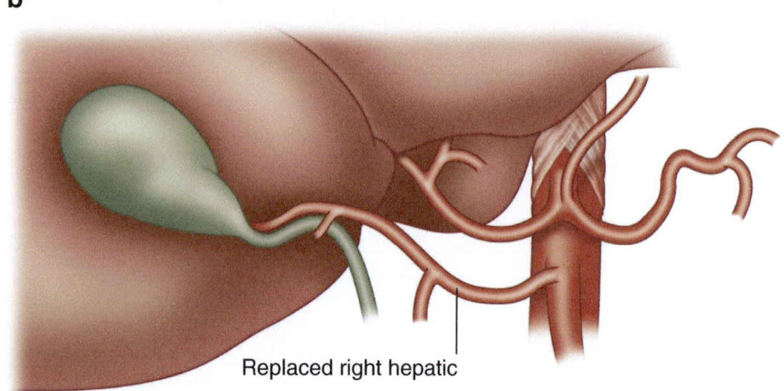

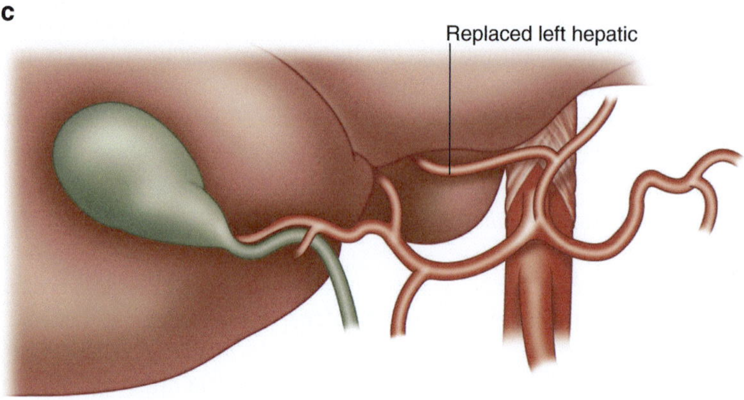

and result in an intrahepatic abscess [2]. Actually, most bleeding from the through-and-through liver wound arises from liver parenchyma within 2 cm of the capsule; the authors have successfully closed both ends of a through-and-through tract with a good hemostasis and without having the above complications [2]. In patients in whom both ends of the missile tract have been closed with liver sutures, rebleeding through the liver sutures from the unopposed deeper structures will be readily apparent within five minutes of tying the liver sutures. When this occurs, the liver suture must be removed and some other hemostatic technique employed.

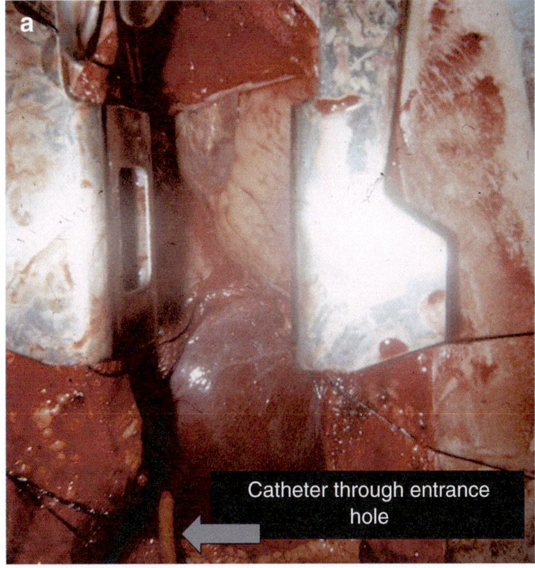

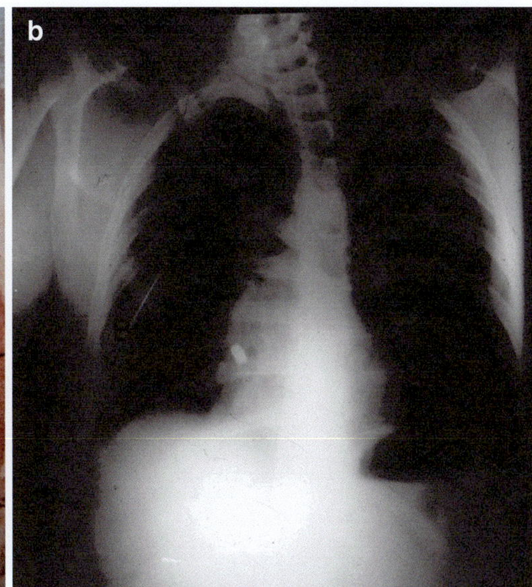

Fig. 2.10 When a missile passes through the substance of the liver with the tract depicted by the catheter (**a**) and ends up being embolized to the heart or lung (**b**), penetration of the anterior wall of the IVC is confirmed. This perforation along the anterior wall of the IVC should not be explored if there is no bleeding, whereas the bullet embolus can be dealt appropriately depending on its final location

Hepatotomy

The next step for this type of wound is tractotomy or hepatotomy, which is achieved by cutting through the normal liver down to the through-and-through tract [2, 8, 12]. This is performed by a combination of electrocoagulation, finger fracture, and ligation of the cross-linking vessels that are encountered while doing the tractotomy (Fig. 2.13) [2, 8]. Hemostasis along the two "cliffs" of the tractotomy is best achieved by gauze compression until the bottom of the tract is reached, by which time one usually will see a partially severed artery and/or vein at the bottom of the crevice. The partial severance of an intra-hepatic artery prevents retraction, contraction, and formation of a platelet plug. These vessels are best treated with simple ties or suture ligation depending upon the depth and accessibility. There are a number of instruments that may help in hepatic dissection. A long GIA stapler may be useful in providing quick division of the uninjured liver while doing a tractomy [8, 12]. Likewise, the argon beam laser can provide excellent access for parenchymal division, although the authors tend

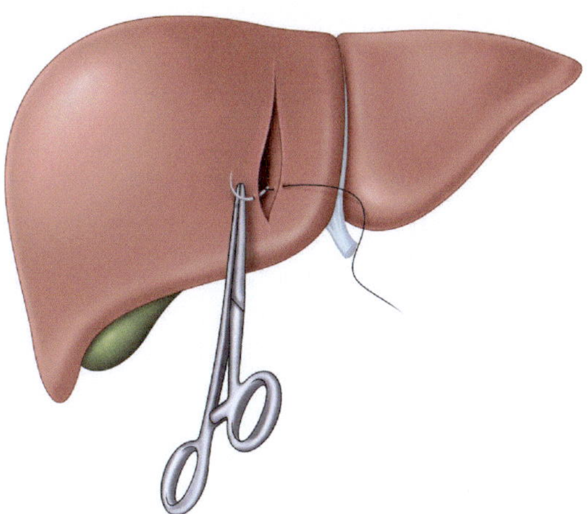

Fig. 2.11 Hepatorrhaphy or suture ligature of the liver is best achieved by using the 2″ blunt-tipped needle swedged onto a 2-O chromic suture. The sutures are placed well away from the wound and deep into the liver substance in order to obtain compression hemostasis of those vessels which are within 3 cm of the liver capsule

to rely on electrocoagulation for this purpose. Likewise, the cross-linking vessels that have to be divided in order to get to the bottom of the tract are best secured with ties or suture ligatures

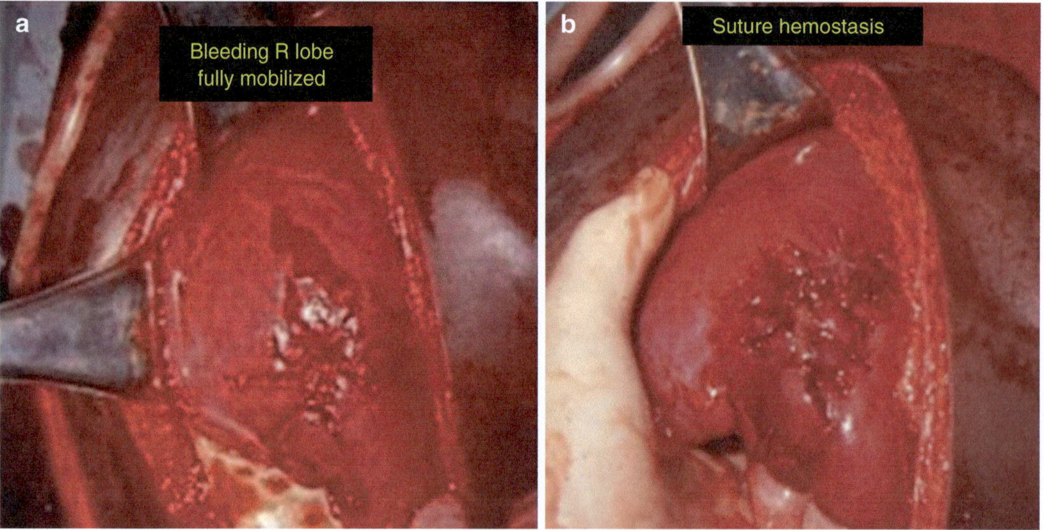

Fig. 2.12 After full mobilization of an actively bleeding right lobe of the liver (**a**), deep liver sutures usually achieve complete hemostasis without causing parenchymal ischemia (**b**)

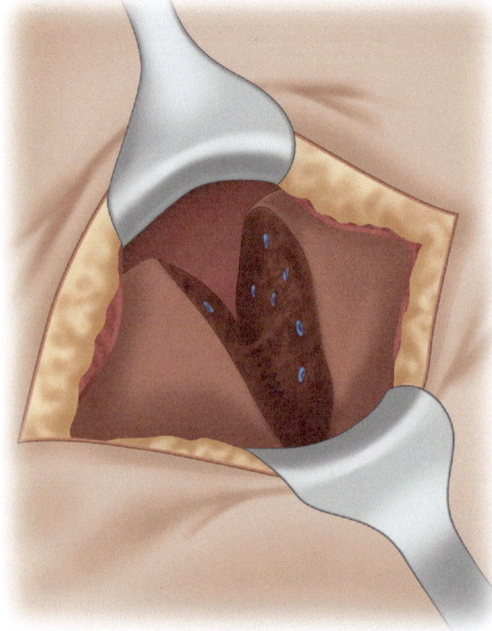

Fig. 2.13 Hepatotomy or tractotomy is often indicated in patients with deep through-and-through gunshot wounds when hemostasis cannot be obtained by suture ligature of the entrance and/or exit wound. Hemostasis along the tract margin is obtained by a combination of electrocoagulation, suture ligature, and ties of cross-linking vessels until the bottom of the tract is reached

rather than clips, which may get attached to the gauze sponges and pulled off when removing the gauze sponges (Fig. 2.13) [2]. Once hemostasis has been achieved in the deep tract or crevice and the visible vessels have been ligated along the two sides leading to the tract, the divided liver is best re-approximated using the same liver suture technique described above (Fig. 2.14) [2].

Resectional Debridement

Some wounds do not lend themselves well to suture ligation or tractotomy. Examples would be patients who have a rifle wound or shotgun blast to a peripheral portion of the liver [3, 8, 9]. The extent of parenchymal damage in this setting is usually too excessive for containment by suture ligatures (Fig. 2.15) [2]. These patients are best treated by resectional debridement or wedge resection of that portion of the liver that is severely damaged. The margins of the resectional debridement should be carried out through the relatively uninvolved portion of the liver so that all of the ragged, shredded fragments get removed. The margins of resection are then contained with the liver suture technique after the ragged,

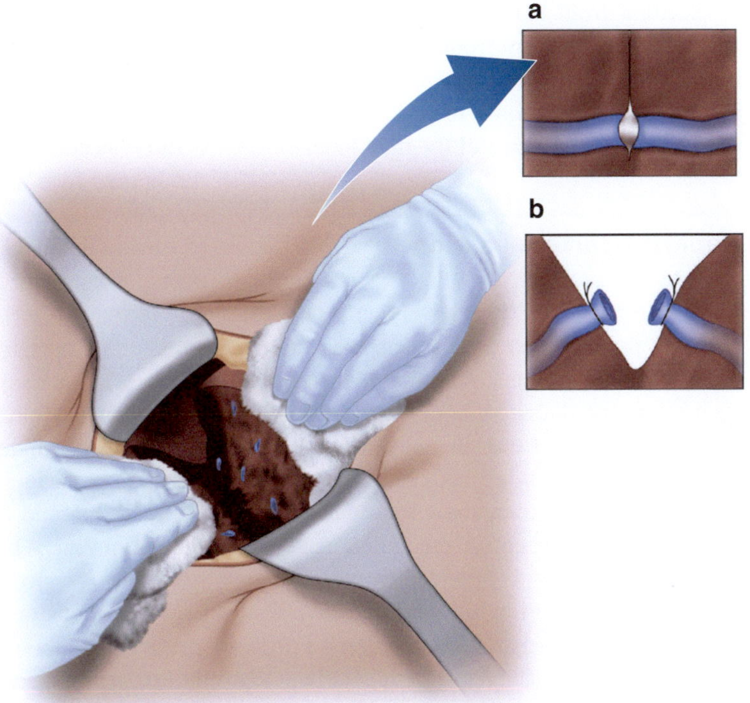

Fig. 2.14 When hemostasis has been achieved in the deep tract and all visible cross-linking vessels have been ligated (**b**), the divided liver is best re-approximated using the same liver suture technique described above (**a**)

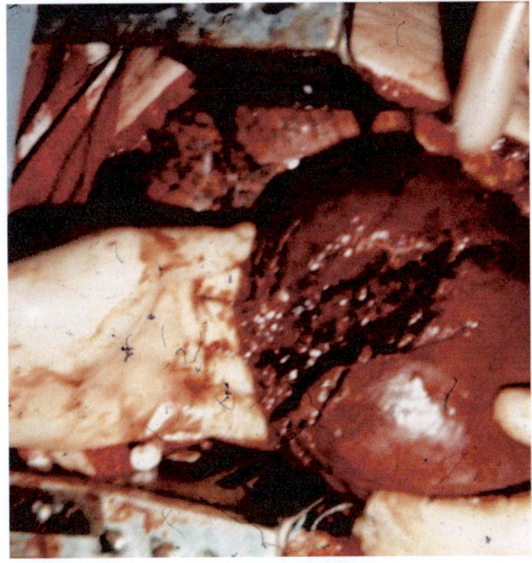

Fig. 2.15 Rifle wounds or short-range shotgun blasts often causes extensive parenchymal damage which is not amenable to suture ligation. These patients are best treated by resectional debridement or wedge resection of the severely injured tissue

shredded portion of the liver is removed. During the period of resection or debridement, digital pressure applied to both the anterior and posterior surfaces of the liver will usually help contain bleeding and may also assist in applying the liver sutures after the damaged portion of the liver has been removed. Often, the decision to perform nonanatomic hepatic resection rather than anatomic resection is determined by the injury whereby patients with obvious devitalized tissue require the so-called resection or debridement without formal anatomic lobectomy [2, 9, 15].

This type of resectional debridement is not easily implemented in patients with superior central liver injuries. An extension of the resection debridement type of incision proximally to the opposite surface will result in a so-called nonanatomic hepatic resection where a significant portion of liver is removed without following the typical anatomic plains. Hemostasis in this setting is usually achieved by manual compression of either the right lobe or left lobe proximal to that portion of the liver that is being removed in a nonanatomic manner [8, 15]. The Pringle maneuver is also helpful in this setting (Fig. 2.8). Hepatic arterial and portal venous injury can be distinguished from hepatic venous injury by the Pringle maneuver, which will cause cessation of bleeding from the hepatic artery and portal venous injuries but not from the hepatic venous injuries [2, 8]. Two mature surgeons should be present when nonanatomic resection is performed through the thick portion of the right lobe.

Hepatic Dearterialization

The use of hepatic artery interruption is not only useful in providing temporary hemostasis while performing nonanatomic resection but may also be used as the definitive hemostatic technique. This is particularly true in patients who have deep wounds, which are not readily accessible to suture ligation, tractotomy, or nonanatomic resectional debridement. A prediction about the likelihood of success is provided by cessation of bleeding with the Pringle maneuver (Fig. 2.8) [2, 8]. If hemostasis is achieved with the Pringle maneuver, then one can move peripherally along the branches of the hepatic artery to find the specific branch that, when occluded, stops bleeding [16]. The hepatic artery provides about 500 ml of blood flow per minute to the liver in comparison to about 1,000 ml of blood flow by way of the portal vein. Since the hepatic artery has a higher oxygen content, it supplies about 40 % of the hepatic oxygen consumption compared to 60 % by the portal vein. Thus, ligation of the hepatic artery should not produce liver necrosis [2]. When, however, there is an associated portal venous injury, the ligation of both will certainly produce necrosis to that segment of the liver. Maintaining good knowledge about the anatomy of the hepatic artery helps implement this technique. When the right hepatic artery is ligated, the gallbladder should be removed since the cystic artery branches of the right hepatic artery; ligation may cause a calculus cholecystitis and necrosis.

Anatomic Resection

Anatomic liver resection should be looked upon as a last resort in achieving hemostasis from the injured liver. Again, knowledge of hepatic artery anatomy is vital (Fig. 2.9) [2, 7]. The liver is divided into two lobes by the bilobar plane, which extends from the middle of the gallbladder fossa to the inferior vena cava. Anatomic hepatectomy is rarely needed for control of the bleeding from the injured liver and should be implemented by surgeons who are experienced with the handling of liver tissue and knowledgeable about the segmental divisions of the liver [9, 13, 15]. Although 70 % hepatic resection is compatible with life in a controlled operative situation, the combination of major liver resection for severe hemorrhage that insults the remaining liver is associated with significant morbidity and mortality. Anatomic resection in the injured patient requires appropriate occlusion and division of the hepatic artery and portal venous branches that are supplying the area to be resected. Patients who undergo major liver resection for a severe hemorrhagic shock insult will likely have impaired liver function in the early postoperative period and require additional fresh frozen plasma to restore procoagulants until the hepatic function improves.

When doing a left hepatectomy, control of ongoing hemorrhage can usually be achieved by digital pressure surrounding the liver after the left triangular ligament has been taken down [2, 8, 12]. One can also use an oval-shaped liver clamp to provide compression to the left of the bilobar plane and the IVC. Anatomic right hepatic lobectomy requires much more extensive mobilization as described. Dividing the right triangular ligament and mobilizing the right lobe away from the right adrenal is necessary for digital compression for the oval liver clamp to be effective [2, 8]. When a patient is actively bleeding, control of either the right hepatic vein or left hepatic vein is always dangerous and certainly more complicated in comparison to doing a standard right or left hepatectomy for metastatic cancer [8, 12, 15]. The operation, when done for cancer, is usually being achieved in a relatively avascular field, whereas when the operation is being done for injury, the first assistant is trying to contain the bleeding as much as possible while the surgeon does the anatomic resection. When doing an anatomic resection, the authors like to leave a margin of 1–2 cm from the bilobar plane in order to help contain digital control of bleeding during resection and to bring about approximation of the anterior and posterior surfaces of the liver following completion of anatomic resection [2]. The liver sutures are used for this purpose. This is achieved after any cross-linking vessels that are observed in the base of resection are ligated.

Damage Control

The observation that temporary liver packs will often provide control of bleeding while attention is directed to the treatment of other injured organs led the way for the pack to be left in place as the definitive part of the first operation [1, 2]. This is especially true in patients who have had the triad of acidosis, hypothermia, and coagulopathy as a result of a severe hemorrhagic shock insult requiring multiple transfusions [8, 9]. Damage control from the bleeding liver is more easily achieved with injuries to the right lobe in that the lap packs or Kerlix gauzes can be placed between the liver and the diaphragm and also between right rib cage and the diaphragm (Fig. 2.3) [2, 11]. This allows for there to be pack hemostasis by providing external pressure on the liver. These packs are then left in place while the patient is taken to the critical care area for correction of coagulopathy, acidosis, and rewarming. Packing of the liver is excellent in selected cases for hemostasis, but the pack serves as a tampon and compromises egress of associated bile leakage [2]. Drains outside or away from the pack are beneficial to provide egress of associated bile leakage. The timing of reoperation should be determined by the patient's degree of improvement but can usually be performed within 24 h. At the time of reoperation, the packs are slowly and sequentially removed. When the last pack is removed, the surgeon may be pleasantly surprised to see that there is no further bleeding [2, 6, 10]. When this occurs, the surgeon needs to simply get out of the abdomen and leave the liver alone. When rebleeding occurs following removal of packs, the pack is reapplied while the surgeon goes through the appropriate steps at mobilization and prepares to use whatever hemostatic technique is most appropriate for the injury. When the hemostatic technique fails and the patient is getting into trouble again, the liver can be repacked and plans can be made for a third operation. Rarely, when bleeding is not controlled by packs, the Pringle maneuver, and digital hepatic compression, vascular isolation of the liver may be necessary. This is achieved by combining the Pringle maneuver with placement of a retrohepatic shunt that extends from the IVC to the right atrium (Fig. 2.16) [2, 12, 16]. This provides a bloodless field in which one hopefully can identify and repair the injured vessels whether they be portal venous, hepatic venous, or IVC. Vascular isolation of the liver is achieved by combining the Pringle maneuver with a retrohepatic shunt extending from the IVC to the right atrium (Fig. 2.16) [8, 12, 16]. Application of this procedure is carried out in desperate situations; there are likely more published authors who have written about this technique than there are patient survivors.

The technique for packing varies, but the authors prefer to use either fluff or Kerlix gauzes [2, 11]. Some authors place rayon cloth between the packs of the liver with the hopes that the removal of the packs will not cause damage to the underlying macerated liver causing rebleeding [6, 10, 12]. Damage to the underlying liver can be avoided by carefully removing the packs in a very slow manner and removing that portion of the pack that yields to gentle tension. If this technique of pack removal is used, rayon cloth under the pack is not needed.

Different types of packs can be used to treat unusual injuries [11]. For example, a gauze plug may be used to fill up a through-and-through gunshot wound tract; a condom may be inflated with saline and placed in a through-and-through gunshot wound tract; additional saline inflations provide lateral compression against the intrahepatic bleeding sites (Fig. 2.17) [2]. An omental plug may be placed in a wound when the liver has been split open; the liver is sutured over the omentum. The authors do not prefer this omental pack technique in that omentum necrosis requiring subsequent omentectomy has been encountered. The pack can also be placed in an intrahepatic position

Fig. 2.16 The retrohepatic shunt with vascular isolation can also be achieved by way of the right atrium to the IVC (**a**) or from the IVC to the right atrium (**b**)

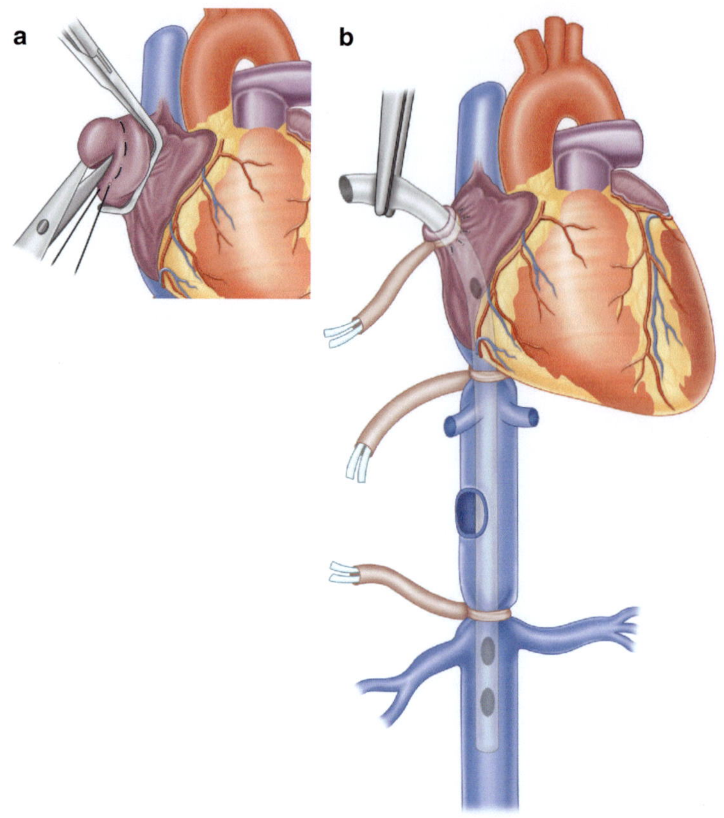

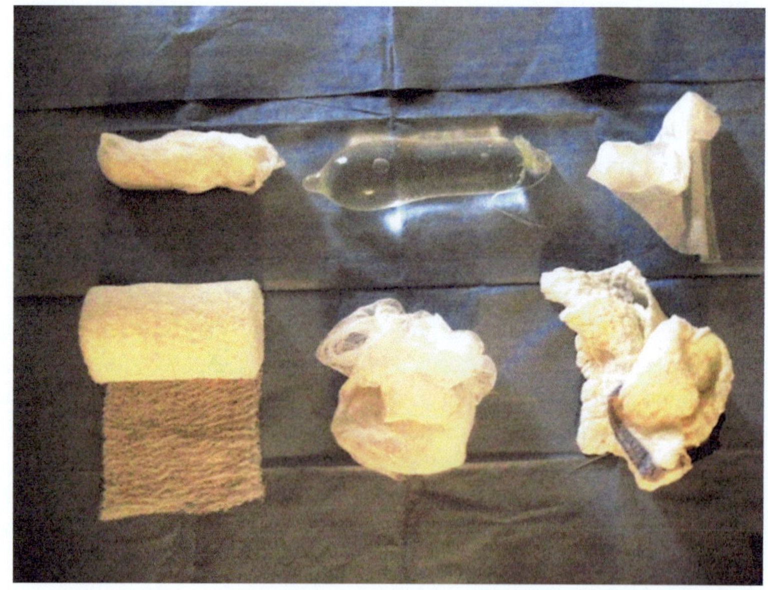

Fig. 2.17 Materials used to achieve hemostasis by liver packing include the gauze plug, the condom plug, fluff gauze, Kerlix roll, fine mesh gauze, and lap sponge

whereby the pack is actually sewed into the middle part of the liver with the liver closed around the pack. This has special merit for patients with left lobe injuries where there is no natural anatomic boundary to provide pressure against the oozing liver [2, 12]. When reoperation and removal of a pack leads to recurrent bleeding, which could not be readily contained by the techniques described above, the liver should be repacked and consideration then should be given to interventional radiography in order to determine whether there is a branch of one of the hepatic arteries that can be embolized [8, 12].

Dearterialization and Liver Packing

The combination of dearterialization and liver packing is hazardous. Once hepatic arterial flow has been interrupted, liver viability is dependent upon portal venous flow. The portal venous flow, in turn, is a low-pressure circulatory system so that a pack will tend to occlude portal venous flow and, thereby, eliminate oxygenation to that portion of the liver. This results in liver necrosis [17].

Nonoperative Therapy

The observation that hepatic bleeding commonly stops in patients who are no longer bleeding at the time of laparotomy led to the implementation of nonoperative therapy in patients with both blunt and penetrating wounds [2, 12, 18]. Following the success of early studies of nonoperative treatment of blunt splenic injury, the authors extended this principle to liver injuries. The authors predicted in 1983 that there would be "increased acceptance of expectant therapy for liver injuries over the next decade" [2]. Currently, most minor (AIS 1,2,3) injuries receive nonoperative management, whereas stable patients with major injuries (AIS 4,5) are treated nonoperatively (Fig. 2.18) [2, 12, 13]. This, of course,

leads to less operative experience with getting hemostasis from the bleeding liver; this creates an educational crisis [19, 20]. Likewise, nonoperative treatment is excellent for non-bleeding intrahepatic hematomas; patients using street drugs, however, may feed the hematoma leading to a hepatic abscess.

Hepatic Injury with Blush

When treating a patient nonoperatively for major liver injury (AIS 4–5), there will often be a blush identified on the contrast CT of the liver. Although it is tempting to have interventional radiography embolize these blushes, one should remember that there are no free lunches and that hepatic necrosis may result from the embolization. The authors recommend that the stable non-bleeding patient with a hepatic blush on contrast CT be observed without intervention.

Hemobilia

Hemobilia is an unusual complication of liver injury [21]. This classic presentation includes a history of recent major trauma, followed some time later by the triad of right upper quadrant abdominal pain, hematemesis, and relief of abdominal pain. Hemobilia is due to the formation of a fistula between a branch of the hepatic artery and the bile duct. Intermittent bleeding into the injured parenchymal causes the right upper quadrant pain due to a intrahepatic rise in pressure within the false aneurysm [2, 19]. When the pressure rises, there will be decompression through the connecting bile duct and the blood rapidly exits through the ampulla at such a rate that the patient has hematemesis and simultaneous relief of pain, which is due to the high intrahepatic pressure. This sequence should make one think immediately of hemobilia, especially after a patient has sustained a major blunt injury.

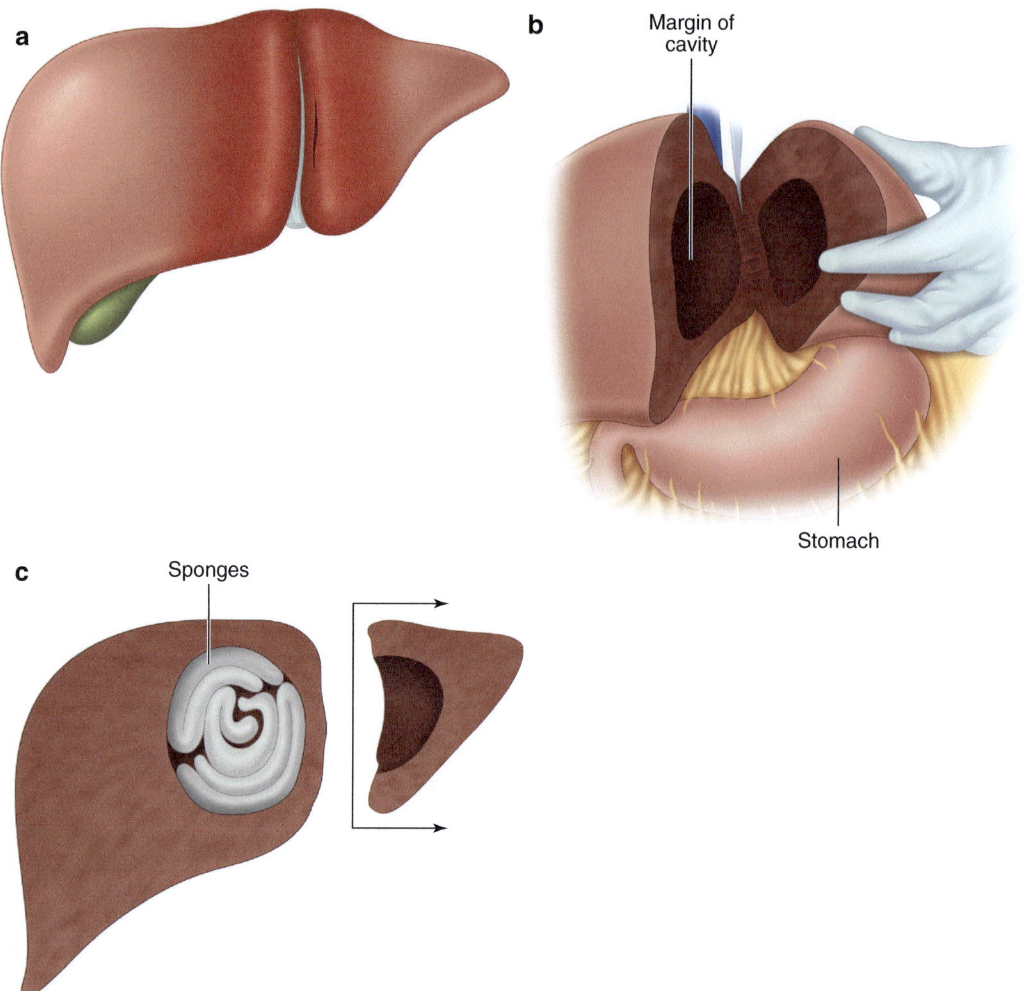

Fig. 2.18 Following severe blunt injury a large intrahepatic hematoma was continually oozing from a full-thickness crack (**a**) which was treated by left lateral segmentectomy and packing of the left medial segment and medial portion of the right lobe (**b**) with closure of the liver over the pack (**c**)

The first diagnostic test should be hepatic angiography and not upper endoscopy [2]. This confirms the suspected hepatic pseudoaneurysm.

The treatment for hemobilia may include embolization, hepatotomy with ligation of the partially severed cross-linking artery, or in unusual situations hepatic resection [21]. During exploration for patients with hemobilia, the diagnosis will be confirmed by the presence of a blood-filled gallbladder and extrahepatic bile ducts (Fig. 2.19) [2]. One can then ligate the hepatic artery which is feeding the false aneurysm and perform the hepatotomy by the techniques described above (Fig. 2.20) [2]. The source of the bleeding will almost invariably be a partially severed branch of the hepatic artery, which can be ligated and divided, after which the extrahepatic arterial occlusion can be released. If the patient has problems with recurrence or if there is evidence of hepatic necrosis due to an unrecognized portal venous injury, reoperation with hepatic resection is needed [21].

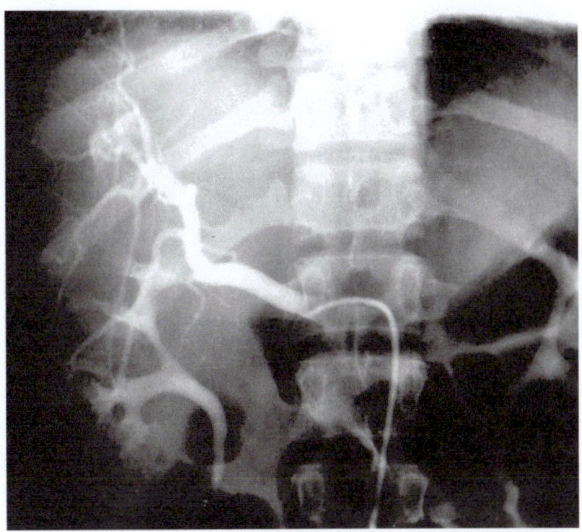

Fig. 2.19 Hepatic arteriography shows the early extravasation from a branch of the right hepatic artery

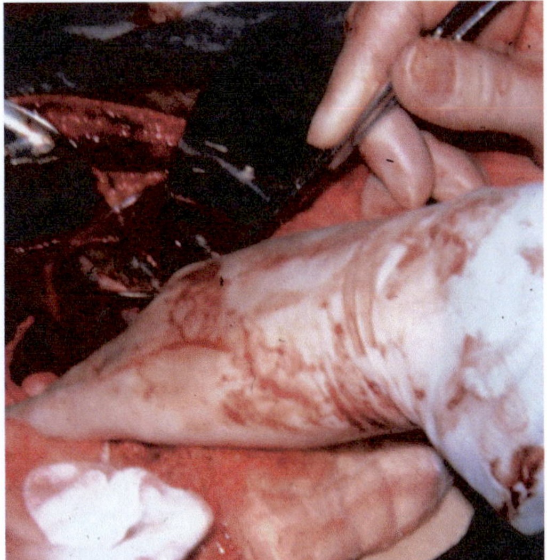

Fig. 2.20 During exploration for patients with hemobilia, the gallbladder and extrahepatic bile ducts will be observed to be full of blood

Hepatic Drainage

Minor liver injuries (AIS 1,2,3) that are promptly made hemostatic by hepatic suture technique usually do not require any hepatic drainage [2, 3]. Major injuries (AIS 4,5), however, often have associated biliary radical severance with

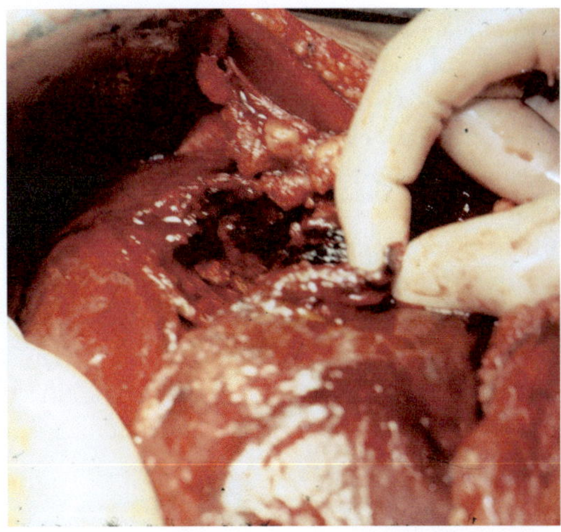

Fig. 2.21 When a liver crack is dissected down to the area of the false aneurysm causing hemobilia, there will be a pseudo-capsule which when entered will identify a partially severed artery which is communicating with the biliary system

the result that there is potential for bile leakage. These patients are best treated with external drainage, which can typically be provided by the closed external drains, namely, the Jackson-Pratt drains. The use of extrahepatic bile duct drainage as a means of decreasing intrahepatic biliary pressure should be avoided since the bile fistulae in patients with major liver injuries are coming from bile radicals peripheral to the extrahepatic biliary system and are, therefore, not effectively decompressed by placement of extrahepatic biliary drains such as a T-tube drain (Fig. 2.21) [2, 22]. Controlled extrahepatic biliary drainage was assessed in a prospective randomized study of 119 patients treated for severe liver injury. The type of drainage, dictated by a double-sealed envelope drawn at the time of operation, included standard drainage alone in 37 patients, standard drainage plus cholecystostomy in 38 patients, and standard drainage plus t-tube choledochostomy in 54 patients. The morbidity consisting of intra-abdominal or subphrenic abscess, septic jaundice, cholangitis, wound sepsis, and erosive gastritis was significantly increased in the patients with t-tube choledochostomy. The mortality was insignificantly increased in this same group. The presence of controlled extrahepatic biliary drainage did not prevent hemobilia, reduce the output of a biliary cutaneous fistula, or reduce the likelihood of postoperative rebleeding from the injured liver [22, 23]. The same principle applies for the placement of extrahepatic biliary stents as a means of treating established bile fistulae [23]. Simple local care of the external bile fistula will result in slow but sure closure as collateralization develops and as fibrosis plugs the point of biliary leakage. A tincture of patience in this setting is a virtue.

Video Captions

Video 1   Initial hemorrhage control (MOV 48398 kb)
Video 7   Liver suture (MOV 39685 kb)
Video 11   Digital compression (MOV 16750 kb)
Video 14   Case 01. A 16-year-old boy was a victim of gunshot wound through the right flank (MOV 35988 kb)

References

1. Lucas CE, Ledgerwood AM. Prospective evaluation of hemostatic techniques for liver injuries. J Trauma. 1976;16:442.
2. Lucas CE, Ledgerwood AM. Treatment of the injured liver. In: Nyhus LM, Baker RJ, editors. Mastery of surgery. 2nd ed. Boston/Toronto/London: Little, Brown & Co; 1992. p. 850.
3. Feliciano DV, Mattox KL, Jordan GL, et al. Management of 1000 consecutive cases of hepatic trauma (1979–1984). Ann Surg. 1986;204:438.
4. Lucas CE, Ledgerwood AM. Factors influencing morbidity and mortality after liver injury. Ann Surg. 1978;44:106.
5. Moore EE, Cogbill TH, Jurkovich GJ, et al. Organ injury scaling: spleen and liver (1994 revision). J Trauma. 1995;38:323.
6. Feliciano DV. Surgery for liver trauma. Surg Clin North Am. 1989;69:273.
7. Kozar RA, Feliciano DV, Moore EE, et al. Western Trauma Association/Critical decisions in trauma: operative management of blunt hepatic trauma. J Trauma. 2011;71:1.
8. Peitzman AB, Marsh JW. Advanced operative techniques in the management of complex liver injury. J Trauma Acute Care Surg. 2012;73:765.
9. Trunkey DD. Hepatic trauma: contemporary management. Surg Clin North Am. 2004;84:437.
10. Feliciano DV, Mattox KL, Burch JM, et al. Packing for control of hepatic hemorrhage. J Trauma. 1986;26:738.
11. Lucas CE, Ledgerwood AM. Perihepatic packing. In: Vincent JL, Hall JB, editors. Encyclopedia of intensive care medicine. Berlin/Heidelberg: Springer; 2011.
12. Leppaniami AK, Mentula PJ, Streng MH, et al. Severe hepatic trauma: nonoperative management, definitive repair or damage control surgery. World J Surg. 2011;35:2643.
13. Pachter HL. Prometheus bound: evolution in the management of hepatic trauma – from myth to reality. J Trauma. 2012;72:321.
14. Chen RJ, Fang JF, Lin BC, et al. Factors determining operative mortality of grade V blunt hepatic trauma. J Trauma. 2000;49:886.
15. Polanco P, Leon S, Pineda J, et al. Hepatic resection in the management of complex injury to the liver. J Trauma. 2008;65:1264.
16. Abdalla EK, Noun R, Belghiti J. Hepatic vascular occlusion: which technique? Surg Clin North Am. 2004;84:563.
17. Lucas CE, Ledgerwood AM. Liver necrosis following hepatic artery transection due to trauma. Arch Surg. 1978;113:1107.
18. Meyer AA, Crass RA, Lim RC, et al. Selective nonoperative management of blunt liver injury using computerized tomography. Arch Surg. 1985;120:550.
19. Lucas CE, Ledgerwood AM. Changing times and the treatment of liver injury. Am Surg. 2000;66:337.
20. Lucas CE, Ledgerwood AM. The academic challenge of teaching psychomotor skills for hemostasis of solid organ injury. J Trauma. 1009;66:636.
21. Sandblom P. Hemobilia: biliary tract hemorrhage. Springfield: Thomas; 1972.
22. Lucas CE, Ledgerwood AM. Controlled biliary drainage for large injuries of the liver. Surg Gynecol Obstet. 1973;137:585.
23. Lucas CE. Endoscopic retrograde cholangiopancreatography for bile leak after severe liver trauma (letter to the editor). J Trauma. 2012;72:537.

Resuscitation Maneuvers for "Extremis"

3

Thomas M. Scalea

Introduction

Inflow control is one of the basic principles in the management of vascular injury or solid organ injury with substantial hemorrhage. In the case of an injury to a blood vessel, vascular control should be obtained proximally and distally as close to the injury as possible to limit bleeding from collateral vessels and provide a dry field. The injury can then be repaired. Nonessential organs such as the spleen can simply be resected. Therefore, inflow control is only important to maintain some degree of cardiovascular stability while a rapid splenectomy is performed. Splenic artery occlusion can be done digitally while the spleen is rapidly mobilized and a clamp placed across the splenic artery and vein. This is not as helpful with the liver. Total hepatectomy is a last ditch desperation effort and, thus, it is almost never the wisest choice.

Certainly the most direct inflow occlusion in the liver is the Pringle maneuver. While it is described elsewhere, a brief discussion is appropriate. A vascular clamp placed across the port of hepatis occludes the hepatic artery and portal vein. This has the advantage of decreasing flow to the liver. In high-grade injuries there is virtually always some component of hepatic venous injury.

T.M. Scalea, MD
R Adams Cowley Shock Trauma Center,
University of Maryland, 22 S. Greene Street,
Baltimore, MD 21201, USA
e-mail: tscalea@umm.edu

The Pringle maneuver does nothing to stem blood loss from the large posterior vein.

Aortic Occlusion

Sometimes the patients are in profound hemorrhagic shock and/or have other injuries that may be bleeding. In that case, inflow control via aortic occlusion has many advantages. If the aorta is occluded above the level of the celiac axis, flow to the liver is markedly reduced. There may be some small amount of flow via collaterals, such as via the intercostal arteries, but for the most part bleeding from the liver should be controlled, at least as effectively as it is with the Pringle maneuver. In addition, flow to the more distal viscera is interrupted, preserving flow to the most essential organs in the body, the heart and the brain. This allows time for rapid volume infusion and transfusion of blood and blood products to replete intravascular volume. Hopefully, the period of aortic occlusion that is necessary is relatively brief. If aorta occlusion is prolonged, the abdominal viscera, particularly the small bowel and colon, will develop ischemia. When occlusion is released, the washout of toxic metabolites can produce cardiovascular collapse, often called declamp shock.

Until recently, aortic occlusion could only be obtained via an open approach. The infradiaphragmatic aorta can be approached several ways. Certainly one of the most popular maneuvers is the left-sided medial visceral rotation.

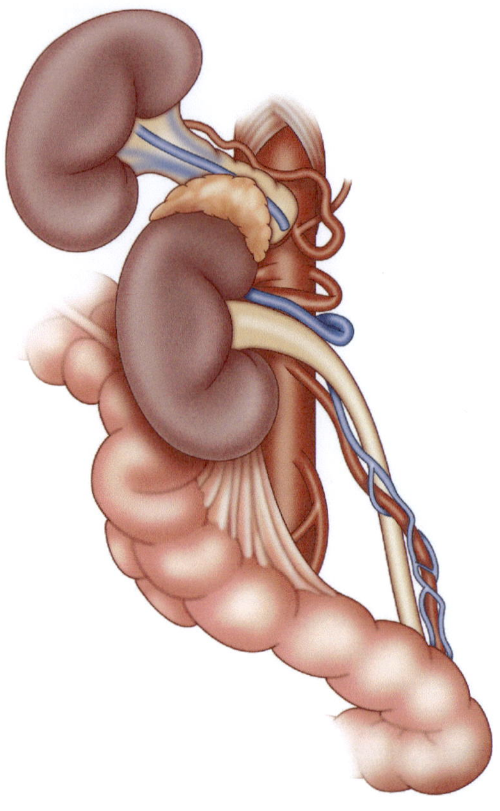

Fig. 3.1 The Mattox maneuver of left-sided visceral rotation to expose the proximal abdominal aorta

This maneuver mobilizes the left colon, the pancreas, the spleen, and the stomach. This brings the operating surgeon directly onto the aorta at the level of the diaphragmatic hiatus. The esophagus is then dissected free from the aorta and the aorta encircled. A cross clamp can then be applied (Fig. 3.1).

Alternatively, the aorta may be approached through the lesser sac. The lesser omentum is widely opened and the left lobe of the liver retracted. This provides a window to the gastroesophageal junction. Again, the esophagus is mobilized and the aorta can be clamped (Fig. 3.2).

Some have advocated aortic compression be accomplished with compression devices, either a sponge stick or a more formal device known as an aortic compressor (Fig. 3.3). This allows aortic compression and presumed occlusion without requiring any other maneuvers. These devices are applied to the aorta anteriorly, hopefully occluding aortic flow. Unfortunately, these devices often migrate, slipping off the aorta. The task of holding these devices is often left to the junior member of the team, who may not be able to maintain true aortic occlusion.

Each of these operative maneuvers has significant disadvantages. They each require time.

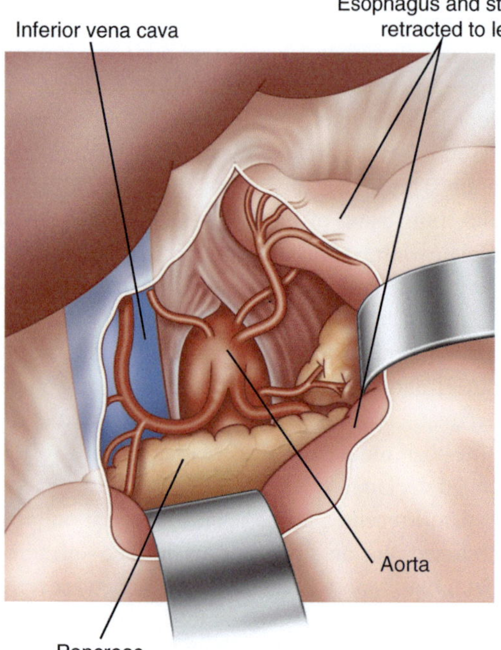

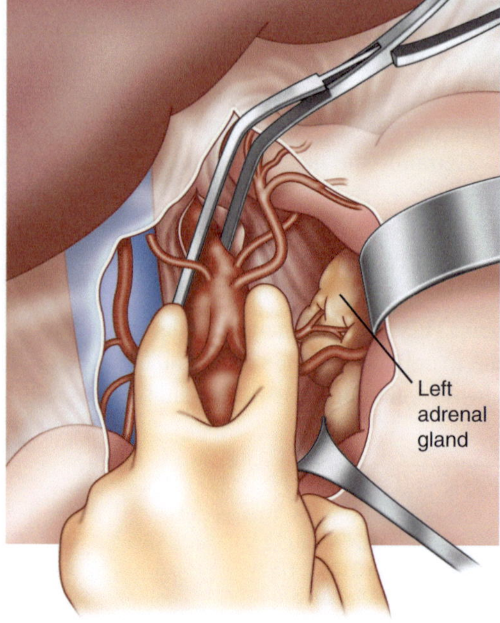

Fig. 3.2 Access to the proximal aortic aorta through the lesser sac

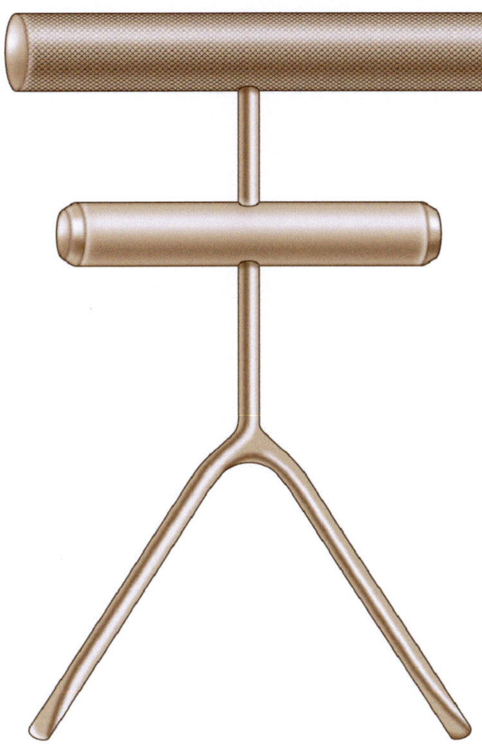

Fig. 3.3 Aortic occlusion clamp

While philosophically and conceptually simple, either of the operative maneuvers to obtain aortic occlusion takes at least several minutes to accomplish. This is, of course, valuable time that could be spent directly attacking the hepatic hemorrhage. As there is no aortic occlusion achieved until the clamp is applied, the liver simply continues to bleed. In addition, either of the two operative maneuvers requires manipulation of an area close to the liver. If there is a hemostatic clot, which may have formed on the liver during hypotension, it can be misplaced by this manipulation, worsening the hepatic bleeding.

An alternative is to occlude the aorta in the chest [1]. This requires a left anterolateral thoracotomy. The lung is retracted anteriorly and the aorta dissected free just above the diaphragm. Once again, the esophagus must be identified and care taken to positively identify the aorta. A cross clamp is then applied. This has the advantage of being somewhat remote from the liver. Thus, the planes are not obscured by ongoing hepatic hemorrhage. In addition, it would be difficult to worsen the liver bleeding, manipulating the aorta in the chest. This has the downside, however, of requiring the surgeon to open an uninjured body cavity. The thoracotomy itself, when performed rapidly, can be a source of substantial blood loss, as it is usually not possible to obtain meticulous hemostasis of the chest wall musculature. In addition, the open chest serves as a source of heat loss, worsening the possibility of hypothermia.

Resuscitative Endovascular Balloon Occlusion of the Aorta

Resuscitative endovascular balloon occlusion of the aorta (REBOA) is a new technique which can be attractive as an adjunct to hepatic hemorrhage. The REBOA is placed via the common femoral artery. A standard femoral arterial line is placed, an Amplatz wire is placed via the femoral arterial catheter and the catheter removed. A 12 French introducer is then placed over the guidewire and threaded up into the iliac artery (Fig. 3.4). The guidewire is left in place. The balloon occluder is then threaded over the guidewire, through the introducer system, and up into the aorta. In the case of hepatic hemorrhage, the balloon must be positioned in the distal thoracic aorta, in order to provide inflow occlusion. Placement of the balloon can be confirmed via plain X-ray or fluoroscopy, particularly if some contrast has been instilled into the balloon (Fig. 3.5). Clinicians facile enough with the ultrasound probe may be able to identify the balloon ultrasonographically. There are a number of technical tips important for safe placement of the REBOA. It must be placed into the common femoral artery. The 12 French introducer system simply is too large to be inserted via the superficial femoral artery. If it is to be inserted percutaneously, care must be taken to access the common femoral artery. Ultrasound guidance can be helpful in ensuring that the common femoral artery is in fact accessed.

One alternative is to place the device via femoral artery cutdown. I find this attractive, as that allows me to positively identify the junction

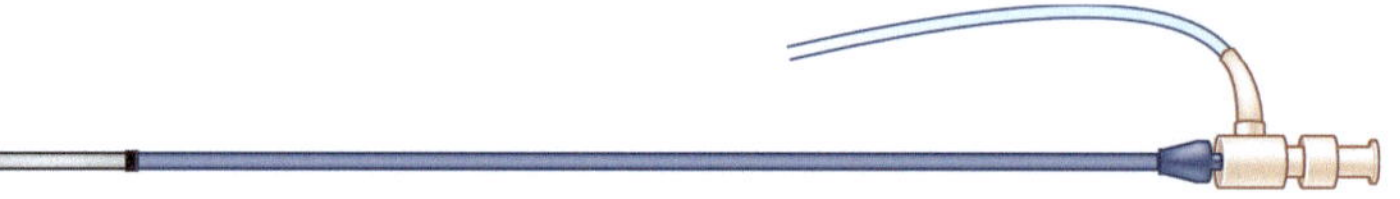

Fig. 3.4 A 12 French introducer placed in the femoral artery

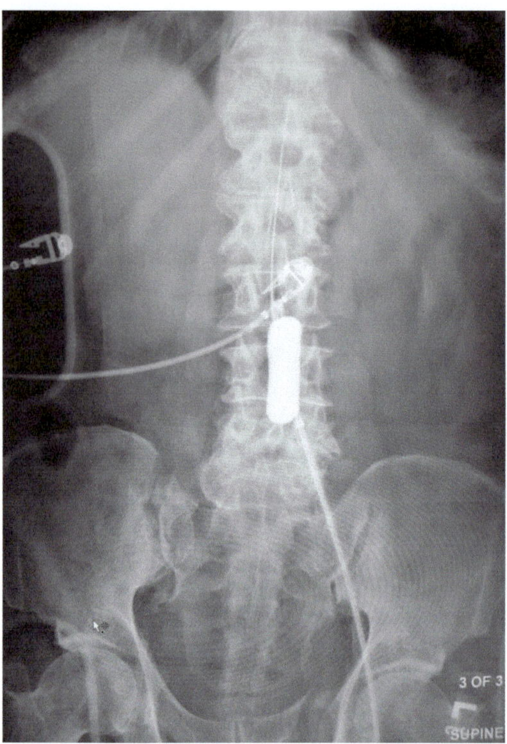

Fig. 3.5 A plain X-ray, after placement of the balloon, can confirm the position, if some contrast has been instilled into the balloon

between the common femoral and superficial femoral artery. Typically, I then place a tie or a loop underneath the common femoral artery and retract it toward the ceiling. This creates a more convenient angle in which to place the femoral arterial line, particularly, in a hypovolemic patient, where the femoral artery may be small and spastic. The introducer is then placed over the guide-wire, similarly as described above. A Rommel tourniquet can be placed around the common femoral artery, to prevent hemorrhage around the introducer system. However, in many cases, the introducer system is large enough that it occupies the majority of the diameter of the femoral artery, limiting blood loss around the vascular site.

Regardless of how the introducer is placed, the femoral artery must be repaired operatively when the introducer is removed. The 12 French introducer leaves an arterial defect that is simply too large to close with simple compression. Most times, the femoral artery can be repaired primarily. Occasionally, in small femoral arteries, a bypass graft may be required.

Early experience with the REBOA has been quite encouraging. This technique championed by Rasmussen et al. has been demonstrated to be quite effective in animal models of hemorrhage [2–4]. A single clinical series exists, recently published by Brenner et al. [5]. This series details the first six patients in which a REBOA was used either at the Shock Center in Baltimore or the University of Texas Houston at Memorial Herman Hospital. There was technical success in all patients. In four of the six patients, the REBOA was used as a bridge to angiographic embolization following blunt trauma, for either solid visceral injury or pelvic hemorrhage. In that series, there were no technical complications of the REBOA.

Dr. Brenner proposes an algorithm describing zones of the aorta (Fig. 3.6). Zone 1 is in the distal thoracic aorta, zone 2 between the esophageal hiatus and the distal aorta, and zone 3 in the distal abdominal aorta, useful for patients with pelvic hemorrhage.

Figures 3.7 and 3.8 demonstrate use of this technique in a patient with a severe liver injury. The patient presented initially hemodynamically stable but developed hypotension. He transiently responded. CT scan (Fig. 3.7) demonstrated a ruptured hepatic hemangioma. The patient developed resistant hypotension and was taken to the operating room, where he had torrential bleeding from the right lobe of his liver. The REBOA was inserted and threaded into the distal aorta. When the balloon was inflated, the patient's blood pressure rose from 60 mmHg to approximately

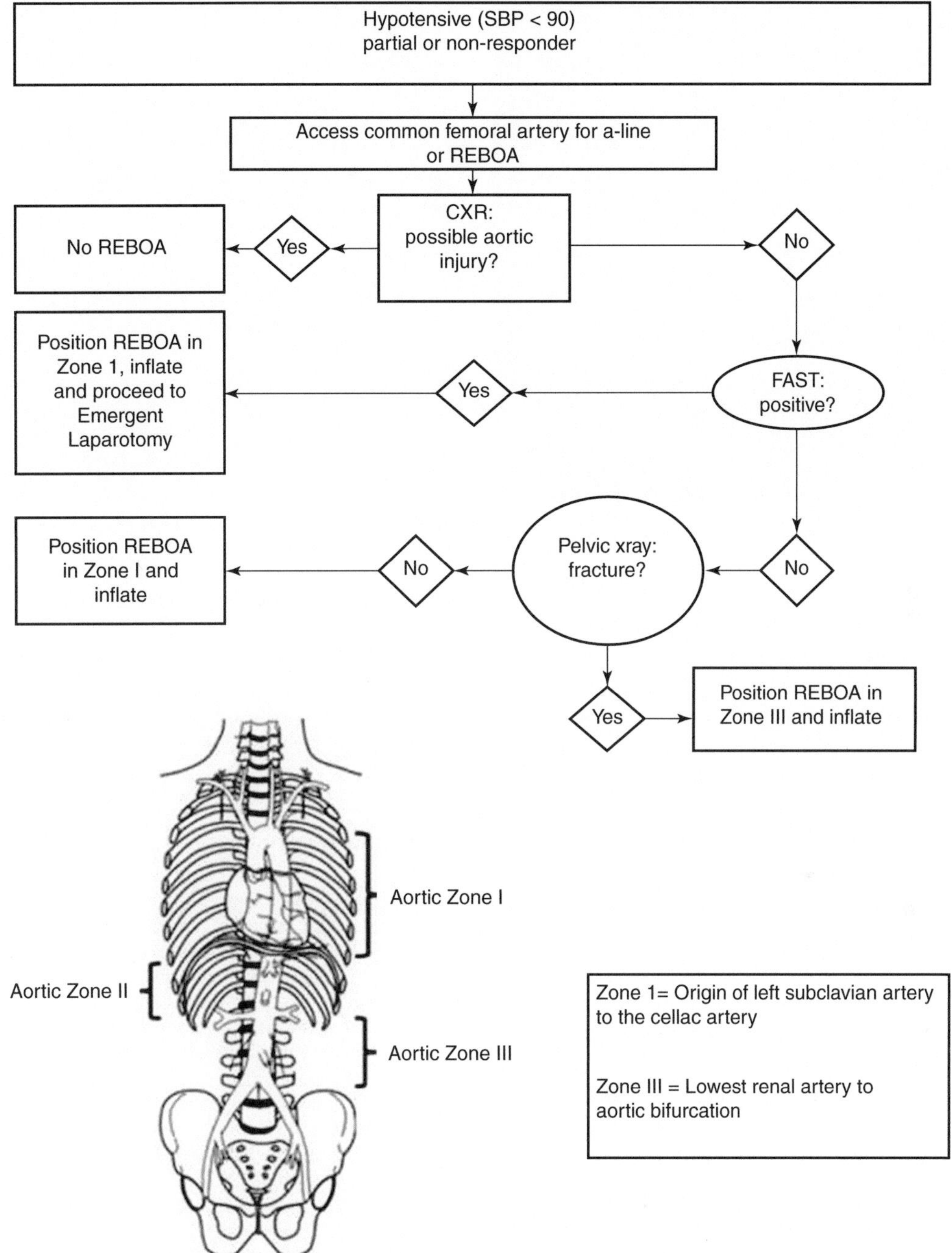

Fig. 3.6 Algorithm showing levels of balloon placement for different levels of aortic occlusion

120/70 mmHg. The patient was then taken to the angiogram suite, where his contralateral femoral artery was accessed using ultrasound guidance. The catheter was introduced up the aorta, into the common hepatic artery. The areas of hemorrhage were identified, the balloon was deflated, and multiple areas of hemorrhage were successfully embolized (Fig. 3.8). The patient ultimately required a right hepatic lobectomy for hepatic necrosis but did well.

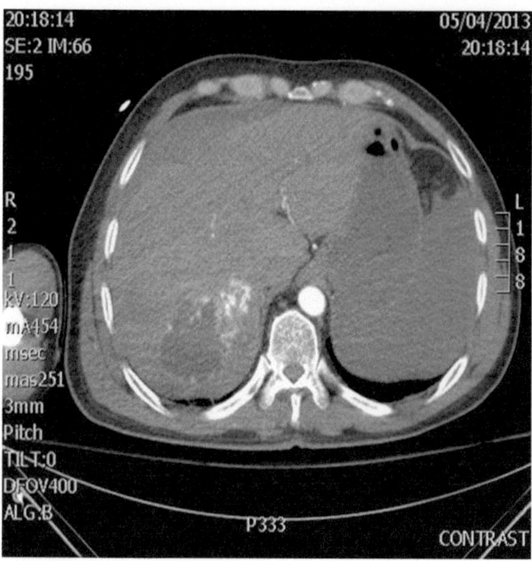

Fig. 3.7 CT scan after blunt trauma demonstrating a ruptured hepatic hemangioma

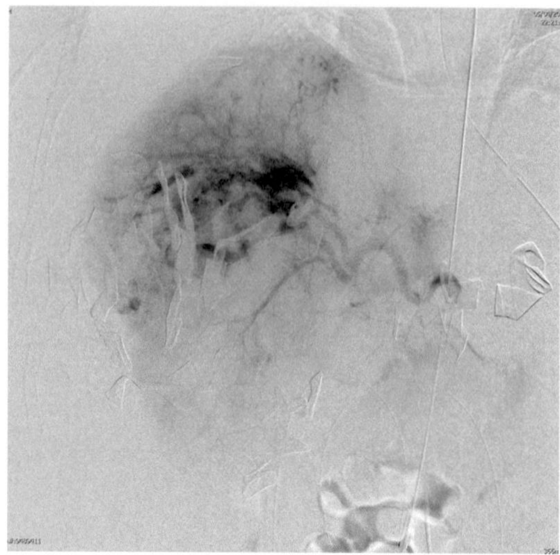

Fig. 3.8 The patient, stabilized after the placement of REBOA in the OR, had hepatic arteriography. The areas of hemorrhage were identified, the REBOA balloon was deflated, and multiple areas of hemorrhage were successfully embolized

The Future

Inflow occlusion is one of the basic principles used to treat vascular injury and/or bleeding from major visceral structures. Some structures such as the spleen and/or the kidney are expendable and can simply be resected. This, however, is virtually never a good idea in the liver. In patients in profound hemorrhagic shock, inflow occlusion of the aorta both helps to control hepatic inflow and improve central hemodynamics. The REBOA is an attractive alternative to traditional open techniques. The technology is beginning to improve. A six and/or seven French introducer system is currently being developed and should be available soon. This will allow easier placement and will likely not require open repair when the sheath is removed. Issues such as training must be addressed with adequate training; the REBOA could conceivably be placed either in the field or in a referring hospital which does not have the capability to provide definitive hemostasis for major liver injuries. The patient could be rapidly transferred with the REBOA in place, deflating the balloon occasionally to prevent declamp shock. This could be used as a bridge to definitive hemostasis in a regional center.

References

1. Ledgerwood AM, Kazmers M, Lucas CE. The role of thoracic aortic occlusion for massive hemoperitoneum. J Trauma Acute Care Surg. 1976;16(8):610–5.
2. White JM, Cannon JW, Stannard A, et al. Endovascular balloon occlusion of the aorta is superior to resuscitative thoracotomy with aortic clamping in a porcine model of hemorrhagic shock. Surgery. 2011;150(3): 400–9.
3. Morrison JJ, Percival TJ, Markov NP, et al. Aortic balloon occlusion is effective in controlling pelvic hemorrhage. J Surg Res. 2012;177(2):341–7.
4. Scott DJ, Eliason JL, Villamaria C, et al. A novel fluoroscopy-free, resuscitative endovascular aortic balloon occlusion system in a model of hemorrhagic shock. J Trauma Acute Care Surg. 2013;75(1): 122–8.
5. Brenner ML, Moore LJ, DuBose JJ, et al. A clinical series of resuscitative endovascular balloon occlusion of the aorta for hemorrhage control and resuscitation. J Trauma Acute Care Surg. 2013;75:506–11.

Massive Hepatic Hemorrhage: Identification

Adrian W. Ong, Vicente Cortes, and Aurelio Rodriguez

Management in the Emergency Room

The patient who presents to the emergency department (ED) with ongoing hemorrhage will show signs of shock such as altered mental status, anxiety, pallor, tachycardia, and tachypnea. Hypotension is commonly defined as a systolic blood pressure (SBP) of less than 90 mmHg. However, an initial SBP greater than 90 mmHg should not give the surgeon a false sense of security. In fact, a redefinition of hypotension as being a systolic blood pressure less than 110 mmHg may be more appropriate based on a recent study of outcomes from a large database that showed increasing mortality associated with a systolic blood pressure less than 110 mmHg [1]. These cutoff values of SBP may not be applicable especially in the older trauma victim who may have baseline systolic hypertension.

Within 1–2 min of arrival, patients who have massive hemorrhage should be identified and the trauma team activated if not already done. The key is to have rapid deployment of adequate personnel and also effective division of labor in the resuscitation process. Team members should know their respective roles during the resuscitation process so as not to exacerbate an often chaotic scene in the emergency room. A focused assessment of sonography in trauma (FAST) should be done within minutes of the patient's arrival and usually concurrently with the primary survey. In the hemodynamically normal patient with a negative FAST after blunt trauma where intra-abdominal injury is possible based on the mechanism of injury, hemodynamic profile, and physical examination, a computed tomography (CT) scan of the abdomen and pelvis should be obtained. In the patient who is not responding to rapid crystalloid infusion, or showing only a transient response, a positive FAST indicates the need for immediate laparotomy (Fig. 4.1), while a negative FAST might indicate an extraperitoneal source of blood loss or that the examination was suboptimal or that the hemodynamic instability was not due to blood loss. In any case, an attempt should be made to stabilize the patient and a CT

A.W. Ong, MD (✉)
Department of Surgery, Reading Hospital,
Sixth Ave and Spruce Street, West Reading,
PA 19611, USA
e-mail: adrian.ong@readinghealth.org

V. Cortes, MD, FACS
Department of Surgery, Reading Hospital,
Sixth Ave & Spruce St, West Reading,
PA 19611, USA
e-mail: vicente.cortes@readinghealth.org

A. Rodriguez, MD
Division of Trauma/Critical Care, Department of
Surgery, Conemaugh Memorial Hospital,
1086 Franklin Street, Johnstown, PA 15905, USA
e-mail: arod@zoominternet.net

Electronic supplementary material Supplementary material is available in the online version of this chapter at 10.1007/978-1-4939-1200-1_4. Videos can also be accessed at http://www.springerimages.com/videos/978-1-4939-1199-8.

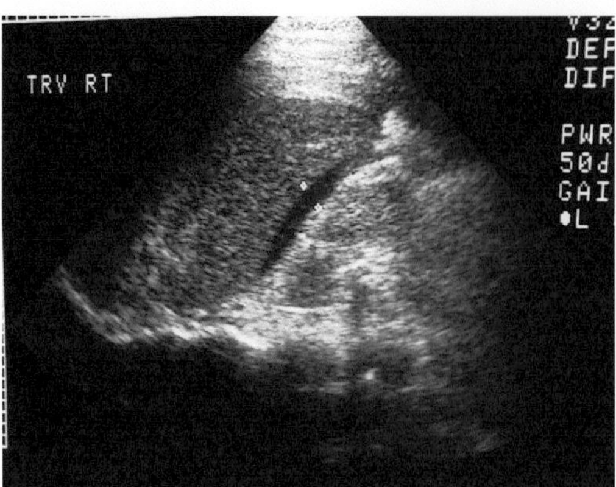

Fig. 4.1 Positive FAST showing fluid in the hepatorenal space

obtained. It is advisable to repeat the FAST prior to leaving the trauma room for CT. Diagnostic peritoneal lavage or laparotomy should be considered if the patient cannot be stabilized.

In patients with penetrating trauma, FAST is less sensitive, and a negative FAST should not be used as the sole criterion to determine need for and urgency of intervention [2]. Gunshot wounds with peritoneal traverse are associated with an extremely high probability of resulting in an injury that requires surgical intervention and the same consideration applies to missile injuries that traverse the upper abdominal quadrants with respect to liver injuries. Stab wounds are associated with a significantly lower probability of intra-abdominal injury, but the presence of shock, signs of peritoneal irritation, or a positive FAST confirms penetration of the peritoneal cavity and high likelihood of intra-abdominal injury requiring surgical intervention.

After ascertaining that there is ongoing intra-abdominal hemorrhage, patients with penetrating abdominal trauma must be transported to the operating room without delay. In these patients, delaying massive fluid resuscitation prior to definitive control of bleeding may improve survival [3]. They are better served by intubation and placement of large-bore vascular access and arterial line by the anesthesiology team in the operating table while the surgical team is assembling for surgical control of hemorrhage.

In the blunt trauma patient with associated significant traumatic brain injury, however, resuscitation to a systolic blood pressure above 90 mmHg is more important, in order to preserve cerebral blood flow and avoid the potential for secondary brain injury associated with hypotension.

In the patient with penetrating torso trauma who loses detectable blood pressure and/or pulses within few minutes of presentation, immediate left anterolateral thoracotomy should be carried out in the emergency department concurrent with orotracheal intubation [4]. After open cardiac massage and addressing the intrathoracic injuries, if there is an organized cardiac rhythm, we favor cross clamping the descending thoracic aorta to minimize abdominal blood loss before proceeding to the operating room. In the patient with blunt trauma who loses blood pressure and/or pulses within few minutes of presentation, ED resuscitative thoracotomy in the emergency room is generally discouraged because of the dismal survival rate, but there have been rare survivors [5].

Assessing Need for Further Radiologic Imaging

The decision to obtain a CT depends on the mechanism of injury, the response to initial fluid resuscitation, and the surgeon's judgment of whether or not information gained from CT would be useful or would alter the management plan.

In the hemodynamically normal patient with a gunshot wound on physical examination, if estimation of trajectory on biplanar plain radiographs suggest peritoneal traverse and there is no evidence of intrathoracic or spinal injury, a preoperative CT is usually not required or helpful. As mentioned before, a negative FAST does not rule out active hemorrhage. In the hemodynamically normal patient with a suspected tangential trajectory, CT may give enough information to the surgeon to avoid laparotomy. In the hemodynamically normal patient with a transmediastinal trajectory or a suspected thoracic vascular injury, CT scanning may also be helpful.

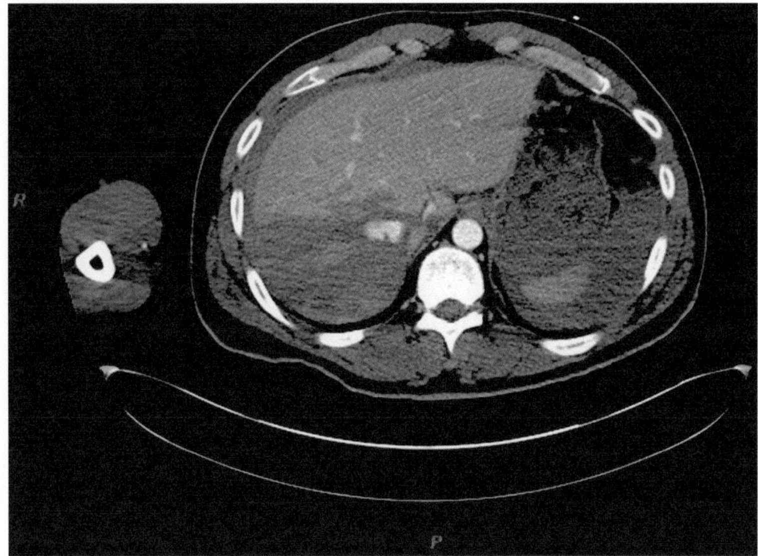

Fig. 4.2 CT showing active liver bleeding with intravenous contrast extravasation and hemoperitoneum. Patient became hypotensive requiring laparotomy shortly after the CT. Bleeding was controlled intraoperatively and no further therapeutic adjunctive measurers were needed

In the blunt trauma patient with a positive FAST, the decision to obtain a CT scan is based on the response to initial fluid resuscitation. Although the imaging time has been reduced with the new generation of multi-detector spiral CT scans to the point of being insignificant, the time and effort required to transport and position the patient remains unchanged and is long enough that the patient may deteriorate with resulting increased morbidity and mortality (Fig. 4.2). If there is suspicion of ongoing bleeding based on information gathered in the trauma room, it is important that a trauma team member continues to direct the resuscitation process in CT. While not a widespread practice, quick bedside estimation of the degree of hemoperitoneum on FAST can be a useful adjunct for the surgeon to decide if there is a need to rapidly transport a patient to the operating room without CT (Table 4.1) [6, 7].

Preparation for the Operating Room

The operating room staff will need to (1) prepare instruments for laparotomy, thoracotomy, midsternotomy, vascular control, and appropriate mechanical retractors; (2) prepare an autologous

Table 4.1 Estimation of hemoperitoneum

Location of blood	Estimated blood volume (ml)
1. Morrison's pouch and/or splenorenal space	150
2. 1 + pelvic cavity	400
3. 2 + left subphrenic space	600
4. 3 + bilateral paracolic gutters	800
5. 4 + right anterior subphrenic space	
Thickness of fluid at right anterior subphrenic space	
0.5 cm	1,000
1.0 cm	1,500
1.5 cm	2,000
2.0 cm	3,000

Adapted with permission from Matsumoto and Ohshiro [7]

blood recovery system and two large capacity suction systems; and (3) secure instruments and materials appropriate for liver hemostasis, i.e., argon beam coagulator, multi-clip appliers, and topical hemostatic agents and carriers.

The trauma surgeon or anesthesiology staff should activate the hospital "massive transfusion protocol" which mandates the delivery of predetermined quantities of uncrossmatched packed RBCs, fresh frozen plasma, and platelets.

Laparotomy and Identification of Massive Liver Bleeding

The patient should be positioned with his upper limbs abducted and extended over arm boards and the anterior torso should be prepped and draped from the base of the neck to the knees and from table top to tablet top to optimize exposure. If there are femoral intravascular catheters already in place for ongoing resuscitation, or previously placed chest drains, they should be securely sutured without overlying dressings, to allow prepping them into the field. It is also a good idea to secure central venous access above the diaphragm concurrently.

In the profoundly hypotensive trauma patient with massive abdominal distention, a possible consideration is left anterolateral thoracotomy for aortic cross clamping and proximal vascular control because sudden decompression may result in cardiac arrest before the alternative supraceliac aortic compression may be established.

A midline incision is the preferred trauma laparotomy incision. In the presence of a tense hemoperitoneum, a midline incision extending from the xyphoid to the pubis is made and the fascia is opened for the entire length of the skin incision exposing the intact peritoneum, prior to opening the peritoneum. If the peritoneum is opened prior to complete division of the midline fascia, the eruption of blood and small bowel loops that could follow might make it impossible to safely use any sharp instruments to rapidly complete the incision without injuring the visceral contents or the hands of the operating surgeons. Once the peritoneum is fully exposed, it may be opened by tearing it digitally from the xyphoid to the pubis.

After the abdomen is entered through a midline incision, the four quadrants of the abdomen are rapidly packed using heavy handheld abdominal retractors and many folded laparotomy packs. The packs are removed, starting with the quadrant where there is the least amount of visible blood loss. After removing the right upper quadrant packing last, the liver injury is assessed. The round ligament is divided and the falciform ligament is taken down all the way up to the hepatic

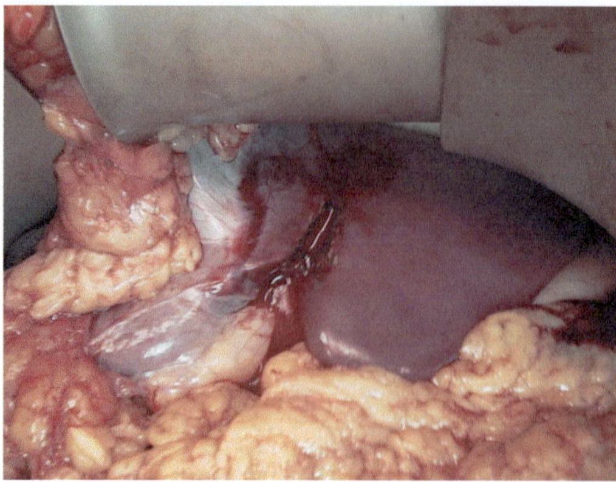

Fig. 4.3 Bleeding from torn liver edges that is obvious without mobilization

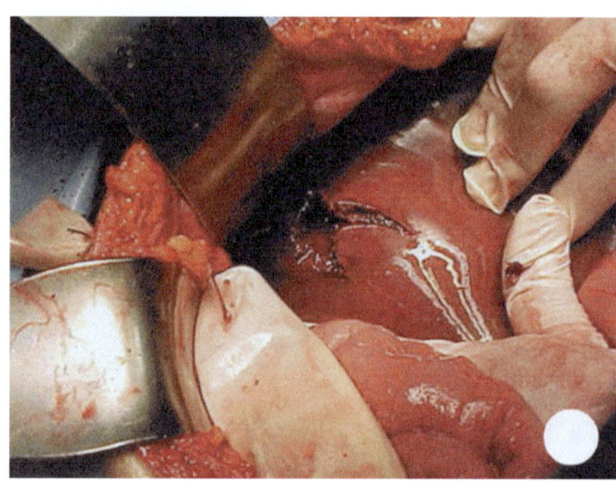

Fig. 4.4 Manual compression to slow down brisk bleeding (Courtesy of Dr Pablo Otolino)

coronary ligament. Bimanual pressure is applied compressing the liver in lateral-to-medial and anterior-to-posterior directions. The organ may be packed again in the right upper quadrant under folded laparotomy pads and handheld retractors. Video 10 demonstrates these maneuvers.

Brisk bleeding from the liver may be evident even without mobilization (Fig. 4.3). The next step is manual compression (Fig. 4.4). All crushed, devitalized liver tissue is resected and bleeding is controlled by individual vessel ligation (debridement-resection). Diffuse bleeding from the raw surface can be controlled by topical hemostatic products such as fibrin glue or argon beam coagulation (Fig. 4.5). If bleeding is brisk and obscures the surgeons view, it is

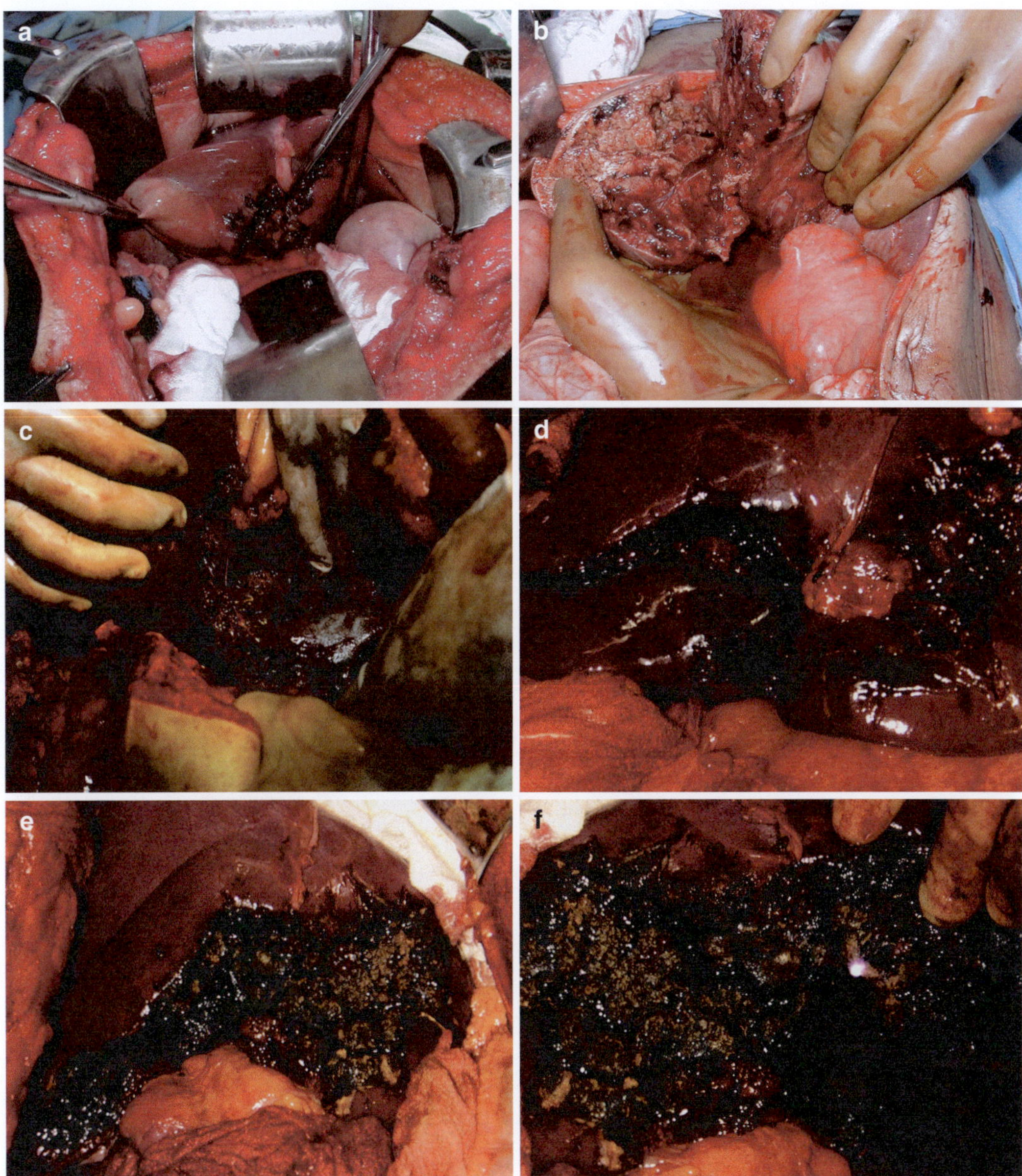

Fig. 4.5 Major lobar injury to the liver. All crushed, non-viable liver tissue is exposed (**a**), gross bleeding is controlled by ligation (**b**), resection of devitalized liver tissue, debridement-resection (**c**). Hemostasis from the raw areas of the liver is secured by local applications of coagulants (**d**). Argon beam coagulator is also very helpful for controlling bleeding from the raw area of the debrided liver (**e, f**) (Courtesy of Dr. Rao Ivatury)

advisable to carry out occlusion of the vascular inflow via the Pringle maneuver. Once the hepatoduodenal ligament is exposed, the foramen of Winslow is found digitally. The left index finger inserted via the foramen into the lesser sac is encircled around the liver pedicle bluntly making an opening in the usually thin lesser omentum. At this point a Penrose drain may be placed around the liver pedicle in preparation for Pringle maneuver: occlusion of the pedicle using a Rummel tourniquet or alternatively a vascular clamp (see Video 6).

It is usually not necessary to mobilize the liver. Manual compression, aided by the Pringle maneuver, is sufficient to allow suturing and clipping in most cases.

If bleeding does not stop, and dark non-pulsatile blood is welling up from behind the liver or through the liver parenchyma despite the above measures, a very real possibility is juxtahepatic venous bleeding. Manual compression of the liver should be resumed, the liver repacked, and the Pringle maneuver reapplied, followed by reassessment to see if the bleeding slows.

If there is no cessation of bleeding with the above, there is a very real possibility of subsequent exsanguination. The surgeon should consider obtaining help from another (experienced) surgeon. The rate of juxtahepatic venous bleeding sometimes is difficult to judge. The bleeding may alternate between brisk and slow depending on the patient's fluctuating volume status. If bleeding wells up rapidly, simple perihepatic packing will not be sufficient to achieve hemostasis. The liver should then be mobilized by dividing the triangular ligament and taking down the bare area and coronary ligament to the level of the IVC on the right and by dividing the triangular ligament and taking down the coronary ligament to the level of the IVC on the left. Mobilization usually requires extension of the midline incision to include the xyphoid and the use of mechanical retraction. To aid in exposure of the suprahepatic inferior vena cava, a right thoracoabdominal incision with takedown of the right hemidiaphragm can be quickly done. Alternatively, a median sternotomy can be done, especially if atrio-caval shunting or venovenous bypass is contemplated. The objective is to achieve hepatic vascular isolation by controlling the supra- and infrahepatic vena cava and occluding the liver pedicle (Video 9). Since the patient might not tolerate total vascular isolation without sufficient infusion of fluids and blood products above the diaphragm, one should consider adding supraceliac aortic occlusion to avoid cardiac arrest.

Video Captions

Video 2   Right hepatic lobe rotation (MP4 42120 kb)

Video 3   Right hepatic lobe rotation (3-D animation) (MP4 33079 kb)

Video 6   Pringle maneuver (MP4 14015 kb)

Video 7   Liver suture (MP4 39685 kb)

Video 9   Hepatic vascular exclusion (MP4 99239 kb)

Video 10   Omental pack (MP4 32585 kb)

Video 11   Digital compression (MP4 16750 kb)

References

1. Eastridge BJ, Salinas J, McManus JG, Blackburn L, Bugler EM, Cooke WH, et al. Hypotension begins at 110 mm Hg: redefining "hypotension" with data. J Trauma. 2007;63(2):291–9.
2. Quinn AC, Sinert R. What is the utility of the Focused Assessment with Sonography in Trauma (FAST) exam in penetrating torso trauma? Injury. 2011;42(5): 482–7.
3. Bickell WH, Wall Jr MJ, Pepe PE, Martin RR, Ginger VF, Allen MK, et al. Immediate versus delayed fluid resuscitation for hypotensive patients with penetrating torso injuries. N Engl J Med. 1994;27(17):1105–9.
4. Seamon MJ, Fisher CA, Gaughan JP, Kulp H, Dempsey DT, Goldberg AJ. Emergency department thoracotomy: survival of the least expected. World J Surg. 2008;32:604–12.
5. Moore EE, Knudson MM, Burlew CC, Inaba K, Dicker RA, Biffl WL, et al. Defining the limits of resuscitative emergency department thoracotomy: a contemporary Western Trauma Association perspective. J Trauma. 2011;70(2):334–9.
6. McKenney KL, McKenney MG, Cohn SM, Compton R, Nunez DB, Dolich M, et al. Hemoperitoneum score helps determine need for therapeutic laparotomy. J Trauma. 2001;50(4):650–4.
7. Matsumoto H, Ohshiro K. Ultrasound in abdominal trauma. In: Machi J, Sigel B, editors. Ultrasound for surgeons. New York/Tokyo: IGAKU-SHOIN Medical Publishers; 1997. p. 72–9.

Massive Hepatic Hemorrhage: Initial Steps in Hemostasis

Juan A. Asensio, Juan Manuel Verde,
Patrizio Petrone, Alejandro J. Pérez-Alonso,
Corrado Marini, and Anthony Policastro

Introduction

Despite the continued advances in the areas of Trauma Surgery and Surgical Critical Care, the mortality of complex hepatic injuries remains extremely high. Similarly, their surgical management poses a formidable challenge to even the most experienced trauma surgeons. Uncontrolled hemorrhage leading to exsanguination is the leading cause of hepatic mortality, accounting for over 50 % of hepatic injury induced mortality [1–3, 5, 6].

American Association for the Surgery of Trauma Organ Injury Scale (AAST-OIS) grade IV and V complex hepatic injuries remain among the most formidable injuries confronting trauma surgeons, as the vast majority of these patients present in shock with multiple associated injuries and most have already embarked in the cycle of acidosis, hypothermia, and coagulopathy that often leads to the lethal tetrad of fatal cardiac dysrhythmias and death. The severity of these injuries requires that trauma surgeons select complex techniques not commonly utilized from their vast surgical armamentarium. The overall incidence of AAST-OIS grade IV and V hepatic injuries is approximately 5 %; therefore, few trauma surgeons and trauma centers have developed significant expertise with their management. The purpose of this chapter is to outline the steps and provide a detailed approach to achieve initial hemostasis in the presence of massive life-threatening hepatic hemorrhage [1–5, 8–13].

J.A. Asensio, MD, FACS, FCCM, FRCS (England) (✉)
Department of Surgery, New York Medical College,
Valhalla, NY, USA

Division of Trauma Surgery and Acute Care Surgery,
Joel A. Halpern Trauma Center, International
Medicine Institute, Research Institute, Westchester
Medical Center, Taylor Pavilion, 100 Woods Rd,
Suite E-137, Valhalla, NY 10595, USA
e-mail: asensioj@wcmc.com

J.M. Verde, MD • A.J. Pérez-Alonso, MD
Westchester Medical Center,
Taylor Pavilion, 100 Woods Rd, Suite E-144,
Valhalla, NY 10595, USA

P. Petrone, MD, MPH
New York Medical College/Westchester
Medical Center, Taylor Pavilion, 100 Woods Rd,
Suite E-140, Valhalla, NY 10595, USA

C. Marini, MD, FACS
New York Medical College/Westchester
Medical Center,
Taylor Pavilion, 100 Woods Rd, Suite E-131,
Valhalla, NY 10595, USA

A. Policastro, MD
Westchester Medical Center,
Taylor Pavilion, 100 Woods Rd, Suite E-136,
Valhalla, NY 10595, USA

Electronic supplementary material Supplementary material is available in the online version of this chapter at 10.1007/978-1-4939-1200-1_5. Videos can also be accessed at http://www.springerimages.com/videos/978-1-4939-1199-8.

R.R. Ivatury (ed.), *Operative Techniques for Severe Liver Injury*,
DOI 10.1007/978-1-4939-1200-1_5, © Springer Science+Business Media New York 2015

Initial Operating Room Management

Any patients suspected as harboring an AAST-OIS grade IV and V hepatic injuries (Fig. 5.1) must be rapidly transported to the operating room (OR). Prior notification of the patient's impending transport to the OR is of the utmost importance, given the fact that special instruments and adjunct technology are often required for the management of these injuries. Prompt notification will immediately set forth in motion protocols for the management of critically injured patients. These patients should be directed to the selected trauma operating room which should be pre-warmed and adequately equipped with rewarming technologies including fluid warmers, warming mattresses, and rapid infusers. Furthermore, the argon beam coagulator must be available as well as instrument trays specifically designed to manage abdominal, thoracic, and vascular trauma.

The massive transfusion protocol (MTP) must also be activated. Activation must proceed expeditiously by the leader of the trauma team, preferably the attending trauma surgeon, trauma fellow, or chief surgical resident, and the blood products must also be present in the operating room at the time the patient's arrival [1–8, 32].

All trauma patients must be placed on the operating table in a cross position with arms extended at a 90° angle. Clearly all patients must be prepped from the neck to the mid-thighs and from side of table to side of table, thus making the thoracic cavity easily accessible if a left anterolateral thoracotomy is required for aortic cross-clamping and open cardiopulmonary resuscitation. Should this be necessary, the standard approach is used. We personally prefer to utilize a Crafoord-DeBakey aortic cross-clamp. Similarly, a median sternotomy may also be performed in the standard fashion.

Among the operating room equipment considered vital are large Poole suction devices (Fig. 5.2) in order to be able to rapidly aspirate blood contained within the abdominal cavity.

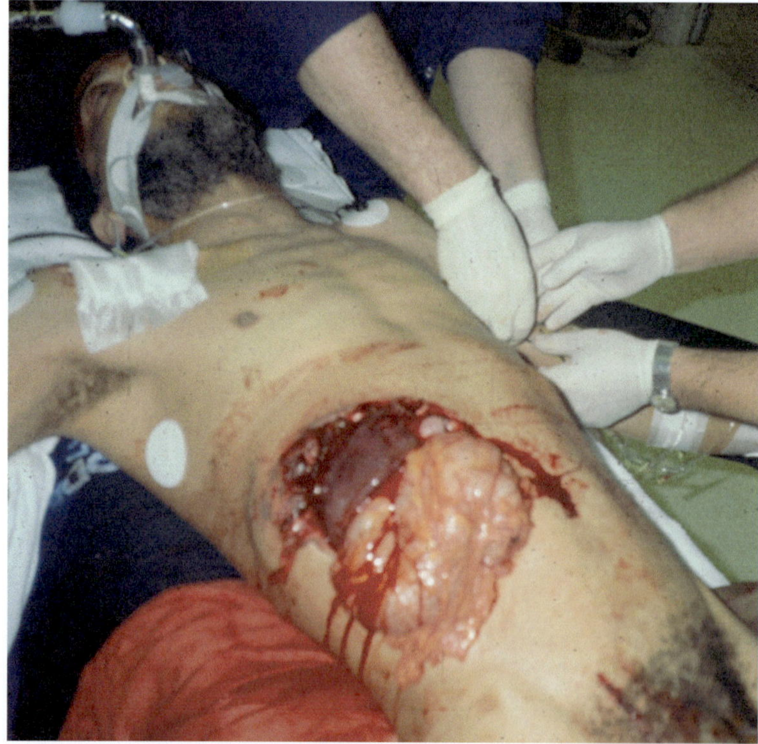

Fig. 5.1 Patient that sustained a close range shotgun blast with an AAST-OIS grade V hepatic injury and significant loss of the abdominal wall. Patient was rapidly transported to the OR and required right hepatic lobectomy

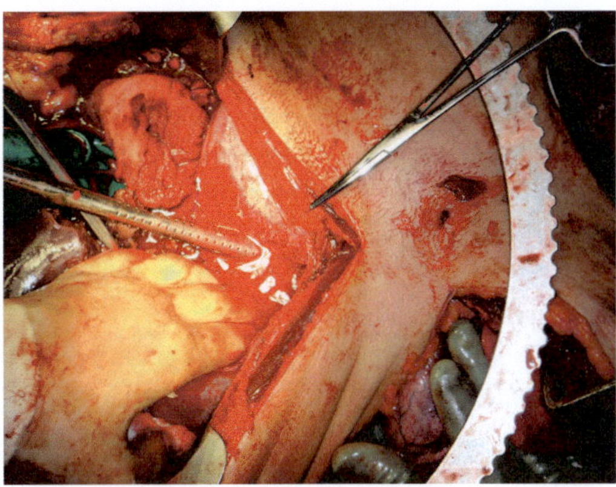

Fig. 5.2 Patient that sustained multiple gunshot wounds requiring a left anterolateral resuscitation thoracotomy and aortic cross-clamping. He recovered an excellent cardiac output and blood pressure. An exploratory laparotomy was carried out. Notice large Poole suction devices required to rapidly remove blood and temporary packing of the liver

Similarly, if a blood scavenging autotransfusion system is available, this must be previously set up and managed by the perfusionists so that autotransfused blood may be administered to the trauma patient intraoperatively. The trauma surgeon must work closely with the attending anesthesiologist and the anesthesia team; however, the trauma surgeon must guide the intravascular volume replacement and select the formula for replacement.

Regardless of the choice of formulas, whether it is 1:2 or 1:1, it is clear that ample quantities of blood and blood products including fresh frozen plasma, platelets, and cryoprecipitate must be available. It is also important that the patient be monitored intraoperatively and his or her end points of resuscitation be followed by continuous point of care (POC) testing with arterial blood gases, so that the pH, bicarbonate, base deficit, and lactic acid levels can be monitored along with coagulation parameters and platelet counts. Electrolytes must also be measured including the ionized calcium, magnesium, and phosphorous while also monitoring the patient's temperature and end-tidal CO_2. If available, thromboelastography (TEG) should be used as a guide for intravascular volume replacement [1–8, 32].

Laparotomy: Initial Steps

Exposure

All trauma patients must be approached via a midline laparotomy incision extending from the xyphoid process to the symphysis pubis. The incision must be rapidly carried through into skin and subcutaneous tissue while controlling hemostasis from the transected subcutaneous vessels. We prefer to utilize either Halsted Mosquitos or Kelly clamps sequentially. This is important since many of the patients are already coagulopathic or will become coagulopathic and subcutaneous vessels are a source of fastidious bleeding. The midline fascia is sharply transected and the peritoneum is then grasped with two Schnidt clamps; utilizing a Metzenbaum scissor, it is incised. Attempts must be made to quantitate the blood loss which will be difficult by rapidly placing the two Poole suction devices in the abdominal cavity. It is important to quantitate intra-abdominal blood loss as best as possible. This measurement then serves as an objective guide for intravascular blood volume replacement [1–8].

Once the abdominal cavity is entered, large clots must be manually removed and attempts at direct visualization of the hepatic injury must be carried out. Although it has been traditional surgical lore that all four quadrants of the abdominal cavity must be packed, we do not subscribe to that notion; we prefer to directly approach the bleeding source, in this case, the liver. At this time, simultaneous compression of the injured liver with two laparotomy packs held over the anterior and posterior surfaces of the liver by an assistant will allow the operating surgeon to rapidly place a Bookwalter or Balfour retractor to allow for exposure. This allows the hands of the surgical assistants to be freed to assist the operating surgeon. Many surgical textbooks recommend that the primary operating surgeon be positioned on the left side of the patient. We do not have any strong preference as to whether we position ourselves on the right or left hand side of the table, but clearly exposure of the injured liver is of paramount importance [1–8].

Mobilization

In order to be able to assess and operatively manage complex hepatic injuries AAST-OIS grades IV and V, the liver must be adequately mobilized. To that extent, the trauma surgeon must be familiar with hepatic anatomy to promptly mobilize the liver by sharply transecting the ligaments that hold the liver in place. The first maneuver is to break the suction that exists between the dome of the right lobe of the liver and the diaphragm which is performed manually and then proceed to sharply transect the falciform ligament utilizing two Schnidt clamps while ligating the transected ligament with suture ligatures of 0 or 2-0 Silk. After the falciform ligament has been transected between clamps and ligated, we then utilize electrocautery to transect the ligament in a cephalad direction toward the dome of the liver. One notable exception is the patient with a cirrhotic liver, in which this maneuver should be avoided if at all possible.

Other important maneuvers in mobilizing the liver, depending on which lobe has been injured, include sharply transecting the triangular ligaments of either the right lobe or left lobe of the liver. Transecting the triangular ligament of the right lobe of the liver is accomplished by placing downward traction on the right lobe while digitally locating this ligament. If it is feasible, placement of an index finger under the ligament serves as a guide; Metzenbaum scissors are then utilized to transect this ligament while the liver is simultaneously rotated from right to left in the abdominal cavity. Meticulous attention must be exercised not to extend the transection of the triangular ligament into the two leaflets of the right coronary ligament without proper visualization, as the right hepatic vein is found in close proximity and may be inadvertently injured.

Similarly, to mobilize the left lobe, downward traction must be placed in the left lobe identifying the left triangular ligament which is then sharply transected in the previously described fashion. Again, caution is required so that the transection of the left triangular ligament is not extended to the left coronary ligament without visualization, as the left hepatic or the common trunk of the left and middle hepatic veins is found in close proximity and may be inadvertently injured. Similarly, the left phrenic vessels, but particularly the left phrenic vein, may be iatrogenically injured. To fully mobilize the right lobe of the liver, it is recommended that a series of folded laparotomy packs be placed behind the right lobe of the liver.

Another important maneuver which is part of mobilization consists of identifying the gastroepiploic foramen of Winslow and assessing whether it is fused or not. This is important if the trauma surgeon anticipates performing a Pringle maneuver which would be facilitated if the foramen were open.

Temporary Hepatic Packing and Compression

After the liver has been fully mobilized, compression is required to allow the anesthesiology team to restore intravascular volume losses which must be replaced. Once the injury has been identified, direct compression of the injured lobe or segment of the liver must be carried out with folded laparotomy packs (Fig. 5.3). Compression must be bimanually applied. However, should there be other intra-abdominal injuries, it is judicious to pack the liver to arrest hepatic hemorrhage temporarily while other life-threatening injuries are addressed.

If there are large bleeding parenchymal lacerations, intrahepatic packing must be considered. This can be performed temporarily by placing sheets of hemostatic agents such as Surgicel™ Nu Knit or plain Surgicel™ which can be applied to the denuded and injured surfaces of the intrahepatic parenchyma directly and be covered with a laparotomy pack. Alternatively, gel foam and thrombin patches may also be used during temporary closure of the hepatic laceration. To achieve closure, its edges are coapted by placement of several separate horizontal mattress Halsted sutures with 2-0 chromic sutures on a CT-1 needle to secure this intraparenchymal pack. Similarly, the liver can then be externally packed by applying several folded laparotomy

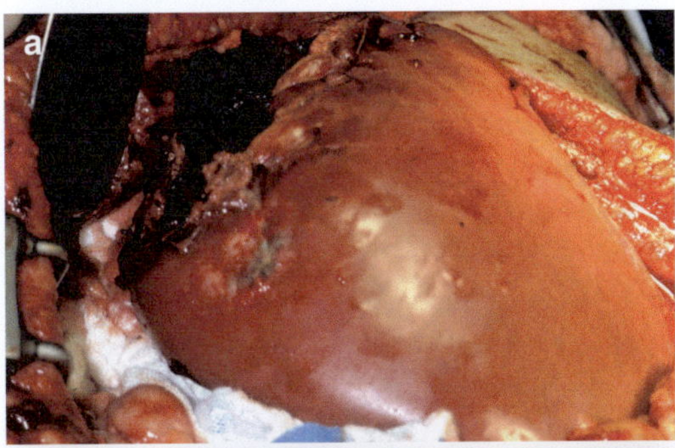

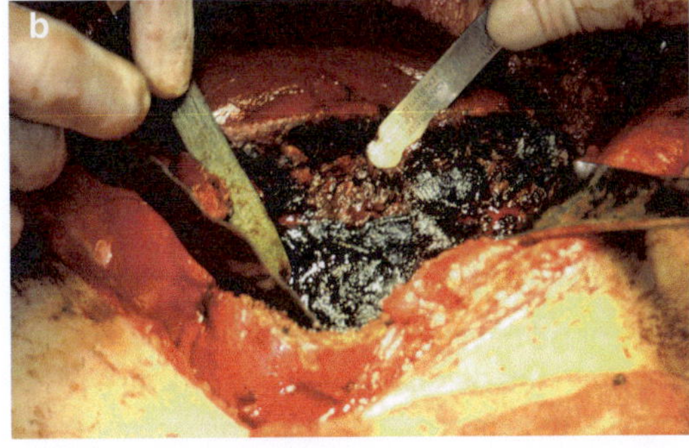

Fig. 5.3 Patient that sustained an abdominal gunshot wound resulting in a grade IV liver injury (**a**). Temporary intrahepatic packing was done along with an external hepatic compression (**b**). Notice the malleable retractors

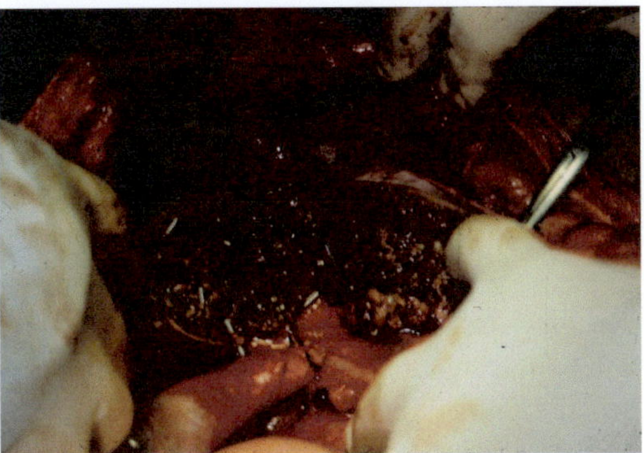

Fig. 5.4 Cantlie's line showing the delimitation between the right and left liver, exposing the retrohepatic inferior vena cava (IVC). Notice the several clips applied in order to control hemostasis. Falciform ligament is also seen marking the left segmental fissure to the lobar fissure

packs compressing the dome of the liver superiorly and inferiorly and by placement of laparotomy packs in the subhepatic pouch of Morison while simultaneously wrapping laparotomy packs around the left lobe of the liver. These maneuvers will allow for temporary control of hemostasis while other life-threatening injuries are addressed and gastrointestinal spillage is controlled [1–8, 14–32].

Injury Identification

It is important for the trauma surgeon to identify and appropriately grade hepatic injuries utilizing the AAST-OIS. It is also important that the trauma surgeon be familiar with Couinaud's description of hepatic segmental anatomy in order to describe accurately the location of the injury (Fig. 5.4).

At times, injuries to Couinaud's segment I, the caudate lobe (Spiegel's lobe), can be challenging to evaluate as they are often associated with a significant zone I supra-mesocolic and right zone II retroperitoneal hematomas. In order to identify injuries in this segment, a right-sided medial visceral rotation must be performed by sharp transection of the avascular line of Toldt which holds the right colon in place. This is carried out by a meticulous combination of blunt and sharp dissection with Metzenbaum scissors while extending this maneuver above the hepatic flexure. Gentle sweeping from the right to left of the colon, digitally or utilizing sponge sticks, will expose the infrarenal inferior vena cava (IVC).

Meticulous attention must be directed to identifying the right ureter and the right gonadal vein which drains in the anterior surface of the infrarenal IVC. An extensive Kocher maneuver must be added, also utilizing a meticulous combination of blunt and sharp dissection mobilizing the first through the third portion of the duodenum from medial to lateral which can be performed while the assistant holds gentle traction on the duodenal C-loop. These maneuvers will expose injuries to the caudate (Spiegel's lobe). In addition, suprarenal dissection of the IVC can then be carried out utilizing a meticulous combination of blunt and sharp dissection. We prefer to separate the blood suffused tissues of the retroperitoneum utilizing either Kittner dissectors or sponge sticks while preserving the integrity of the very delicate IVC [1–8, 17–32].

After the liver has been mobilized and exposed, it is important to carefully observe and visualize the injury in order to assign an AAST-OIS injury grade. This is important, as intraoperative injury grading will lead to appropriate technique selection from the vast armamentarium of surgical techniques that a trauma surgeon must possess in order to deal with these injuries. Trauma surgeons must be cognizant of the fact that only the most complex surgical techniques will be required for the management of complex hepatic injuries grade IV or V; however, these techniques are infrequently utilized.

We prefer to grade the depth of the injury by placing the end of a scalpel which has a ruler in order to measure the depth of the injury. This must be done gently and not to cause any further bleeding. Alternatively, a sterile metal ruler can also be utilized to measure depth. Once this maneuver has been performed, the surgeon will have all the necessary information required to assign an injury grade and select the appropriate surgical technique to control the hemostasis [1–8, 17–32].

Decisions

Thoracotomy

The decision to perform a left anterolateral resuscitative thoracotomy is easy and usually dictated by the patient's hemodynamic compromise or the onset cardiopulmonary arrest. The standard incision is utilized commencing at the fifth intercostal space from the left sternocostal margin and extending it laterally to the medial border of the left latissimus dorsi. All patients should have their left arm elevated in a cephalad direction to open the intercostal spaces. Similarly, in female patients, the left breast must be also elevated cephalad to avoid iatrogenic injury [33–42].

The incision is sharply carried through into skin and subcutaneous tissues utilizing a 10 or 21 scalpel blade. The intercostalis muscle is then identified and sharply incised for approximately 2 cm. Insertion of the index finger will allow guidance to sharply transect the three slips of this muscle utilizing Metzenbaum scissors. This incision is sharply carried through from the medial to the lateral border with simultaneous transection of the parietal pleura.

Placement of a Finochietto retractor follows completion of the incision to access the left hemithoracic cavity. At that time, evacuation of any blood is carried out. Inspection of the left lung and pericardium is also carried out. Whether or not there is an associated cardiac injury, the pericardium is then grasped with two Allis clamps anterior to the left phrenic nerve and, utilizing either a 10 or 15 scalpel blade, a 1–2 cm incision is created as the two Allis clamps lift the pericardium off the heart to avoid iatrogenic injury. At that time, Metzenbaum scissors are then inserted and the incision extended in a cephalad direction with the upper limits being the root of the ascending aorta. Similarly, the incision is then extended in a caudad direction toward the apex of the heart and any clots located are evacuated. This is an important maneuver if open cardiopulmonary resuscitation is required [33–42].

Attention is then shifted toward cross-clamping the descending thoracic aorta, another vital maneuver, to be able to redistribute the remaining blood volume to perfuse both the carotid and coronary arteries as the patient's intravascular blood volume is rapidly replaced.

The descending thoracic aorta is located against the spinal column. The NG tube placed during the initial assessment and resuscitation will serve to identify the esophagus which crosses in the lower aspect of the left hemithoracic cavity from the right to the left. Having identified the esophagus, the aorta is palpated and then utilizing a meticulous combination of blunt and sharp dissection with Metzenbaum scissors, the circumference of the aorta is dissected. At that time, the aorta may be digitally occluded or clamped with a Crafoord-DeBakey aortic clamp to allow the anesthesiologists to replace lost intravascular blood volume. With this maneuver, the patient's blood pressure should rise to between 80 and 100 systolic; if this occurs, it serves as a positive indicator of outcome. Similarly, this maneuver will also help in arresting arterial subdiaphragmatic hemorrhage.

The decision to perform a right anterolateral thoracotomy is more difficult. It is indicated in the presence of significant hemorrhage from the right dome of the liver especially if there has been an associated destructive injury to the right hemidiaphragm. The same previously described technique for a left anterolateral thoracotomy applies.

The decision to perform median sternotomy is a difficult one and should be considered when there is extensive injury to the dome of the liver which may involve the hepatic veins draining into the retrohepatic vena cava or an injury to the retrohepatic vena cava itself. A median sternotomy must be rapidly performed with the incision commencing at the sternal notch and ending in the xyphoid process utilizing a 10 or 21 scalpel blade and transecting the skin and subcutaneous tissues. It is important to remain in the midline of the sternum. This incision is sharply carried through skin and subcutaneous tissue and electrocautery is used to achieve hemostasis [33–42].

A meticulous combination of blunt and sharp dissection at the sternal notch must be carried out in order to open a plane to place the sternal saw. This can be carried out with Mixter right angle or Schnidt clamps. The trauma surgeon must be aware that both the innominate artery and vein are in close juxtaposition with the posterior surface of the upper sternum in order to avoid iatrogenic injury. Once this plane has been sufficiently opened, the sternal saw is placed and the anesthesiologists are asked to temporarily cease ventilation. The sternal saw is then directed from a cephalad to caudad direction [33–42].

Once the sternum is open, two Army-Navy retractors are used to elevate the transected right and left portions of the sternum while electrocautery is utilized to secure hemostasis. Electrocautery must be used directly under the border of the sternum at a depth of no more than 0.5 cm in order to avoid iatrogenic injury to the internal mammary arteries. A Finochietto retractor is then placed and gradually opened. At times, it is important to place several laparotomy packs and folded surgical towels to buttress and support this retractor inferiorly. The thymus in young patients is identified in the upper portion of this incision and should be swept in both cephalad

and lateral directions utilizing either sponge sticks or Kittner dissectors. The fibrous tissues of the pericardium are then identified and grasped between two Allis clamps and are then incised from a cephalad to caudad direction in a linear fashion to expose the heart. We prefer utilizing radial incisions in the inferior borders of the pericardium in order to provide wider exposure for visualization of the heart. The pericardium is then secured with stay sutures of 0 Silk to the flanges of the Finochietto sternal retractor. The heart is then identified and attention is then directed toward locating the space of Gibbon which defines the entrance of the suprahepatic cava through the diaphragm into the right atrium. Frequently this space is fused. This space should not be dissected as it is easy to injure the very delicate intrapericardial portion of the IVC. Enough space exists for the placement of a Craafoord-DeBakey aortic clamp at the IVC should this be necessary [33–42].

Median Sternotomy

Median sternotomy was frequently used in the past when trauma surgeons utilized Schrock's atrio-caval shunt. In our opinion, median sternotomy should now be infrequently used and only for very selective cases. Similarly, we as well as the vast majority of trauma surgeons have abandoned the use of the atrio-caval shunt. Nevertheless, the trauma surgeon must be facile in performing either a thoracotomy or median sternotomy in selected cases of grade IV and V hepatic injuries.

Injury Grading

Since the advent of the AAST Liver Injury Scale (Table 5.1), the injury grading system for the liver has undergone several modifications. Consistent hepatic injury grading has proven to be a great advancement in the management of hepatic injuries (Fig. 5.5), as it allows the trauma surgeon to select the appropriate surgical technique from their vast armamentarium to

Table 5.1 The American Association for the Surgery of Trauma (AAST) liver injury scale (1994 revision)

Grade[a]	Type of injury	Description of injury
I	Hematoma	Subcapsular, <10 % surface area
	Laceration	Capsular tear, <1 cm parenchymal depth
II	Hematoma	Subcapsular, 10–50 % surface area
		Intraparenchymal <10 cm in diameter
	Laceration	Capsular tear 1–3 parenchymal depth, <10 cm in length
III	Hematoma	Subcapsular, >50 % surface area of ruptured subcapsular or parenchymal hematoma; intraparenchymal hematoma >10 cm or expanding
	Laceration	>3 cm parenchymal depth
IV	Laceration	Parenchymal disruption involving 25–75 % hepatic lobe or 1–3 Couinaud's segments
V	Laceration	Parenchymal disruption involving >75 % of hepatic lobe or >3 Couinaud's segments within a single lobe
	Vascular	Juxtahepatic venous injuries, i.e., retrohepatic vena cava/central major hepatic veins
VI	Vascular	Hepatic avulsion

From Moore et al. [7]

[a]Advance one grade for multiple injuries up to grade III

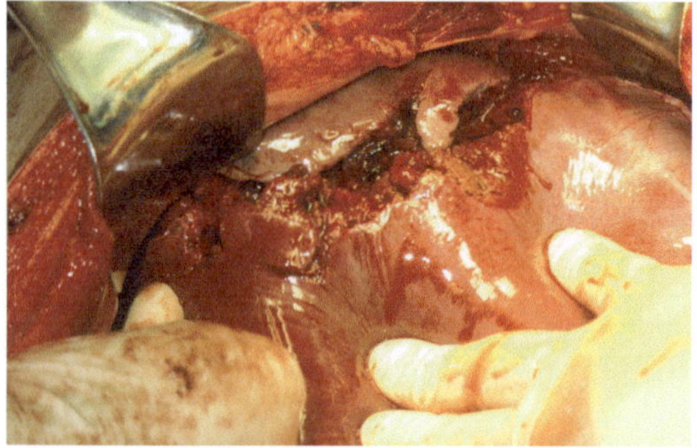

Fig. 5.5 Case of a hepatic complex injury AAST-OIS grades IV–V

manage injuries appropriately stratified to injury grade, thus reserving the most complex surgical techniques for the most complex injuries. Similarly, establishing uniformity in the description of these injuries has advanced research as means of comparing outcomes for these injuries [1–4, 7].

Maneuvers to Control Hemorrhage

The Pringle Maneuver and Initial Decision Making

Since this maneuver was described in 1908 by J. Hogarth Pringle [38], it has proven to be a significant and valuable adjunct in the surgical armamentarium for the management of hepatic injuries (Fig. 5.6). Although originally described in animals, specifically in rabbits, its use was extended to patients. This maneuver was utilized by Madding and Kennedy [44] in their classical paper from their experiences based in the European theater of combat during World War II and subsequently emphasized by the same authors in their classical 1965 monograph *Trauma to the Liver* [45].

Although the Pringle maneuver is often discussed in many hepatic injury series, it is very difficult to estimate the frequency with which it is utilized. Asensio and colleagues [1, 2] have described its use in up to 59 % of the patients with AAST-OIS hepatic injuries grades IV and V. Safe occlusion time for the portal triad has not been established and has been variably reported in the literature to range from 5 to 90 min [1–4, 17–31]. It is difficult to determine at which point portal triad occlusion results in ischemic injury to the liver. It is well known that repeated clamping and de-clamping of the portal triad should not be performed, as this definitely produces reperfusion injury to the liver [1–4, 17–31].

The Pringle maneuver has both diagnostic and therapeutic functions. Upon entering the abdominal cavity and after determining if the patient has sustained an AAST-OIS grade IV or V hepatic injury, portal triad occlusion is indicated [1–3]. We prefer to perform this with a 60° angled Glover clamp, although a 60° angled DeBakey clamp is also suitable. After application of the Pringle maneuver, the trauma surgeon should determine if hepatic hemorrhage has ceased.

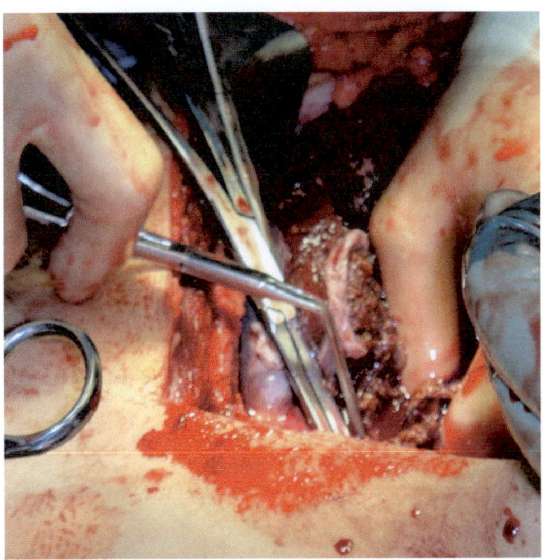

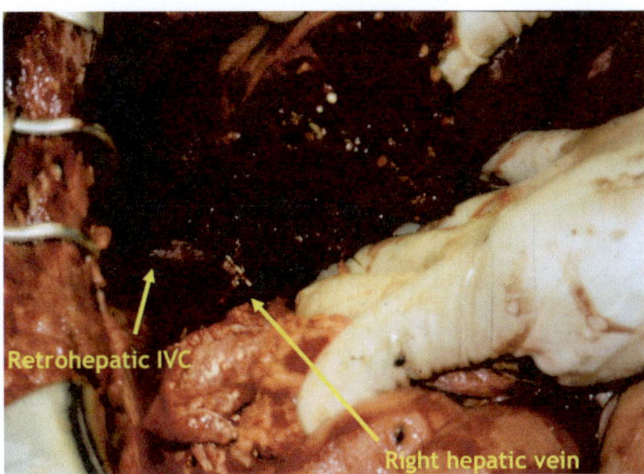

Fig. 5.7 In order to expose the retrohepatic inferior vena cava (IVC) the trauma surgeon must identify Cantlie's line, and it can be found at the left of the falciform ligament, as is shown in this picture. Also notice the right hepatic vein

Fig. 5.6 The Pringle maneuver is shown with a 60° angled DeBakey clamp. This maneuver has both diagnostic and therapeutic functions. Portal triad occlusion is indicated when the trauma surgeon has determined that the patient has sustained an AAST-OIS grade IV or V hepatic injury

Although this maneuver does not necessarily and completely arrest hepatic hemorrhage, it definitely decreases it significantly. After application of the Pringle maneuver, the trauma surgeon should communicate with the operating room nursing and house staff to note the time of portal triad occlusion which should not exceed 15 min. This maneuver allows the trauma surgeon to then initiate the necessary steps to control hepatic hemorrhage and secure the initial hemostasis.

If application of the Pringle maneuver does not arrest hepatic bleeding and active hemorrhage continues, this signals that the majority of bleeding is secondary to an injury of the retrohepatic vena cava and/or hepatic veins and, as such, the trauma surgeon must then initiate the appropriate maneuvers to deal with these extremely severe injuries [1–4, 43].

Approach to the Retrohepatic Cava

Rarely, securing the initial hemostasis requires a direct approach to the retrohepatic IVC (Fig. 5.7). We have personally abandoned the utilization of the Schrock's atrio-caval shunt in favor of such direct approach to the retrohepatic cava at Cantlie's line [1–3]. Generally, the utilization of Schrock shunt is fraught with pitfalls; it requires immediate median sternotomy as well as a right atriotomy and passage of the shunt, a Pringle maneuver, as well as encirclement of the vena cava in several locations such as the supra- and infrarenal IVC. This is time consuming and it involves opening a second cavity in a patient that has already embarked in the bloody vicious cycle of "acidosis, hypothermia, and coagulopathy." More often than not, this maneuver is performed very late when there is little hope for survival. Furthermore, it is well known that there are more anecdotal cases of the utilization of the shunt than there are survivors [1–3, 17–31].

If we are dealing with a retrohepatic vena cava injury, we identify Cantlie's line which is a line that starts in the gallbladder fossa and angles at 35° all the way to the dome of the liver; it is generally found approximately 5–10 cm to the left of the already transected falciform ligament. This represents the true dividing line between the right and left lobes of the liver and it is an avascular plane. We prefer to rapidly incise this line utilizing electrocautery and then proceed to utilize digitally fracturing of the hepatic parenchyma until the retrohepatic cava is reached. The depth of the hepatic parenchyma Cantlie's line may range anywhere from 10 to 15 cm. At that time, the right and left lobes of the liver can be separated [1–3]. It helps to utilize narrow malleable retractors in order to separate the parenchyma and identify the retrohepatic cava. It is also important to note that the hepatic venous drainage of the caudate's lobe may include anywhere from 12 to 50 very small veins that drain directly in the surface of the retrohepatic cava. Direct attempts at repair should be carried out utilizing 3-0 polypropylene vascular sutures, as either simple interrupted or running. Similarly, if there has been a large longitudinal laceration of the retrohepatic cava, a partial occlusion Satinsky or Cooley clamp can be utilized to control hemorrhage. This longitudinal laceration should then be repaired utilizing a running suture of the same material [1–4].

Hepatotomy, Hepatorrhaphy, and Selective Intrahepatic Vascular Ligation

This is a very important principle as intraparenchymal bleeding is the culprit for massive hepatic hemorrhage. To that extent, hepatotomy must be performed. To secure initial hemostasis, although it may initially offend the sensibilities of a trauma surgeon to consider extending the laceration in an already injured liver, however, it is important to note that the bleeding is found generally within the intraparenchymal substance of the liver. Generally, the subcapsular Glisson's plexus is not contributory to massive hepatic hemorrhage with the exception of ruptured large subcapsular hematomas of the liver. Our approaches to hepatotomy consist in scoring Glisson's capsule while utilizing the electrocautery unit and proceed to digitally fracture the hepatic parenchyma [1–4, 17–31].

At that time, the utilization of very narrow malleable retractors (Fig. 5.3b), of either the converse type or cerebellar malleable retractors utilized to elevate the brain, is very important, as they provide gentle separation and excellent exposure to retract the injured hepatic parenchyma. Alternative, even the back end of 8' DeBakey forceps may be utilized [1–4].

Once hepatotomy has been performed, digital fracturing will identify vessels that must be

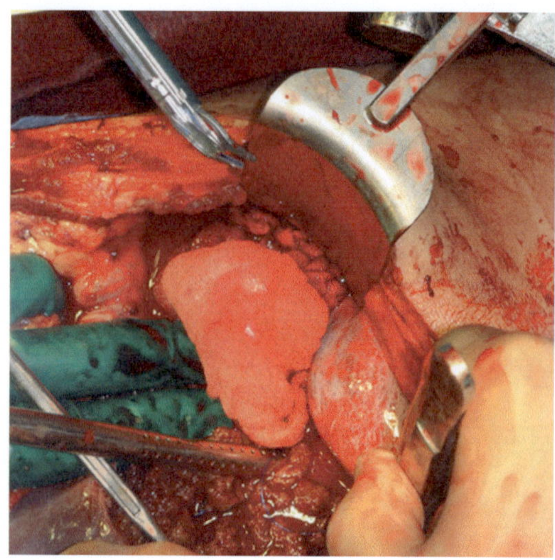

Fig. 5.8 Once hepatotomy is performed, clipping the intrahepatic transected vessel must be done rapidly. Notice the clip applier at the top of the picture

transected. We prefer to rapidly clip these vessels (Fig. 5.8) with handheld Weck™ clip appliers. We suggest utilizing either medium or large clips, as this generally allows for rapid transection of vessels to access the depths of the hepatic parenchyma. Similarly, clip appliers can also control transected bleeding vessels. It is helpful for the surgeons to utilize broad based 8' DeBakey forceps to actually grasp the bleeding vessels which may be either totally or partially transected with the left hand while utilizing the clip applier with the right hand. The commercially available handheld clip appliers with multiple clips may be useful to some; however, we find that often they do not control hemorrhage.

Alternatively, the surgeon may utilize 2-0 chromic sutures on a CT-1 needle to control bleeding vessels within the hepatic parenchyma (Fig. 5.9). We prefer to utilize either single interrupted or figure of eight sutures. Similarly, the utilization of the electrocautery unit or the argon beam coagulator is of the utmost importance in controlling the denuded or raw surfaces of the hepatic parenchyma which can also bleed significantly.

Hepatic venous injuries are the most difficult injuries to control on patients that have sustained higher-grade hepatic injuries. Mortality is even higher than that of the retrohepatic cava. A direct

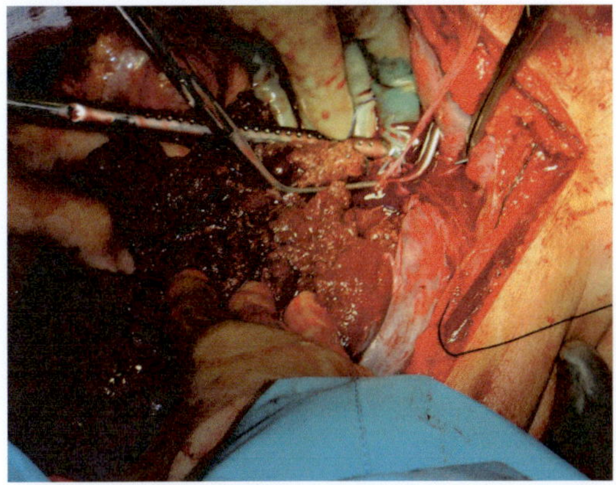

Fig. 5.9 Chromic sutures are utilized to control bleeding vessels as are shown in the picture, utilizing either single interrupted or figure of eight sutures

approach through Cantlie's line accompanied by simultaneous dissection of the anterior leaflets of the right and left coronary ligaments utilizing Metzenbaum scissors in the previously described fashion will allow for exposure of the hepatic veins. Once they are exposed, they should rapidly be controlled either temporarily with a straight 6' DeBakey clamp or, alternatively, they may be transected with an endostapler (Endo GIA™) which will rapidly control hemorrhage. This approach will generally allow the trauma surgeon to access the common trunk consisting of the middle and left hepatic veins that generally drain into the retrohepatic cava or alternatively the most proximal portions of the middle or left hepatic veins [1–4].

To control the right hepatic vein, this approach may also be utilized alternatively. Mobilization of the right lobe of the liver in the previously described fashion will expose the right hepatic vein which may be either controlled as previously described or transected with an endostapler (Endo GIA™) [1–4].

Nonanatomic Resection and Debridement

The vast majority of higher-grade hepatic injuries will require some means of nonanatomic resection and debridement (Fig. 5.10). This is performed after extensive hepatotomy and hepatorrhaphy

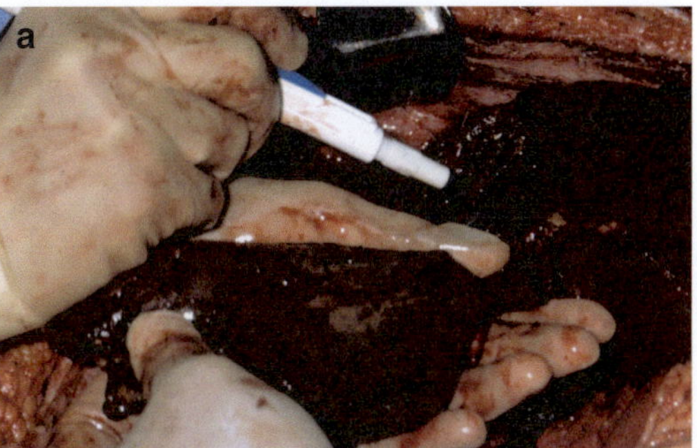
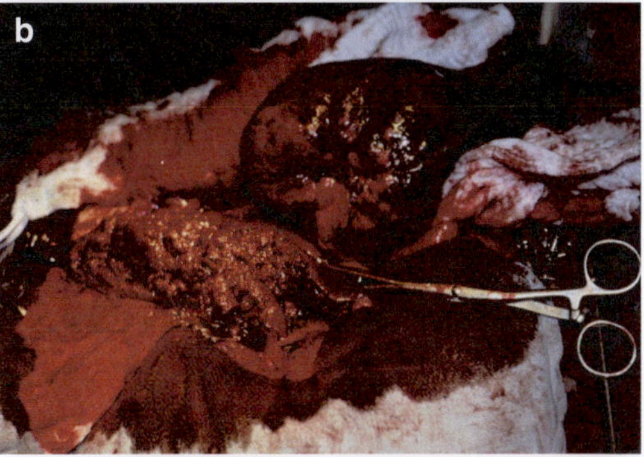
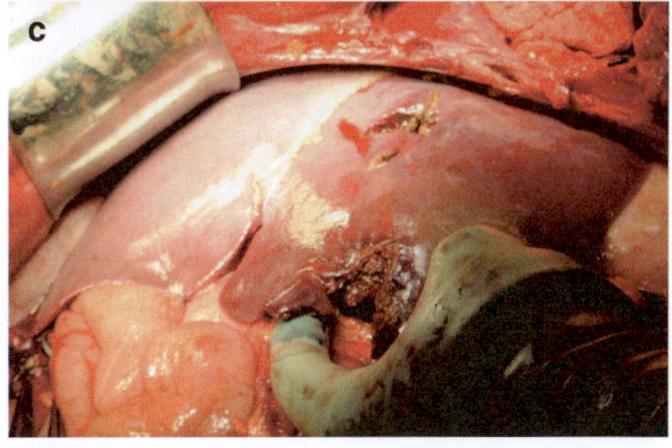

Fig. 5.10 (**a–c**) Debridement and nonanatomic resection in a patient who sustained a gunshot wound to the liver. An important number of cases of higher-grade hepatic injuries will require some kind of nonanatomic resection and debridement

with selective intraparenchymal vascular ligation for hemorrhage control and is often required to control the initial hemostasis. At that time, we prefer to score the capsule of the nonanatomic segment to be resected by first transecting Glisson's capsule, utilizing electrocautery. Similarly, the argon beam coagulator can also help as a valuable adjunct to control hemorrhage (Fig. 5.11). At that time, the surgeon may continue with digital fracture and simultaneous control of bleeding either with direct suturing utilizing

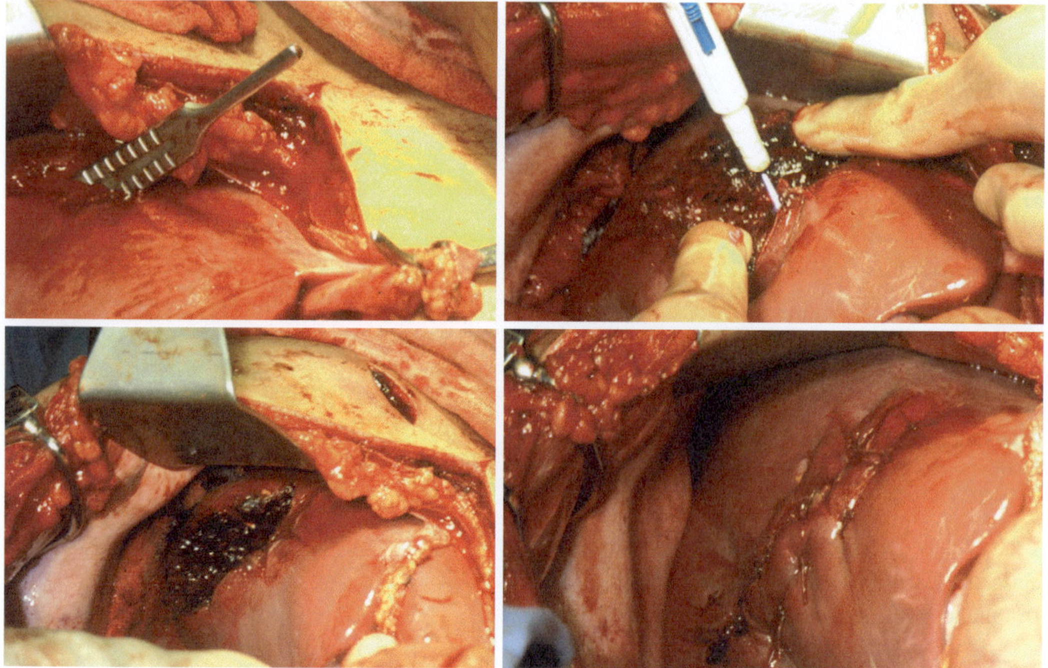

Fig. 5.11 After initial hemostasis control of a patient who sustained a gunshot wound to the liver, the argon beam coagulator serves as a valuable adjunct to control bleeding from the denuded or raw surfaces of the injured hepatic parenchyma

2-0 chromic sutures or handheld clip appliers. Alternatively, an endostapler may be utilized to transect portions of the hepatic parenchyma. After resection has been accomplished, the argon beam coagulator serves as a valuable adjunct to control bleeding from the denuded or raw surfaces of the resected hepatic parenchyma [1–4].

Fibrin glue is also an important adjunct and should be utilized. Similarly, if the hepatic laceration can be closed, this is performed by coapting the hepatic parenchyma utilizing 2-0 chromic sutures with a CT-1 needle in a horizontal Halsted mattress sutures (Fig. 5.12) [1–4]. *We do not recommend* the utilization of blunt hepatic needles as they tend to cause significant additional injury to the liver. We realize that our personal approach is a departure from this old and outmoded dictum in hepatic injury management [1–4], but we believe that the vast majority of trauma surgeons that have significant experience with complex hepatic injury management also do not utilize these needles. Similarly, we recommend that closure of hepatic parenchymal lacerations be achieved by placement of sutures 1 cm away from each

transected edge and 1 cm deep and definitely recommend that deep occlusive hepatic sutures be *abandoned* as they produce significant ischemia, strangulate hepatic tissue, and lead to hepatic necrosis. The famous *Liver Sews* as originally described by Mays *do not* have any room in the modern trauma surgeons armamentarium [1–4].

Lobectomy

The principals of hepatic lobectomy are well known to trauma surgeons. They still carry a significant mortality that may range anywhere from 50 to 100 % as reported in large series with a preponderance of hepatic injuries AAST-OIS grade IV or V; rarely they must be performed to secure the initial hemostasis. If a trauma surgeon has to perform hepatic lobectomy to secure hemostasis, he must perform it rapidly. This would entail rapid dissection of the portal triad extending to the hepatic plate utilizing a meticulous combination of blunt and sharp dissection. The utilization of Kittner's dissectors is also very important.

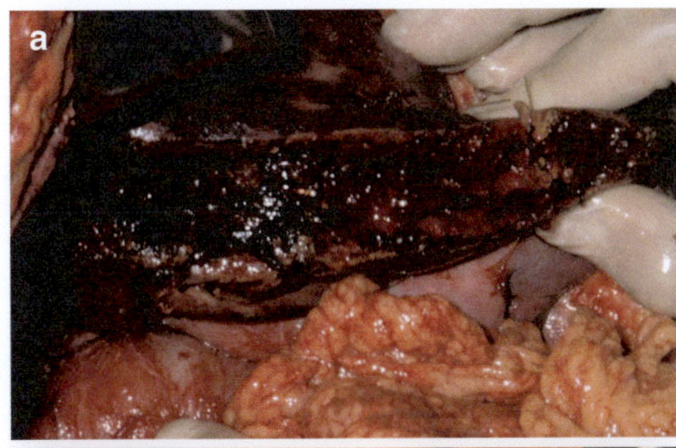

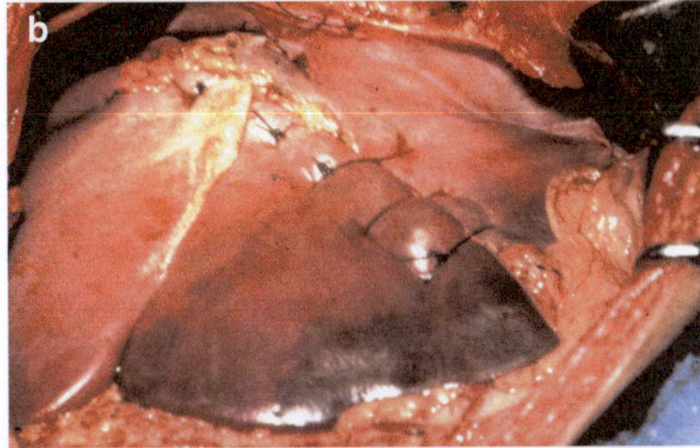

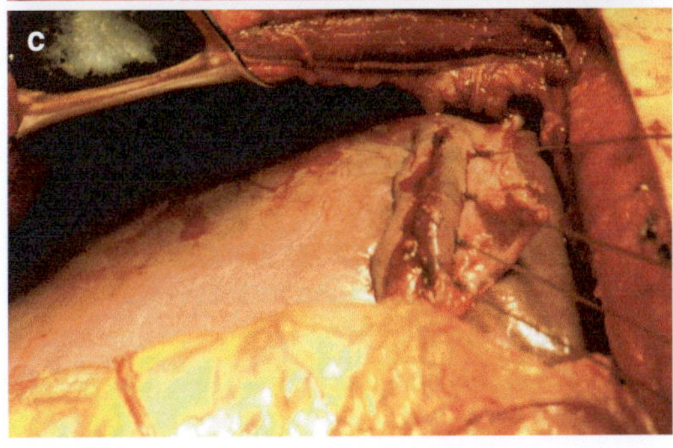

Fig. 5.12 If the hepatic laceration can be closed, it can be achieved by coapting the hepatic parenchyma, (**a**) utilizing 2-0 chromic sutures with a CT-1 needle in a horizontal Halsted mattress suture (**b**) and interposing omentum in-between (**b, c**)

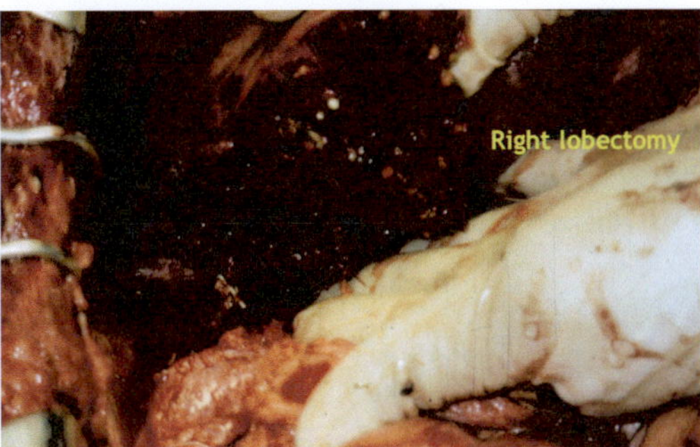

Fig. 5.13 After digital fracturing of Cantlie's line, removal of the right lobe of the liver must be performed from medial to lateral

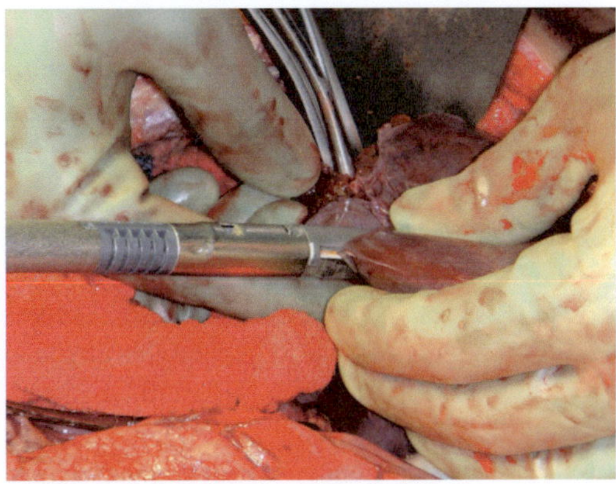

Fig. 5.14 Endostaplers have been used to transect and control arterial or venous supply to the liver, as well as hepatic ducts, and then transfixion suture ligatures have been utilized

Both the common and right and left hepatic arteries must be identified and encircled utilizing the vessel loops. Similarly, the common bile duct which is lateral to the hepatic arteries must also be dissected in a cephalad and caudad directions up to the hepatic plate where identification of either the right main hepatic duct or left main hepatic duct must be carried out and again encircled utilizing the vessel loops [1–4, 17–31].

Finally, the portal vein which lies posterior to both of these structures must be identified and traced to identify its division into the right and left portal veins. Depending on which lobe the surgeon

is to resect, the appropriate hepatic vein must be located and also controlled. Selective clamping of the right hepatic artery, right branch of the portal, as well as the right hepatic duct are carried out in anticipation to then transecting the right hepatic vein with an endostapler. This is then followed by digital fracturing of Cantlie's line in order to remove the right lobe of the liver (Fig. 5.13), which must be performed from medial to lateral [1–4].

The same maneuvers are applied for a rapid left hepatic lobectomy by controlling and transecting the structures that provide the arterial, portal venous, and hepatic venous blood supply to the left lobe of the liver. Similarly, the left hepatic duct must then be transected and ligated. We prefer to utilize the endostaplers for transection of these vascular structures (Fig. 5.14) or similarly doubly ligating them in continuity utilizing sutures of 2-0 Silk on each side, transecting the vascular structure utilizing a 60° angle Potts scissors, and then utilizing single transfixion suture ligatures of 2-0 Silk on the portion that is to remain [1–4].

Conclusion

The management of complex hepatic injuries AAST-OIS grades IV and V requires that the trauma surgeon be a skillful and adept technical operating surgeon that must possess a vast surgical armamentarium as well as be facile in utilizing surgical techniques that are required at best in 5–10 % of the cases. Survival of these very complex injuries requires a team approach and has increased significantly since the implementation of the multidisciplinary approach to the management of complex hepatic injuries described by Asensio and colleagues which includes rapid operative intervention and the selective utilization of "bailout" or "damage control" techniques after control of major hepatic hemorrhage including those previously described in this chapter [1–6].

The young trauma surgeon must realize that all hepatic bleeding does not necessarily stop with hepatic packing, as packing in desperation invariably leads to the patient's demise. The trauma surgeon must do his best in order to be able to control the most significant hepatic bleeding and then use hepatic packing as an adjunct. The patient should then be transported rapidly to the angiography suite where interventional radiologists may then utilize selective hepatic angiography and angioembolization to control the bleeding from the smaller vessels that are constricted and not bleeding at the time of surgery (Fig. 5.15) [1–6].

The patient must then be returned to the Surgical Critical Care Unit (SCCU) and be managed by the trauma surgeon that originally operated on the patient as he must also possess the surgical critical care skills and training required to care for these patients. The multidisciplinary approach to the management of complex hepatic injuries and their complications postoperatively

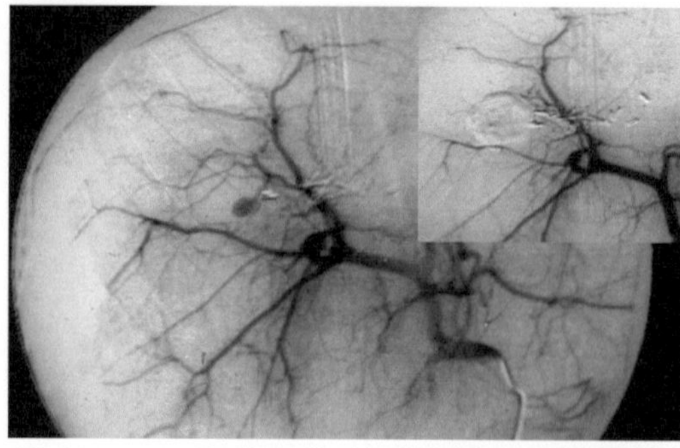

Fig. 5.15 Bleeding from a small intrahepatic vessel and the use of angiography and angioembolization by an interventional radiologist to control it (*inlet*)

utilizing CT-guided drainage and ERCP and highly selective stenting transected hepatic ducts has shown a significant improvement in the mortality rates of these critically injured patients [1, 4, 46–57].

Video Captions

Video 2   Right hepatic lobe rotation (MP4 42120 kb)
Video 3   Right hepatic lobe rotation (3-D animation) (MP4 33079 kb)
Video 4   Left hepatic lobe rotation (MP4 53192 kb)
Video 5   Left hepatic lobe rotation (3-D animation) (MP4 30377 kb)
Video 6   Pringle maneuver (MP4 14015 kb)
Video 8   Finger fracture of the liver (MP4 22289 kb)

References

1. Asensio JA, Demetriades D, Chahwan S, et al. Approach to the management of complex hepatic injuries. J Trauma. 2000;48(1):66–9.
2. Asensio JA, Roldán G, Petrone P, et al. Operative management and outcomes in 103 AAST-OIS grades IV and V complex hepatic injuries: trauma surgeons still need to operate, but angioembolization helps. J Trauma. 2003;54(4):647–53.
3. Asensio JA, Petrone P, García-Núñez L, et al. Multidisciplinary approach for the management of complex hepatic injuries AAST-OIS grades IV-V: a prospective study. Scand J Surg. 2007;96(3):214–20.

4. Demetriades D, Karaiskakis M, Alo K, et al. Role of postoperative computed tomography in patients with severe liver injury. Br J Surg. 2003;90(11):1398–400.

5. Asensio JA, McDuffie L, Petrone P, et al. Reliable variables in the exsanguinated patient which indicate damage control and predict outcome. Am J Surg. 2001;182(6):743–51.

6. Asensio JA, Petrone P, O'Shanahan G, Kuncir EJ. Managing exsanguination: what we know about damage control/bailout is not enough. Proc (Bayl Univ Med Cent). 2003;16(3):294–6.

7. Moore EE, Cogbill TH, Jurkovich GJ, et al. Organ injury scaling: spleen and liver (1994 revision). J Trauma. 1995;38(3):323–4.

8. Asensio JA, Chahwan S, Hanpeter D, et al. Operative management and outcome of 302 abdominal vascular injuries. Am J Surg. 2000;180(6):528–33.

9. Asensio JA, Petrone P, Kimbrell B, Kuncir E. Lessons learned in the management of thirteen celiac axis injuries. South Med J. 2005;98(4):462–6.

10. Asensio JA, Berne JD, Chahwan S, et al. Traumatic injury to the superior mesenteric artery. Am J Surg. 1999;178(3):235–9.

11. Asensio JA, Britt LD, Borzotta A, et al. Multiinstitutional experience with the management of superior mesenteric artery injuries. J Am Coll Surg. 2001;193(4):354–65.

12. Asensio JA, Petrone P, Garcia-Nuñez L, et al. Superior mesenteric venous injuries: to ligate or to repair remains the question. J Trauma. 2007;62(3):668–75.

13. Asensio JA, Petrone P, Roldán G, et al. Analysis of 185 iliac vessel injuries: risk factors and predictors of outcome. Arch Surg. 2003;138(11):1187–93.

14. Cogbill TH, Moore EE, Jurkovich GJ, et al. Severe hepatic trauma: a multi-center experience with 1,335 liver injuries. J Trauma. 1988;28(10):1433–8.

15. Feliciano DV, Mattox KL, Jordan GL, et al. Management of 1000 consecutive cases of hepatic trauma (1979–1984). Ann Surg. 1986;204(4):438–45.

16. Beal SL. Fatal hepatic hemorrhage: an unresolved problem in the management of complex liver injuries. J Trauma. 1990;30(2):163–9.

17. Fabian TC, Croce MA, Stanford GG, et al. Factors affecting morbidity following hepatic trauma. A prospective analysis of 482 injuries. Ann Surg. 1991;213(6):540–7.

18. Reed RL, Merrell RC, Meyers WC, Fischer RP. Continuing evolution in the approach to severe liver trauma. Ann Surg. 1992;216(5):524–38.

19. Cué JI, Cryer HG, Miller FB, et al. Packing and planned reexploration for hepatic and retroperitoneal hemorrhage: critical refinements of a useful technique. J Trauma. 1990;30(8):1007–11.

20. Carrillo EH, Richardson JD. Delayed surgery and interventional procedures in complex liver injuries. J Trauma. 1999;46(5):978.

21. Richardson J, Franklin GA, Lukan JK, et al. Evolution in the management of hepatic trauma: a 25-year perspective. Ann Surg. 2000;232(3):324–30.

22. Pachter HL, Spencer FC, Hofstetter SR, et al. Significant trends in the treatment of hepatic trauma. Experience with 411 injuries. Ann Surg. 1992;215(5):492–500.

23. Pachter HL, Hofstetter SR. The current status of nonoperative management of adult blunt hepatic injuries. Am J Surg. 1995;169(4):442–54.

24. Sherman HF, Savage BA, Jones LM, et al. Nonoperative management of blunt hepatic injuries: safe at any grade? J Trauma. 1994;37(4):616–21.

25. Meredith JW, Young JS, Bowling J, Roboussin D. Nonoperative management of blunt hepatic trauma: the exception or the rule? J Trauma. 1994;36(4):529–34.

26. Fang JF, Chen RJ, Lin BC, et al. Blunt hepatic injury: minimal intervention is the policy of treatment. J Trauma. 2000;49(4):722–8.

27. Chen RJ, Fang JF, Lin BC, et al. Factors determining operative mortality of grade V blunt hepatic trauma. J Trauma. 2000;49(5):886–91.

28. Working Group, Ad Hoc Subcommittee on Outcomes, American College of Surgeons-Committee on Trauma. Practice management guidelines for emergency department thoracotomy. J Am Coll Surg. 2001;193(3):303–9.

29. Asensio JA, Murray J, Demetriades D, et al. Penetrating cardiac injuries: a prospective study of variables predicting outcomes. J Am Coll Surg. 1998;186(1):24–34.

30. Asensio JA, Hanpeter D, Demetriades D. The futility of utilization of emergency department thoracotomy. A prospective study. Proceedings of the American Association for Surgery of Trauma. 58th annual meeting. Baltimore; 1998. p. 210.

31. Asensio JA, Tsai KJ. Chapter 25. Emergency department thoracotomy. In: Demetraides D, Asensio JA, editors. Trauma management. Georgetown: Landes Bioscience; 2000. p. 271–9.

32. Asensio JA, Hanpenter D, Gomez H, et al. Chapter 30. Thoracic injuries. In: Shoemaker W, Greenvik A, Ayres SM, et al. editors. Textbook of Critical Care. 4 ed. Philadelphia: Saunders; 2000. p. 337–48.

33. Asensio JA, Gambaro E, Forno W, et al. Penetrating cardiac injuries. A complex challenge. Ann Chir Gynaecol. 2000;89(2):155–66.

34. Asensio JA, Stewart BM, Murray J, et al. Penetrating cardiac injuries. Surg Clin North Am. 1996;76(4):685–724.

35. Buckman RF, Badellino MM, Mauro LH, et al. Penetrating cardiac wounds: prospective study of factors influencing initial resuscitation. J Trauma. 1993;34(5):717–25.

36. Spangaro S. Sulla tecnica da seguire negli interventi chirurgici per ferite del cuore e su di nuovo processo di toracotomia. Clinica Chir; Milan. 1906. As quoted by Beck CS: wounds of the heart. The technic of suture. Arch Surg. 1926;13:205–27.

37. Duval P. Le incision median thoraco-laparotomy. Et Mem Soc de Chir de Paris. 1907. As quoted by Ballana C: Brasdaw lecture. The surgery of the heart. Lancet. 1920;CXCVIII:73–9.

38. Pringle JH. Notes on the arrest of hepatic hemorrhage due to trauma. Ann Surg. 1908;48(4):541–9.
39. Couinaud C. Les enveloppes vasculo-biliaire du foie ou capsule de Glisson leur intérêt dons la chirurgie vésiculaire, les resections hépatiques et l'abord du hile du foie. Lyon Chir. 1954;49:589–607.
40. Madding GF, Kennedy PA. Trauma to the liver, Major problems in clinical surgery, vol. III. Philadelphia/London: WB Saunders Company; 1965.
41. Denton JR, Moore EE, Coldwell DM. Multimodality treatment for grade V hepatic injuries: perihepatic packing, arterial embolization, and venous stenting. J Trauma. 1997;42(5):964–7.
42. Wagner WH, Lundell CJ, Donovan AJ. Percutaneous angiographic embolization for hepatic arterial hemorrhage. Arch Surg. 1985;120(11):1241–9.
43. Johnson JW, Gracias VH, Gupta R, et al. Hepatic angiography in patients undergoing damage control laparotomy. J Trauma. 2002;52(6):1102–6.
44. Madding GF, Lawrence KB, Kennedy PA. Forward surgery of the severely wounded. Second Aux Surg Group. 1942–1945; 1:1307.
45. Moore EE. Thomas G. Orr Memorial Lecture. Staged laparotomy for the hypothermia, acidosis, and coagulopathy syndrome. Am J Surg. 1996;172(5):405–10.
46. Hagiwara A, Murata A, Matsuda T, et al. The efficacy and limitations of transarterial embolization for severe hepatic injury. J Trauma. 2002;52(6):1091–6.
47. Pachter HL, Spencer FC, Hofstetter SR, Coppa GF. Experience with the finger fracture technique to achieve intra-hepatic hemostasis in 75 patients with severe injuries of the liver. Ann Surg. 1983;197(6):771–8.
48. Feliciano DV, Mattox KL, Burch JM, et al. Packing for control of hepatic hemorrhage. J Trauma. 1986;26(8):738–43.
49. Carmona RH, Peck DZ, Lim RC. The role of packing and planned reoperation in severe hepatic trauma. J Trauma. 1984;24(9):779–84.
50. Ivatury RR, Nallathambi M, Gunduz Y, et al. Liver packing for uncontrolled hemorrhage: a reappraisal. J Trauma. 1986;26(8):744–53.
51. Svoboda JA, Peter ET, Dang CV, et al. Severe liver trauma in the face of coagulopathy. A case for temporary packing and early reexploration. Am J Surg. 1982;144(6):717–21.
52. Caruso DM, Battistella FD, Owings JT, et al. Perihepatic packing of major liver injuries: complications and mortality. Arch Surg. 1999;134(9):958–62.
53. Hidalgo F, Narváez JA, Reñé M, Domínguez J, et al. Treatment of hemobilia with selective hepatic artery embolization. J Vasc Interv Radiol. 1995;6(5):793–8.
54. Sandblom P, Saegesser F, Mirkovitch V. Hepatic hemobilia: hemorrhage from the intrahepatic biliary tract, a review. World J Surg. 1984;8(1):41–50.
55. Hagiwara A, Yukioka T, Ohta S, et al. Nonsurgical management of patients with blunt hepatic injury: efficacy of transcatheter arterial embolization. Am J Roentgenol. 1997;169(4):1151–6.
56. Mohr AM, Lavery RF, Barone A, et al. Angiographic embolization for liver injuries: low mortality, high morbidity. J Trauma. 2003;55(6):1077–81.
57. D'Amours SK, Simons RK, Scudamore CH, et al. Major intrahepatic bile duct injuries detected after laparotomy: selective nonoperative management. J Trauma. 2001;50(3):480–4.

Liver Trauma: Parenchymal Repair and Resectional Debridement

6

H. Leon Pachter and S. Rob Todd

Introduction

The liver is one of the most commonly injured organs following abdominal trauma. The management of liver injuries, however, has evolved significantly over the past 25 years. Operative intervention, for the most part, has given way to a nonoperative approach. Nevertheless, surgical intervention is at times required most often for the patient who presents with hemodynamic instability. Once a decision has been made to perform a laparotomy for hepatic trauma, the surgeon must have an extensive armamentarium, in effect, a "toolbox" full of operative techniques at his or her disposal. Perhaps, the most widely utilized of these techniques is hepatic repair and resectional debridement.

En route to the operating theater, the patient should receive antibiotics to cover aerobic and anaerobic microorganisms in case the gastrointestinal tract has been violated as well [1]. Once in the operating theater, one must be careful to avoid hypothermia in hopes of preventing the "bloody vicious cycle" – hypothermia, acidosis, and coagulopathy, often referred to as the "triad of death" [2]. The skin preparation should include the anterior and lateral trunk from the chin to the knees. Such a wide preparation allows the surgeon access to the thoracic cavity should this be necessary. It also provides access to the greater saphenous vein within the thigh should a native vascular replacement be needed.

A midline incision is preferred for all patients undergoing a trauma laparotomy, including those with hepatic trauma. The first step in the operative management of suspected hepatic trauma is to pack all four quadrants of the abdomen with laparotomy pads and to manually compress the liver with both hands (Fig. 6.1). This allows the anesthesiologists time to catch up with the resuscitation. This process must occur in concert with the trauma surgeon, who should dictate the need for the initiation of the massive transfusion protocol or the concomitant use of vasopressors. The packs are then removed in a clockwise fashion starting in the left upper quadrant and ending in the right upper quadrant. At this point in time, the surgeon should be able to assess the extent of the injury.

H.L. Pachter, MD (✉)
Department of Surgery,
New York University School of Medicine,
530 First Avenue, HCC 6C,
New York, NY 10016, USA
e-mail: leon.pachter@nyumc.org

S.R. Todd, MD, FACS, FCCM
Trauma and Emergency Surgery, Bellevue Hospital Center, New York, NY, USA

Department of Surgery and Anesthesiology,
New York University School of Medicine,
550 First Avenue, NB 15 E 9,
New York, NY 10016, USA
e-mail: srtodd@nyumc.org

Electronic supplementary material Supplementary material is available in the online version of this chapter at 10.1007/978-1-4939-1200-1_6. Videos can also be accessed at http://www.springerimages.com/videos/978-1-4939-1199-8.

R.R. Ivatury (ed.), *Operative Techniques for Severe Liver Injury*,
DOI 10.1007/978-1-4939-1200-1_6, © Springer Science+Business Media New York 2015

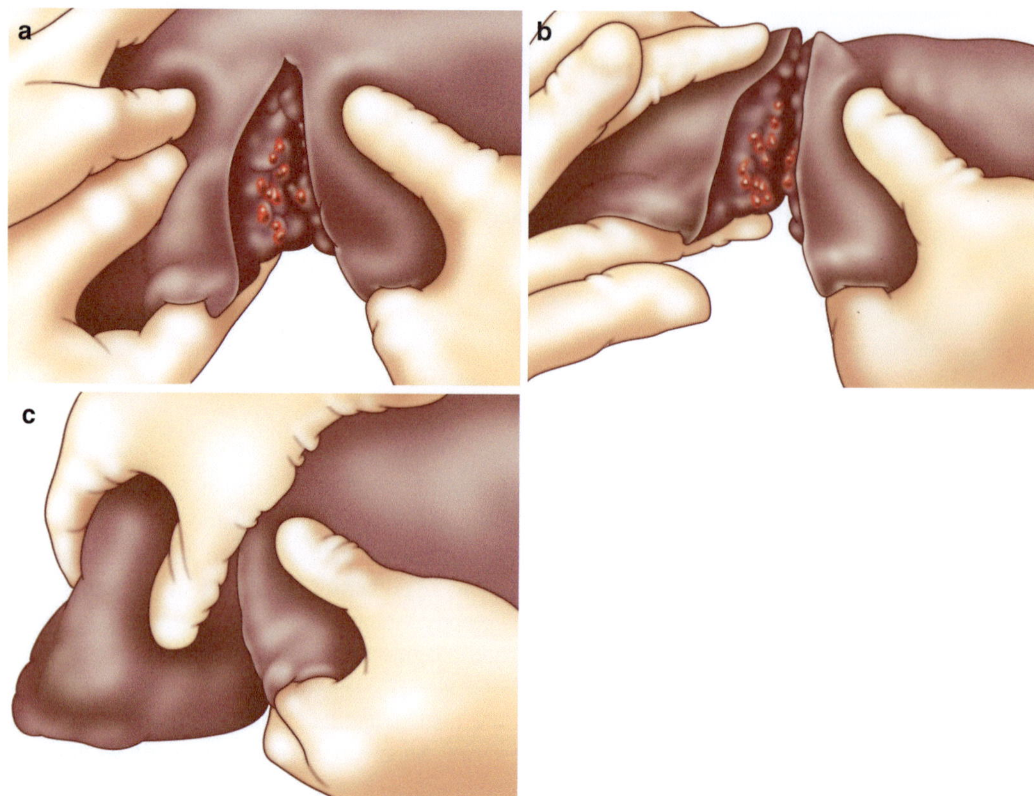

Fig. 6.1 Manual compression of the liver to temporarily control bleeding: by bimanual pressure on either side of the laceration (**a**), pressure between the thumb and fingers (**b**), compressing the liver lobe above and below (**c**), or squeezing together the liver tissue on either side of the injury

This, and the patient's hemodynamic stability, will guide the remainder of the management.

Simple Techniques of Repair

If the source of hemorrhage turns out to be a minor or modest injury (grade I or II) (Table 6.1), which is often the case, simple techniques of repair may be sufficient [3, 4]. Such techniques include drainage alone (for non-bleeding injuries), manual compression, high-energy surgical devices (electrocautery, argon beam plasma coagulation, etc.), topical hemostatic agents, and suture hepatorrhaphy. These basic techniques will suffice in 90 % of penetrating wounds and 60 % of blunt injuries [5, 6]. While these will be discussed individually below, they are often used in conjunction with one another.

Drainage Alone (For Non-bleeding Injuries)

The drainage of minor non-bleeding hepatic injuries is rarely, if ever, required. If a minor capsular tear or laceration is identified, any avulsed biliary ducts should be directly visualized and suture ligated. As such, the vast majority of these injuries will not drain in the postoperative period and thus do not warrant drainage.

Manual Compression

Many minor injuries are associated with rib fractures. Often, a 5–10 min period of manual compression is all that is required to control any hemorrhage. If hemorrhage is controlled in this fashion, then no further therapeutic maneuvers are required, nor is drainage necessary.

Table 6.1 The American Association for the Surgery of Trauma (AAST) liver injury scale (1994 revision)

Grade	Injury description	
I	Hematoma	Subcapsular, <10 % surface area
	Laceration	Capsular tear, <1 cm parenchymal depth
II	Hematoma	Subcapsular, 10–50 % surface area; intraparenchymal, <10 cm diameter
	Laceration	1–3 cm parenchymal depth, <10 cm length
III	Hematoma	Subcapsular, >50 % surface area or expanding. Ruptured subcapsular or parenchymal hematoma; Intraparenchymal hematoma >10 cm or expanding
	Laceration	>3 cm parenchymal depth
IV	Laceration	Parenchymal disruption involving 25–75 % of hepatic lobe or >3 Couinaud's segments within a single lobe
V	Laceration	Parenchymal disruption involving >75 % of hepatic lobe or 1–3 Couinaud's segments within a single lobe
	Vascular	Juxtahepatic venous injuries, i.e., retrohepatic vena cava/central major hepatic veins
VI	Vascular	Hepatic avulsion

Used with permission from Moore et al. [3]

High-Energy Surgical Devices (Electrocautery, Argon Beam Plasma Coagulation)

In addition to manual compression, high-energy surgical devices (electrocautery, argon beam plasma coagulation, etc.) are frequently utilized in minor or modest hepatic injuries, with varying degrees of success. Electrocautery should only be used to stop the bleeding of small vessels (larger vessels being ligated) or raw tissue surfaces. If individual vessels are appreciated, one is prudent to grasp them with tissue forceps and cauterize in this fashion. The argon beam has been utilized effectively to control local bleeding from raw edge surfaces [7]. The argon beam laser is less effective in controlling bleeding emanating from severed blood vessels of any significant magnitude (effective on small vessels only with a depth of penetration of approximately 2.5 mm).

Table 6.2 Topical hemostatic agents

Passive	Active	Tissue sealants
Collagens	Thrombins	Fibrin sealants
Cellulose		Polyethylene glycol
Gelatins		Albumin/glue
Combinations		

Reprinted from Samudrala [9], Copyright 2008, with permission from Elsevier

Topical Hemostatic Agents

Topical hemostatic agents have gained tremendous popularity for use in emergency bleeding control, and that from hepatic trauma is no different. A number of agents are currently available and may be divided into two categories: those that act passively through contact activation and promotion of platelet aggregation and those that act on the clotting cascade in a biologically active manner (Table 6.2) [8, 9]. Such agents are applied directly to the site of bleeding and provide an excellent adjunct when standard means of hemostasis are ineffective or impractical [10]. Sealants function similarly.

The agents should be applied directly to the site of bleeding followed by manual compression for 5–10 min. After releasing compression, remaining bleeders may be cauterized (using tissue forceps). There are several benefits to the topical hemostatic agents. First, they avoid the global effects of systemic hemostatic medications, i.e., unwanted blood clots [11]. Second, they may be titrated to the needed effect, i.e., used liberally with significant bleeding or sparingly with minimal bleeding. Ultimately, there is the prolonged benefit with respect to the postoperative blood loss and the need for excessive transfusions [12].

Suture Hepatorrhaphy

Approximately 50 % of all hepatic injuries managed operatively involve peripheral penetrating wounds or parenchymal lacerations 1–3 cm in depth (grade II). Suture hepatorrhaphy has traditionally been the mainstay therapy of such injuries. In doing so, it is important to initially enter the laceration and identify and ligate all injured blood vessels and bile ducts selectively. This may prove to be difficult if not impossible in coagulopathic patients or those with deeper lacerations. In such cases, it is best to proceed directly to mass closure, with the placement of large sutures through the liver parenchyma to arrest bleeding by coapting the two edges.

The suture of choice is an 0 chromic. If the laceration is 1–3 cm in depth, a standard (CT-21) needle may be used to loosely approximate the edges of the laceration in an interrupted fashion. For deeper lacerations, use a large blunt nose liver needle and perform a horizontal mattress closure. In order to prevent tearing through the liver, throw down two knots without tension. Have the first assistant hold the knots with a tonsil clamp, gently releasing it as the surgeon squares the knots. In this manner, tearing through the liver capsule rarely occurs.

Past personal experience with suture hepatorrhaphy has shown that tightly tied horizontal mattress sutures may result in necrosis of the underlying parenchyma during the postoperative period. For this reason, it is best to proceed with selective vascular and bile duct ligation followed by loose approximation of the liver edges rather than necrosing horizontal mattress sutures. Exceptions to this rule include patients (1) with multiple injuries and (2) who are coagulopathic, such that speed is critical and precise techniques are somewhat precluded.

Advanced Technique of Repair

The incidence of complex hepatic injuries (grades III, IV, and V) has remained stable over the past 25 years at 12–15 % [13]. These account for approximately 10 % of all penetrating injuries and less than 40 % of blunt injuries. Such injuries require a more advanced technique of repair involving the following six critical steps: (1) manual compression and resuscitation, (2) portal triad occlusion, (3) finger fracture of the parenchyma to identify and ligate lacerated blood vessels and bile ducts, (4) resectional debridement of nonviable hepatic parenchyma, (5) insertion of a viable omental pedicle into the injury site, and (6) closed suction drainage for grade III–V injuries.

Manual Compression/Resuscitation

Upon entering the peritoneal cavity, all efforts should focus on intraoperative resuscitation. As previously mentioned, this entails packing all four quadrants of the abdomen with laparotomy pads and manually compressing the liver with both hands (Fig. 6.1). This allows the anesthesiologists time to catch up with the resuscitation, ultimately working to prevent/correct the potentially lethal "bloody vicious cycle." This step is absolutely critical, in that very few injuries cannot be temporized by such a maneuver, and yet few if any patients will survive without adequate resuscitation. It is only after this step that the surgeon should begin to assess the extent of the injury.

Portal Triad Occlusion (The Pringle Maneuver)

In 1908, J. Hogarth Pringle described occlusion of the portal triad for controlling hepatic hemorrhage [14]. Known as "the Pringle maneuver," it entails placing an atraumatic vascular clamp (either a Satinski or curved DeBakey clamp) across the hepatoduodenal ligament (Fig. 6.2) [15, 16]. Prior to doing so, initial finger occlusion of the portal triad gives the operating surgeon an idea of whether or not this maneuver will be successful. It typically controls hemorrhage originating from intrahepatic branches of the hepatic artery and/or portal vein. Failure to do so implies that the site of injury is at the retrohepatic vena cava or hepatic veins.

In order to avoid ischemic injury to the liver parenchyma, the safe cross-clamp time of the portal triad has been thought to be no more than 15–20 min in normothermic conditions [17–19]. In order to minimize this risk, the operating surgeon should clamp and release (for 5 min) the portal triad flow at 15–20 min intervals. Such "warm ischemia" decreases the time the liver is without blood supply, thereby minimizing ischemia.

Two methods examined to extend this time are (1) a bolus infusion of steroids (20–30 mg/kg of

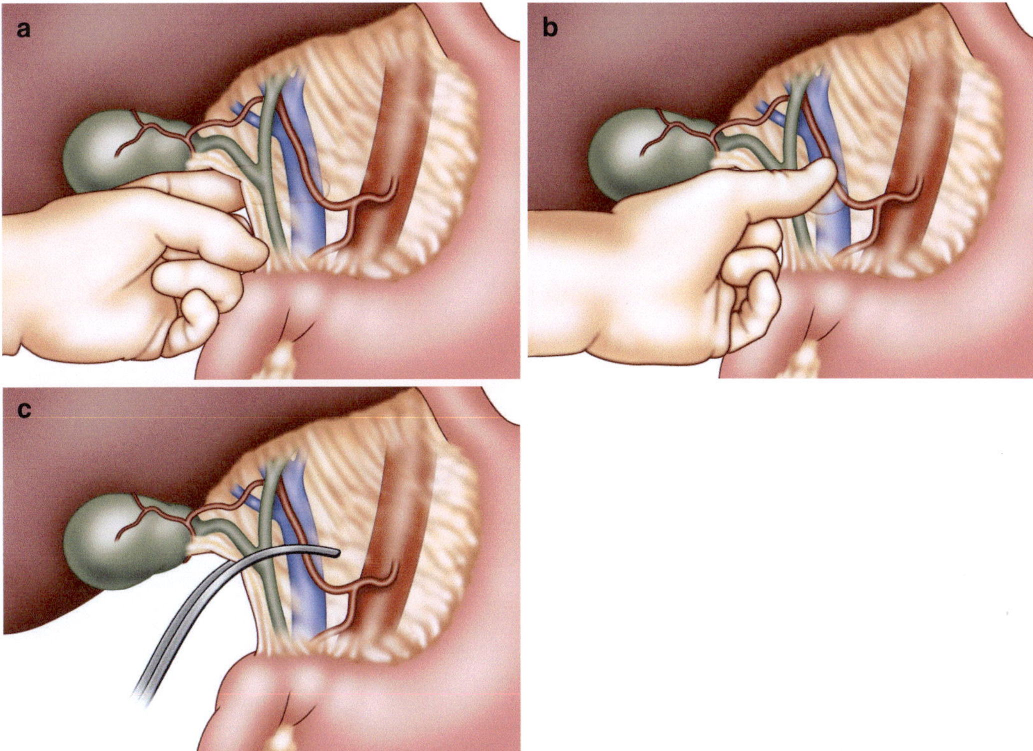

Fig. 6.2 Portal triad occlusion (the Pringle maneuver). (**a**) The surgeon slides his left hand with palm facing up into the foramen of Winslow and with the thumb feels the hepatic arterial pulse. (**b**) The hepatic artery in the free edge of the lesser omentum is compressed between the thumb and the other fingers, reducing hepatic blood flow. (**c**) A curved vascular clamp may now be applied to the lesser omentum

Solu-Medrol) and (2) topical hypothermia (cooling the liver to 30–32 °C). Steroids have been abandoned as experimental data have documented that (1) the percentage of high-energy phosphates within the liver at 60 min is lower than in control animals and (2) the incidence of sepsis is increased in injured patients receiving steroids [19, 20]. Topical hypothermia significantly prevents ischemia/reperfusion injuries to the liver, thus extending the safe cross-clamp time [21]. Using a "slush" solution or iced Ringer's lactate directly applied to the surface of the liver, a temperature of 27–32 °C can quickly be attained. The surface temperature can be measured via a short intrahepatic temperature probe, appreciating that there will be temperature variations within the liver parenchyma. If this method is to be employed, it is essential to initiate a series of steps to prevent systemic hypothermia, such as covering the remaining abdominal viscera with warm laparotomy pads. If the patient becomes hypothermic, topical hypothermia should be abandoned. Likewise, if the patient is hypothermic prior to instituting topical hypothermia, it should not be undertaken.

Finger Fracture Technique

Following the aforementioned steps and adequate intraoperative resuscitation, the liver is brought into the wound by having the first assistant place his/her hand behind the mobilized organ and bringing it forward. A suction apparatus in the first assistant's right hand may then be utilized to better expose the injury. The next critical step is the "finger fracture technique," popularized by Tien Yu Lin [22]. It is an essential maneuver for

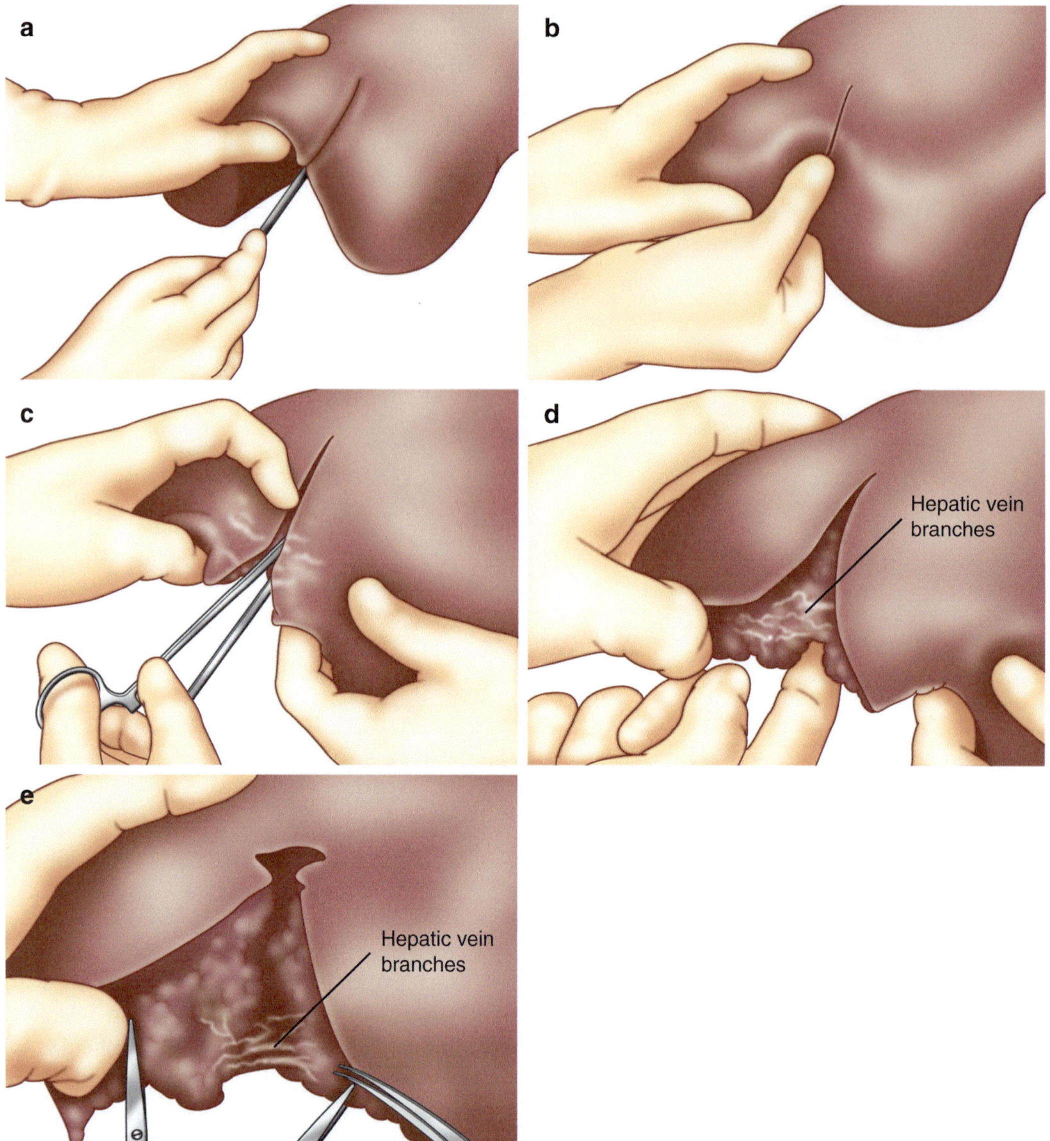

Fig. 6.3 Finger fracture technique: The liver capsule over the injury is incised (if necessary) with the back of a surgical knife (**a**). The liver tissue is teased off between the thumb and index finger (**b**), leaving hepatic vein branches as glistening white structures, bridging across (**c**). These are clamped, clipped, or tied (**d**) and the finger fracture extended (**e**)

rapidly exposing injured blood vessels and bile ducts within the hepatic parenchyma.

With occlusion of the portal triad, Glisson's capsule is incised in the direction of the injury by means of electrocautery. The normal hepatic parenchyma is then crushed between the surgeon's thumb and forefinger ("finger fracture technique"), thus allowing the surgeon to identify the normal blood vessels and bile ducts, which are ligated or clipped as encountered (Fig. 6.3). In doing so, care should be taken to appreciate the normal hepatic anatomy so as not to injure the main, right, or left hepatic ducts. With adequate intrahepatic retraction, lacerated blood vessels and bile ducts may be ligated or repaired under direct visualization. Once the surgeon has achieved "adequate" hemostasis, the cross-clamp on the portal triad is removed to assess the situation at hand. Additional bleeding sites may then be ligated or clipped. If bleeding persists, one must be wary of an injury to the retrohepatic vena cava or hepatic veins.

The oft-mentioned objection to this technique is the belief that incising the liver along nonanatomical planes will lead to uncontrollable bleeding if not preceded by proximal control (hilar dissection and proper ligation of the appropriate inflow and outflow vessels) [23, 24]. This fear has been debunked by the works of Lin (hepatomas), Ton (hepatomas), Pachter (complex hepatic trauma), and Fischer (war wounds of the liver) [25–28].

Resectional Debridement

If there are loose, friable, and/or particularly devascularized regions of hepatic tissue secondary to the injury, these areas should undergo resectional debridement (rather than a formal hepatic resection) in hopes of decreasing perihepatic and intrahepatic sepsis in the postoperative period. To be successful, this must be carried down to healthy hepatic parenchyma. Via the "finger fracture technique," the surgeon should identify a plane of healthy parenchyma just beyond the injured tissue. All of the hepatic tissue just inside of the clips or sutures on the blood vessels and bile ducts is then debrided without significant hemorrhage.

If the patient is coagulopathic, such a deliberate approach is not feasible. In these instances, rapid resectional debridement should be performed. To do so, place large vascular clamps (either a Satinski or DeBakey clamp) to either side of the injury and debride the tissue within the clamps (Fig. 6.4). An 0 chromic suture is then used to ligate the tissue en mass using an interrupted horizontal mattress suture pattern. An alternative approach is to utilize large horizontal mattress sutures for hemostasis. While such rapid resectional debridement is not optimal, it provides a safe, fast means of debridement in dire situations.

Viable Omental Pack

The finger fracture technique followed by resectional debridement inevitably creates a significant dead space within the hepatic parenchyma. This should be managed via a viable omental pedicle (based on the blood supply of either gastroepiploic vessel), first championed by Stone and Lamb [29]. Having fully mobilized the omentum from the greater curvature of the stomach and the transverse colon, it is inserted into the debrided hepatic parenchyma without tension. The free edges of the liver are then loosely approximated over the omental pedicle with a 0 chromic suture. Video 11 illustrates the insertion of omental pack.

Not only does such a pack "fill the dead space," it (1) is also efficient at tamponading minor venous oozing emanating from the raw hepatic parenchymal bed; (2) introduces peritoneal macrophages (the first line of defense in the peritoneal cavity) into a potential area of infection; and (3) is a source of stromal cell-derived factor 1-alpha, which may be crucial to healing via the recruitment of chemokine receptor cells [15, 16, 29]. In using such a technique, Fabian et al. and Pachter et al. reported postoperative abscess rates of 8 and 8.6 %, respectively [17, 30].

Closed Suction Drainage

Following all of the aforementioned maneuvers, the liver should be drained both anteriorly and posteriorly with #10 French Jackson-Pratt drains. Closed suction drainage is superior to open drainage (and no drainage) and as such should be the only means of drainage [30].

Adjunctive Techniques

There are many adjunctive measures often utilized in conjunction with the above. These include perihepatic packing, angioembolization, damage control surgery, hepatic artery ligation, portal vein ligation, and improvised balloon tamponade. These will be discussed elsewhere in the textbook and as such will not be discussed here.

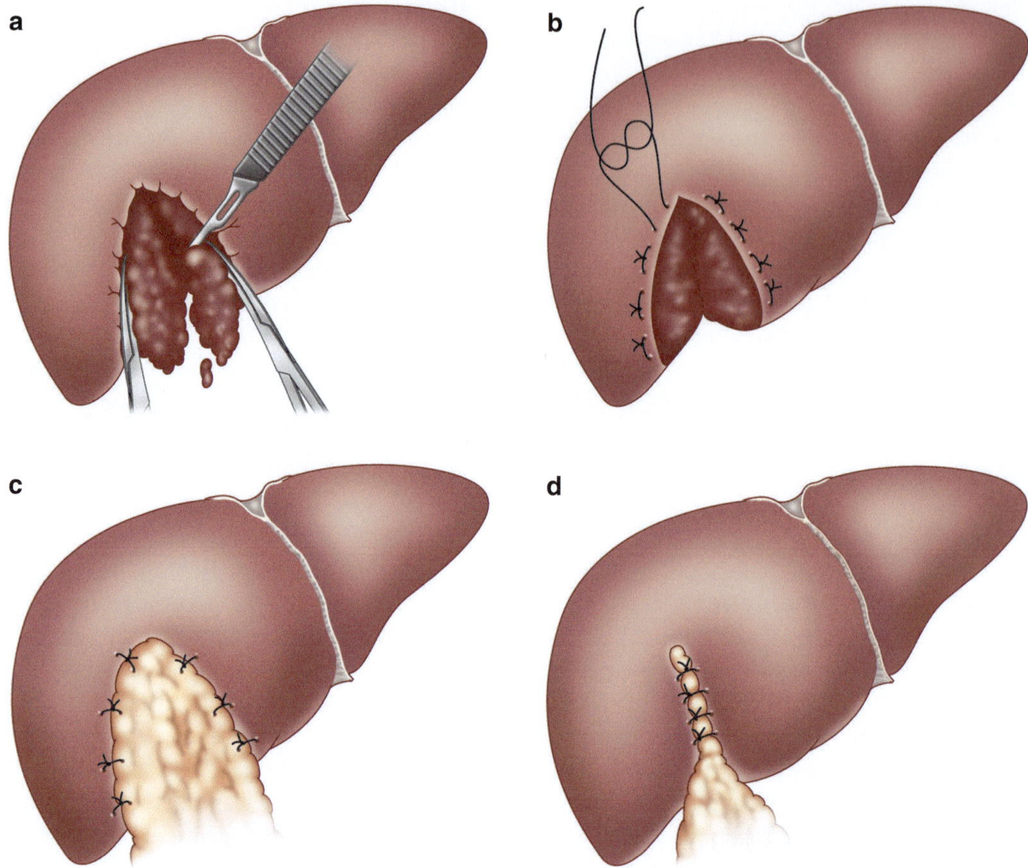

Fig. 6.4 Rapid resectional debridement. Via the "finger fracture technique," a plane of healthy parenchyma just beyond the injured tissue is identified and all of the hepatic tissue just inside of the clips or sutures on the blood vessels and bile ducts is debrided (**a**). Bleeding from the raw surface of the liver can be controlled by mattress sutures (**b**) or a pedicle of viable omentum to fill the dead space. (**c**) A piece of omentum is mobilized, placed into the debrided liver and sutured in place. (**d**) This figure illustrates the use of omentum. Please note that the mobilized and grafted omentum has an intact vascular supply and is well perfused

Potential Pitfalls

Along with such techniques come potential pitfalls, including intra-abdominal abscesses, bleeding, ductal injuries/bilomas, and hemobilia. In all comers, the incidence of such complications is remarkably low.

Intra-abdominal Abscesses

The incidence of intra-abdominal abscesses following hepatic trauma can vary widely (1.9–17 %) depending on the magnitude of the injury, the presence of other intra-abdominal injuries (especially the colon), and the quality of the repair [5, 31]. If an abscess is identified (most commonly by computed tomography [CT]), one can attempt percutaneous drainage via interventional radiology [31]. Reoperation is reserved solely for those in which this is unsuccessful or whose septic picture does not resolve. In such instances, a posterior rib resection approach is preferred.

Bleeding

Bleeding in the early postoperative period is most often secondary to bleeding from discrete vessels within the liver or juxtahepatic vascular injuries.

If possible, one should wait until the "bloody viscous cycle" has resolved prior to returning to the operating theater. It is critical to control all bleeding at this return visit, to include exploring previous repair sites and consideration for perihepatic packing, selective extralobar hepatic artery ligation, and atriocaval shunting.

Only in instances of persistent hypotension or progressive abdominal compartment syndrome should one return to the operating theater sooner. In such instances, perihepatic packing and damage control surgery should be performed (unless a discrete bleeding vessel is appreciated).

Missed Ductal Injuries/Bilomas

Missed ductal injuries (and resultant bilomas) occur in approximately 8–10 % of patients sustaining major hepatic injuries. Primary management involves percutaneous drainage, with most biliary fistulae closing within 3 weeks (and many sooner) if there is no evidence of distal biliary obstruction. Rarely is reoperation required.

Hemobilia

Upper gastrointestinal bleeding within the first several months of hepatic trauma should raise the suspicion of hemobilia [32, 33]. All such patients should undergo an emergent hepatic arteriogram with embolization of the bleeding vessel. One should also consider an upper gastrointestinal endoscopy to evacuate any potential clot in the biliary ducts (with possible stenting).

After the Fact

Dulchavsky et al. have documented the wound healing strength of the healing liver to be 6–8 weeks [34]. Thus, limiting the return to normal activities beyond 8 weeks seems unwarranted. For injuries greater than a grade III, it would seem prudent to repeat a computed tomography scan of the liver at 3 months if the patient is contemplating a return to contact sports.

Video Captions

Video 8   Finger fracture of the liver (MP4 22289 kb)

Video 10   Omental pack (MP4 32585 kb)

Video 11   Digital compression (MP4 16750 kb)

References

1. Feliciano DV, Gentry LO, Bitondo CG, et al. Single agent cephalosporin prophylaxis for penetrating abdominal trauma. Results and comment on the emergence of enterococcus. Am J Surg. 1986;152:674–81.
2. Kashuk J, Moore EE, Milikan JS, Moore JB. Major abdominal vascular trauma – a unified approach. J Trauma. 1982;22:672–9.
3. Moore EE, Cogbill TH, Jurkovich GJ, Shackford SR, Malangoni MA, Champion HR. Organ injury scaling: spleen and liver (1994 revision). J Trauma. 1995;38: 323–4.
4. Pachter HL, Knudson MM, Esrig B, et al. Status of nonoperative management of blunt hepatic injuries in 1995: a multicenter experience with 404 patients. J Trauma. 1996;40:31–8.
5. Feliciano DV, Mattox KL, Jordan Jr GL, et al. Management of 1,000 consecutive cases of hepatic trauma (1979–1984). Ann Surg. 1986;204:438–45.
6. Cox EF, Flancbaum L, Dauterive AH, et al. Blunt trauma to the liver. Analysis of management and mortality in 323 consecutive patients. Ann Surg. 1988;207:126–34.
7. Trunkey D. Hepatic trauma: contemporary management. Surg Clin North Am. 2004;84:437–50.
8. Oz MC, Rondinone JF, Shargill NS. FloSeal Matrix: new generation topical hemostatic sealant. J Card Surg. 2003;18:486–93.
9. Samudrala S. Topical hemostatic agents in surgery: a surgeon's perspective. AORN J. 2008;88:s2–11.
10. Gabay M. Absorbable hemostatic agents. Am J Health Syst Pharm. 2006;63:1244–53.
11. Tomizawa Y. Clinical benefits and risk analysis of topical hemostats: a review. J Artif Organs. 2005;8: 137–42.
12. Block JE. Severe blood loss during spinal reconstructive procedures: the potential usefulness of topical hemostatic agents. Med Hypotheses. 2005;65:617–21.
13. Richardson JD, Franklin GA, Lukan JK, et al. Evolution in the management of hepatic trauma: a 25 year perspective. Ann Surg. 2000;232:324–30.
14. Pringle JH. Notes on the arrest of hemorrhage due to trauma. Ann Surg. 1908;48:546–66.
15. Pachter HL, Hofstetter SR, Liang NG, et al. Liver and biliary tract trauma. In: Feliciano DV, Moore EE, Mattox KL, editors. Trauma. 3rd ed. Stamford: Appleton & Lange; 1996. p. 487.
16. Pachter HL, Spencer FC. Recent concepts in the treatment of hepatic trauma. Ann Surg. 1979;190: 423–8.

17. Pachter HL, Spencer FC, Hofstetter SR, Liang HG, Coppa GF. Significant trends in the treatment of hepatic trauma. Experience with 411 injuries. Ann Surg. 1992;215:492–500.

18. Pachter HL, Spencer FC, Hofstetter SR, Liang HG, Coppa GF. The management of juxtahepatic venous injuries without an atriocaval shunt: preliminary clinical observations. Surgery. 1986;99:569–75.

19. Patel S, Pachter HL, Yee H, Schwartz JD. Topical hypothermia attenuates pulmonary injury after hepatic ischemia reperfusion. J Am Coll Surg. 2000;191:650–6.

20. Demaria EJ, Reichman W, Keney PR, Armitage JM, Gann DS. Septic complications of corticosteroid administration after central nervous system trauma. Ann Surg. 1985;202:248–52.

21. Eidelman Y, Glat PM, Pachter HL, et al. The effects of topical hypothermia and steroids on ATP levels in an in vivo liver ischemia model. In: Presented at the Eastern Association for the Surgery of Trauma. Freeport. 14 Jan 1994.

22. Ty L, Le CS, Chen KM, Chen CC. Role of surgery in the treatment of primary carcinoma of the liver: a 31 year experience. Br J Surg. 1987;74:839–42.

23. Balasegaram DM, Joishy SK, McNamara JJ, et al. Hepatic resection: the logical approach to surgical management of major trauma to the liver. Am J Surg. 1981;142:580–3.

24. Balasegaram DM. Hepatic resection in trauma. Adv Surg. 1984;17:129–70.

25. Lin TY, Hsu KY, Hsieh CM, et al. Study on lobectomy of the liver. Taiwan I Hsueh Hui Tsa Chih. 1958;57:750–69.

26. Ton TT. A new technique for operation on the liver. Lancet. 1963;1:192–3.

27. Pachter HL, Spencer FC, Hofstetter SR, et al. Experience with the finger fracture technique to achieve intra-hepatic hemostasis in 75 patients with severe injuries to the liver. Ann Surg. 1983;197:771–8.

28. Fischer RP, Stremple JF, McNamara JJ, et al. The rapid right hepatectomy. J Trauma. 1971;11: 742–8.

29. Stone HH, Lamb JM. Use of pedicled omentum as an autologous pack for control of hemorrhage in major injuries of the liver. Surg Gynecol Obstet. 1975;1 41:92–4.

30. Fabian TC, Croce MA, Stanford GG, et al. Factors affecting morbidity following hepatic trauma: a prospective analysis of 482 liver injuries. Ann Surg. 1991;213:540–7.

31. Scott CM, Grasberger RC, Heeran TF, et al. Intraabdominal sepsis after hepatic trauma. Am J Surg. 1988;155:284–8.

32. Mays ET. Hepatic trauma. Curr Probl Surg. 1976;13:1–73.

33. Sparkman RS. Massive hemobilia following traumatic rupture of the liver. Report of a case and review of the literature. Ann Surg. 1953;138:899–910.

34. Dulchavsky SA, Lucas CE, Ledgerwood AM, Grabow D, An T. Efficacy of liver wound healing by secondary intent. J Trauma. 1990;30:44–8.

Parenchyma: Formal Lobectomy

Andrew B. Peitzman and James Wallis Marsh

Introduction

Mortality is higher for blunt than penetrating liver injury, due to greater extent of parenchymal injury [1]. Although mortality has decreased, the most common cause of death for major hepatic injury remains exsanguination [2]. The mortality for complex liver injuries remains greater than 50 % in most series, and juxtahepatic caval injury continues to have mortality of 65–100 % [3, 4]. However, our institution reported a series of 215 patients with complex liver injuries (56 of whom underwent nonanatomic or anatomic liver resection) with operative mortality of 9 % associated with major hepatic injury and 25 % for juxtahepatic caval injury [5]. Although extensive hepatorrhaphy or nonanatomic liver resection is often indicated acutely for major hepatic injury, anatomic hepatic lobectomy is uncommonly necessary. Either nonanatomic or anatomic lobectomy at the initial laparotomy for trauma is dictated by the extent and the location of the liver injury. The operative resection is often completion of a resection essentially started by the injury itself. Less commonly, resection is the best or quickest way to gain access to a retrohepatic site of hemorrhage. Equally important is the application of anatomic lobectomy at a later laparotomy after packing and damage control have staunched hemorrhage at the index exploration. Anatomic resection definitively eliminates nonviable liver tissue, removes the potential for delayed hemorrhage, and avoids a bile leak from associated bile duct injury.

Anatomy

One of the major operative risks in both elective and emergency hepatic surgery is injury to the noninvolved portal structures. The surgeon must be familiar with hepatic anatomy and the common variations (see Chap. 1) [6–9]. The liver is divided into two hemilivers by the main portal fissure (Cantlie's line). This line extends from the medial margin of the gallbladder running superiorly to the inferior vena cava (IVC) (Fig. 7.1). The eight segments of the liver are defined by the courses of the portal and hepatic venous systems. The right hemiliver consists of segments V through VIII, supplied by the right hepatic artery and right portal vein. The left hemiliver, nour-

A.B. Peitzman, MD (✉)
Department of Surgery, University of Pittsburgh,
F-1281, UPMC-Presbyterian, 200 Lothrop Street,
Pittsburgh, PA 15213, USA
e-mail: peitzmanab@upmc.edu

J.W. Marsh, MD, MBA
Department of Surgery, University of Pittsburgh
School of Medicine,
7th Floor Montefiore Hospital, 3459 5th Avenue,
Pittsburgh, PA 15213, USA
e-mail: marshw@upmc.edu

Electronic supplementary material Supplementary material is available in the online version of this chapter at 10.1007/978-1-4939-1200-1_7. Videos can also be accessed at http://www.springerimages.com/videos/978-1-4939-1199-8.

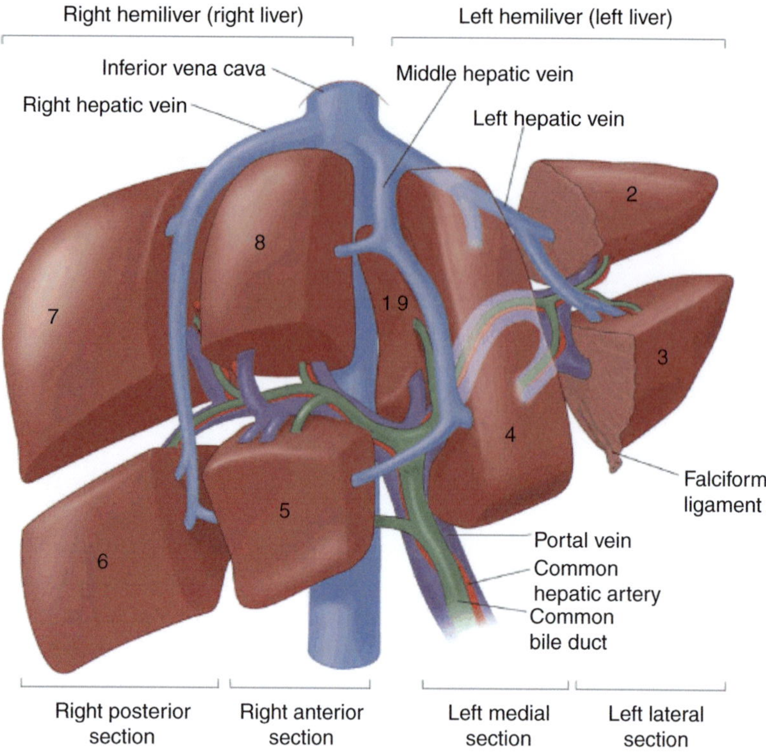

ished by the left hepatic artery and left portal vein, is comprised of segments II–IV. The caudate lobe is distinct from the two hemilivers (segment I). The portal triad (portal vein, hepatic artery, and bile duct branches) to a lobe or segment runs centrally *within the* segments of the liver. In addition, the portal triad is protected by a substantial sheath which is an extension of Glisson's capsule. In contradistinction, the hepatic veins lie in the planes *between* lobes and segments, are not enclosed in a sheath; therefore more likely to tear than the tougher portal triads. The least variable structures are the venous inflow and outflow.

Under most circumstances, the right hepatic vein is the largest of the three and enters the superior surface of the vena cava on the right superior aspect of the vena cava. In 85 % of cases, the middle and left hepatic veins exit the liver separately but then join before entering the left anterior aspect of the vena cava. The extrahepatic segments of the major hepatic veins are only 1–2 cm in length. Each hepatic vein has a long (8–12 cm) intrahepatic segment with multiple branches and runs within a portal fissure.

The short hepatic veins enter the anterior wall of the vena cava posterior to the liver. They vary in number, averaging 5–7, and range up to 1 cm in diameter [10]. If the right hepatic vein is small, any large ($\geq$5 mm) short hepatic veins should be preserved when possible if a resection is not being performed.

The two most common anomalies of the hepatic artery are a replaced right hepatic artery from the superior mesenteric artery which courses posterior to the portal vein (15 %) and replaced left hepatic artery from the left gastric artery (12 %). This artery should be carefully sought, as it can easily be missed and cut. When present, this artery courses under the left lateral segment through the gastrohepatic omentum and always crosses posterior to a vagus nerve branch.

Although highly variable, most anomalies of the bile ducts are intrahepatic and do not normally affect the surgery of the liver. One of the most common surgical anomalies of the biliary system is the right posterior duct which crosses over and enters the left ductal system. When this occurs, the insertion is generally just superior to the main biliary bifurcation. This becomes important when

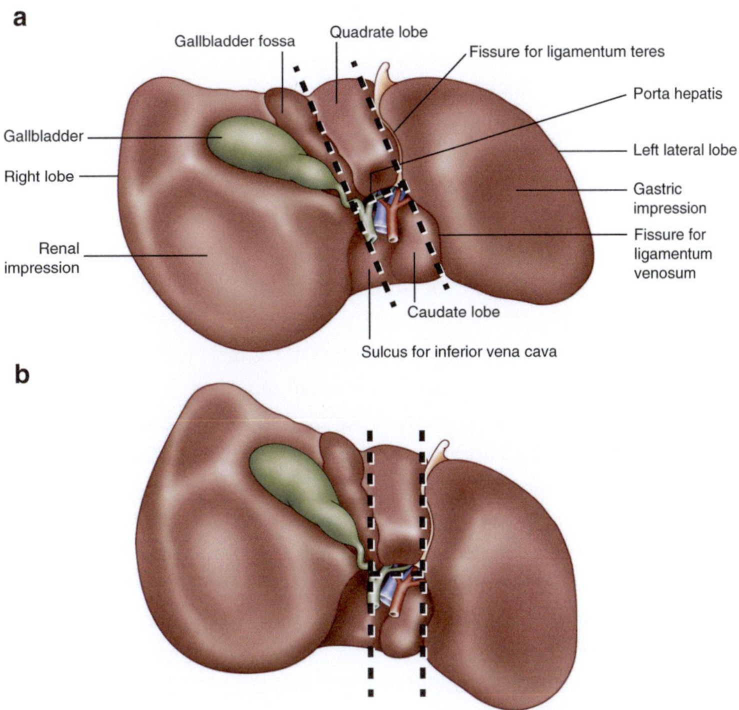

Fig. 7.2 Porta hepatis and features of the visceral surface of the liver. (**a**) Typical orientation of the H configuration of the portal structures. (**b**) Incorrect but common depiction of relationship of H configurations parallel with the midsagittal plane of the body

performing a left hepatic lobectomy requiring division of the bile duct close to the bifurcation. This can be detected by pre-parenchymal division with a cholangiogram taken through the cystic duct. When this iatrogenic injury goes unrecognized, the patient most often develops a significant bile leak postoperatively.

The fissures on the visceral surface of the liver are important landmarks during liver resection. The important fissures run in what can be presented as a "capital H" configuration (Fig. 7.2) [7, 8]. The right limb of the H runs from the gallbladder fossa posteriorly to the inferior vena cava (demarcating separation of right and left lobes). The left limb of the H runs from round ligament to ligamentum venosum, demarcating dividing line between segment IV and segments II and III. The cross of the H is the porta hepatis.

Approach to the Liver

The caudate lobe (segment 1) from the patient's left provides access to all structures of the liver; it often encircles the inferior vena cava posteriorly [11]. Access is gained to the caudate lobe by elevating the left lateral segment and then opening the gastrohepatic omentum. Avoid an aberrant left hepatic artery from the left gastric artery (see above). The left triangular ligament can be taken down quickly. The left triangular ligament can then be divided with the electrocautery or scissors to the insertion of the left phrenic vein into the left hepatic vein. Divide the falciform ligament down to the hepatic veins, which are more posteriorly than most surgeons believe.

It may also be advantageous to elevate the right side of the liver (often not necessary in urgent situations). To do this, the right side of liver should be elevated medially and superiorly exposing the right triangular ligament, cut with electrocautery or scissors. Do not drift into the liver parenchyma as the ligament is divided; superiorly, avoid entering the diaphragm. Detach the right adrenal gland from the underside of the liver. Full mobilization of the right lobe of the liver continues with the assistant retracting the right lobe of the liver to the patient's left; the short hepatic veins are each clipped or tied and divided proceeding from caudal to cephalad until the right hepatic vein is reached. The dorsal ligament must be divided to fully free the liver from the IVC.

Key principles dealing with major hepatic injury in the operating room include the following:

1. The best help possible with you at the operating table.
2. Adequate exposure. A trauma laparotomy will start with a midline incision. A right subcostal extension is often necessary to expose retrohepatic venous injury or posterior right lobe injury. On rare occasion, a median sternotomy will assist in exposure of suprahepatic injury to the IVC. Thoracotomy adds little to operative exposure of the liver.
3. Exposure is achieved with a self-retaining retractor system (many good options available). Retraction in both cephalad and anterior directions is critical; attempt to lift the ribcage off the table with the retractor.
4. Intravenous access above the diaphragm. Low central venous pressure is maintained throughout the case to minimize bleeding—central venous pressure less than 5 mmHg.
5. Pedicle ligation demarcates the liver segment to be resected and controls inflow prior to parenchymal dissection.
6. Minimize blood loss, as excessive blood loss is the major determinant of perioperative outcome. Expertise and technology to minimize blood loss during parenchymal dissection are essential. Operative tools for dissection and coagulation assist in this, such as the tissue link devices, argon beam coagulator, the stapling devices, the LigaSure, and many other advances [12–24]. Many of the instruments available for dissection and coagulation in elective liver resection are not appropriate and essentially ineffective in the patient actively bleeding from a major liver injury.

Stapling Devices

The use of stapling devices has greatly reduced transection time in hepatic surgery and stapling devices are useful in the setting of trauma [25–28]. Crushing staples are best and are fitted with the vascular loads. The capsule of the liver along the intended cutting plane is scored first with the electrocautery, and then the liver parenchyma is crushed and stapled with the stapler.

However, there are a few caveats when using the stapler:

- Once the parenchymal transection is begun with the stapler, there will always be bleeding along the staple line (which is best controlled with bimanual compression until the transection is complete). Complete expeditiously.
- Place the smaller blade of the stapler into the parenchyma.
- The staplers are unaware what they are stapling. What is between the jaws of the stapler will be divided, including the hilar structures and hepatic veins. Thus, the surgeon must be certain of the hepatic anatomy and location of the stapler. In an elective resection, ultrasound can assist with identification of structures. In the trauma setting, a rapid hepatic lobectomy, generally nonanatomic, can be performed with the staplers. Remember the location of the middle hepatic vein running within the main portal fissure. Inadvertent injury to middle hepatic vein will add another major bleeding site. Make certain that the resection line is off-center (Cantlie's line), toward the lobe being resected, relative to the middle hepatic vein.
- The stapler should pass easily into the parenchyma. When it meets resistance, the stapler is either going through the capsule of the liver or into an intrahepatic vascular structure. When this occurs, redirect stapler either deeper or more superficially in the liver. Alternatively, a Kelly clamp can be passed into the liver along the intended transection plane as a guide, before placing the blades of the stapler.

Instruments and Other Techniques

The *argon beam coagulator (ABC)* is useful for surface injuries to the liver and for subcapsular hematomas. *LigaSure* or *Enseal* is useful for division of the liver under controlled circumstances. Salient Surgical Technology devices (formerly

TissueLink) are useful tools for dissection of the liver and for hemostasis on the intrahepatic tissue. These devices link radiofrequency with cool saline at the cone-shaped tip of the device. The Cavitron Ultrasonic Surgical Aspirator (CUSA, Tyco Healthcare, Mansfield, MA) combines ultrasonic energy with aspiration. The CUSA dissects tissue, but does not offer coagulation or hemostasis. The Harmonic Scalpel (Ethicon Endo-Surgery, Cincinnati, Ohio) uses ultrasound energy applied to vibrating ultrasonic shears, sealing and dividing vessels up to 3 mm. The bipolar device (the *Aquamantys*) is useful for hemostasis alone and is quick. However, these devices are not useful for large parenchymal injuries, especially in cracks and crevices that can occur in liver trauma. None of these devices should be used near the main hepatic ducts, as significant thermal injury will occur. If the patient is stable and has undergone any significant resection, the raw liver surface should be treated with one of these devices to minimize the risk of postoperative bleeding or biliary leak.

Thrombin activated factors help seal small bile leaks and stop minor bleeding; they should not be depended upon to stop any significant bleeding.

We do not utilize *aortic clamping* for isolated hepatic trauma. It affords the surgeon nothing and deprives the other abdominal viscera of inflow.

The Operation

The intrahepatic radical to either lobe may be approached from outside or inside the liver. Formal extrahepatic dissection can be time-consuming, with potential risk because of anatomic variability. Intrahepatic hilar division is as safe as extrahepatic hilar division in terms of intraoperative blood requirements, morbidity, and mortality (Figs. 7.3, 7.4, and 7.5) [15, 16, 29–31]. The stapling devices have facilitated this approach [22, 27]. The intrahepatic approach to the pedicles involves dissection of hepatic parenchyma along the hepatic fissures with control of the pedicles within the liver (see Fig. 7.2).

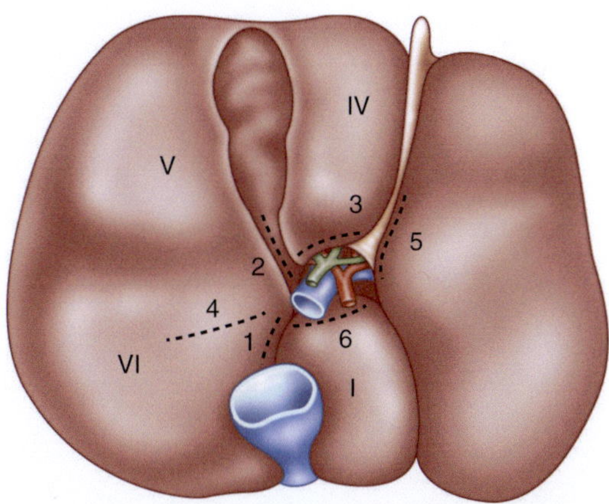

Fig. 7.3 Sites for hepatotomy in portal pedicle isolation. The undersurface of the liver is illustrated. The *dotted lines* indicate sites for hepatotomy if control of the intrahepatic portal pedicles is desired. Incision at 3 allows lowering of the hilar plate. Incisions at 1 and 2 allow control of the right main pedicle. Incisions at 1 and 4 allow control of the right posterior pedicle. Incisions at 2 and 4 allow control of the right anterior pedicle. Incisions at 3 and 5 allow control of the left pedicle (Reprinted Fong and Blumgart [26], with permission from Elsevier)

Intraoperative ultrasound is invaluable in identification of the portal triads or hepatic veins within the liver.

Large blood loss during parenchymal dissection must be avoided. Dissection through the liver parenchyma to the inflow and outflow vessels without prior vascular control avoids erroneous ligation of portal structures, but bleeding from the transected liver surface may be substantial unless the procedure is performed quickly. The Pringle is often applied as an atraumatic clamp across the hilar structures. However, the authors prefer double-looping a wide vessel loop around the hilar structures, pulling up hard on the vessel loop, and clamping the vessel loop just anterior to the hilar structures. This avoids any potential injury to the common bile duct which may occur even with an atraumatic clamp. The Pringle maneuver or selective inflow occlusion may minimize blood loss, but increases the risk of postoperative liver dysfunction. The normal liver can tolerate up to 120 min of ischemia, as long as done intermittently rather than continuously. Ten to fifteen minutes of clamp time of the portal hepatitis, spelled by 5 min of liver perfusion between clamp times [15, 16, 32].

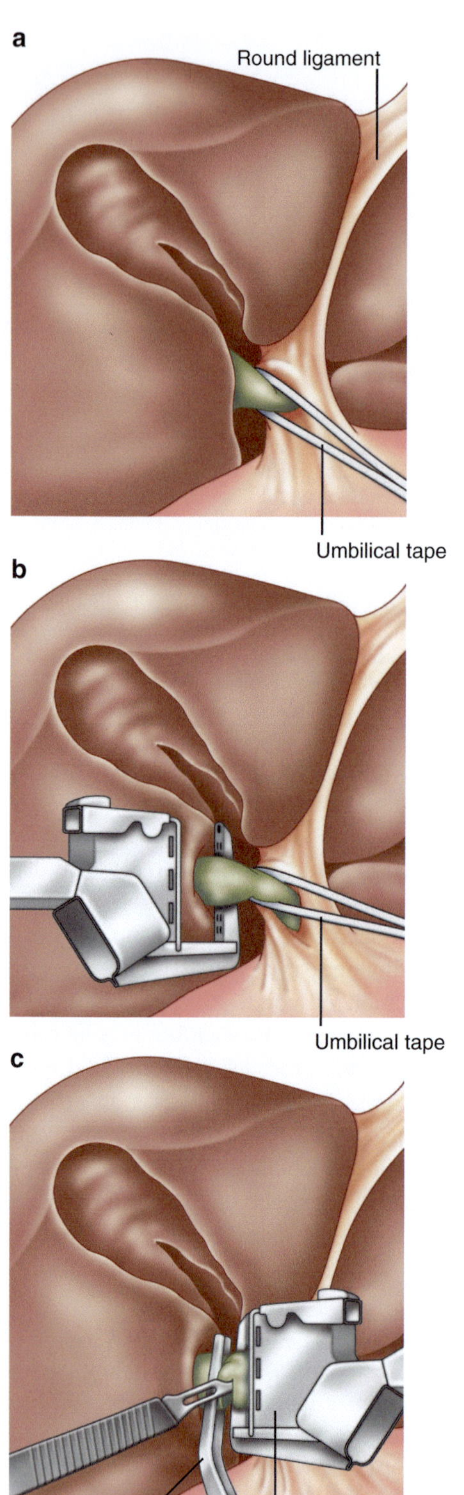

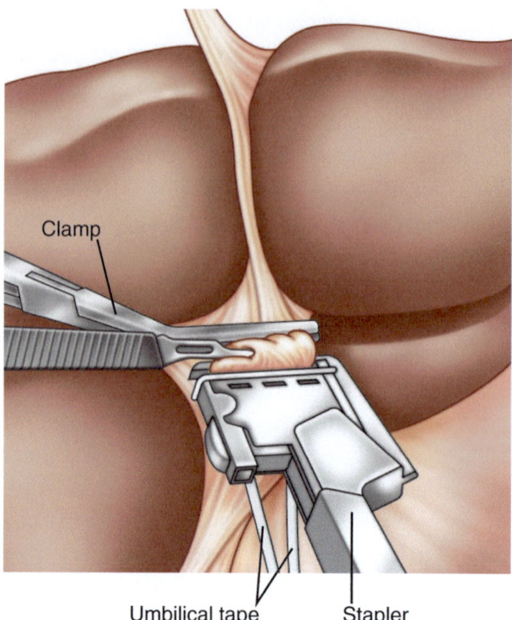

Fig. 7.5 Stapler ligation of left portal pedicle. After incisions into the liver at sites 3 and 5 in Fig. 7.3, the left portal pedicle is delivered into view and an umbilical tape is placed around the pedicle for control. While constant traction is placed on the umbilical tape downward, a vascular stapler is applied on the left main pedicle. The traction of the umbilical tape prevents accidental application of staples too close to the takeoff of the caudate branches. After application of the stapler, a vascular clamp is placed on the specimen side of the portal pedicle. The left portal pedicle is then cut using a scalpel (Reprinted from Fong and Blumgart [26], Copyright 1997, with permission from Elsevier)

Fig. 7.4 Control of the right portal pedicle. After incisions into the liver at sites 1 and 2 in Fig. 7.3, the right portal pedicle is delivered into view. An umbilical tape is placed around the pedicle for control. (**b**) Placement of the stapler. While constant traction is placed on the umbilical tape to the right, a vascular stapler is applied on the main right pedicle. The traction of the umbilical tape prevents accidental application of staples too close to the hilus. (**c**) Division of the right portal pedicle. After application of the stapler, a vascular clamp is placed on the specimen side of the portal pedicle. The right portal pedicle is then cut using a scalpel (Reprinted from Fong and Blumgart [26], Copyright 1997, with permission from Elsevier)

As mentioned, techniques for liver resection include finger fracture technique, clamp crushing, staplers, ultrasonic dissection, such as the Cavitron Ultrasonic Surgical Aspirator (CUSA, Tyco Healthcare, Mansfield, MA), the water jet dissector, the Harmonic Scalpel (Ethicon Endo-Surgery, Cincinnati, OH), the LigaSure (Valleylab, Tyco Healthcare, Boulder, CO), the TissueLink dissecting sealer (TissueLink Medical Inc, Dover, NH), or radiofrequency-assisted liver transection. The clamp-crushing technique is still widely applied because of its effectiveness and low cost. A recent meta-analysis did not indicate a "benefit of any alternative transection technique on patients' perioperative outcome compared with the clamp-crushing technique. The clamp-crushing technique remains the reference technique for transection of the parenchyma in elective hepatic resection" [33–35]. For elective resection, we do utilize much of the newer technology, as we will discuss.

General Principles for Elective Liver Resection

- Supradiaphragmatic intravenous access, blood is available.
- Use a fixed table retractor (Thompson, Buckwalter, etc.). It is important to pull both cephalad and lift the anterior chest wall away from the table for optimal exposure.
- Take down the round and falciform ligaments; expose the anterior surface of the hepatic veins.
- Left hepatectomy → take down the left triangular ligament. Right hepatectomy → mobilize the right lobe from the right coronary and triangular ligaments.
- Open the gastrohepatic ligament and search for replaced hepatic arteries.
- Perform a cholecystectomy late in the case; leave the gallbladder with the cystic duct intact (until end of case). For major nonanatomic or anatomic resections for trauma, a cholangiogram should be performed (assuming the patient is stable). This defines the biliary anatomy and prevents postoperative bile leak. Saline is intermittently injected via the cystic

duct remnant (cholecystectomy performed) to identify and oversew leaking bile ducts in the liver parenchyma or resection margin. This maneuver helps avoid a postoperative bile leak. Often, this is at a delayed operation following damage control at the first procedure.
- Utilize ultrasound to identify intraparenchymal vascular structures.

Right Hepatic Lobectomy [14]

- The assistant retracts the right lobe of the liver to the patient's left; mobilize the liver from the inferior vena cava; ligate the short hepatic veins moving from caudal to cephalad up to the right hepatic vein To free the liver from the inferior vena cava, the dorsal attachment of the liver should be divided with the stapler or cautery.
- Perform a right hilar dissection. Lower the hilar plate, then doubly ligate and divide the right hepatic artery; stay high on the right side of the common bile duct.
- Divide the right portal vein after taking, if necessary, the small lateral portal vein branch off the right portal vein to the caudate/right lobe, followed by division of the right hepatic artery with a vascular stapler (white 2.5-mm cartridge).
- Notch or divide the caudate process crossing to the right hepatic lobe.
- Make a counter incision at the right base of the gallbladder fossa; tunnel a Kelly clamp deep to the hilar plate and emerge anterior to the IVC; place an umbilical tape in the tunnel which runs behind the hilar plate. After checking the inflow to the left side of the liver with the Doppler or ultrasound, divide the right hilar plate with right hepatic ducts using the vascular stapler.
- Confirm the parenchymal transection plane by ultrasound, and then stay 1 cm to the right of the middle hepatic vein.
- Score the liver capsule with electrocautery. Bovie approximately 1 cm into the liver parenchyma; use a LigaSure or stapler to divide the parenchyma.
- Continue parenchymal division with a LigaSure or stapler device until middle hepatic

vein branches to segment V/VIII branches are encountered.

- Pringle maneuver as described earlier.
- Complete the parenchymal slice with sequential crushing vascular stapling (may pretunnel with a large Kelly clamp if desired); parenchymal transection time will be less than 10 min.
- Inspect the cut edge for bleeding; place a figure-of-eight suture on vessels or ducts; may also treat with TissueLink device such as the Aquamantys. Release the Pringle maneuver and dry up the cut edge with a radiofrequency sealant device.
- Inspect the IVC and right retroperitoneal space for hemostasis.
- Perform completion ultrasound to confirm left portal vein and hepatic vein patency.
- Perform a saline cholangiogram via the cystic duct stump and oversew any leaks.
- Reattach the proximal falciform ligament onto the diaphragm with a figure-of-eight suture. Leave a closed suction drain in the subphrenic space.

As mentioned, some liver surgeons advocate a one-step division of the entire intrahepatic Glissonian pedicle with the stapler. However, it is the authors' preference to divide the right hepatic artery and portal vein extrahepatically. We restrict the intrahepatic maneuver for division of the right hilar plate with the right hepatic ducts. Key to a safe transection plane is accurate ultrasound visualization and mapping of the middle hepatic vein; stay to the right of it.

Left Hepatic Lobectomy [14]

- Split the gastrohepatic ligament adjacent to the undersurface of the left lateral section and the caudate lobe.
- If present, double ligate and divide a replaced or accessory left hepatic artery.
- Clamp the round ligament; pull it anteriorly as a handle to expose the left hilum.
- Divide existing parenchymal bridge between segments III and IVB.
- Dissect the left hilum at the base of the umbilical fissure and lower the hilar plate anterior to the left portal pedicle.
- Incise the peritoneum overlying the hilum from the left side and double ligate the left hepatic artery (test to confirm a palpable pulse in the right hepatic artery or check with Doppler or ultrasound—if the patient is hypotensive, a palpable pulse may be undetectable).
- Dissect the portal vein at the base of the umbilical fissure (the vein takes a nearly 90° bend from the transverse to the umbilical portion).
- Divide the left portal vein with a vascular stapler; stay just distal to the takeoff of the caudate inflow branch (if the caudate lobe is being preserved).
- Divide the ligamentum venosum caudally.
- Make a counterincision in segment IVB, 1 cm above the base of the umbilical fissure. Pass a Kelly clamp behind the left hilar plate, aim for the left lower quadrant, and exit just anterior (and superficial) to or through the caudate lobe.
- Place an umbilical tape in the tunnel behind the left hilar plate.
- Confirm inflow to the right hepatic lobe with a Doppler or ultrasound; then divide the left hilar plate and left hepatic duct with a vascular stapler.
- Fold the left lateral segment up and to the right, to expose the window at the base of the left hepatic vein as it enters the inferior vena cava. First, divide any loose areolar tissue overlying the ligamentum venosum which is divided proximally.
- Pass a blunt right-angle clamp in the window between the right hepatic vein and the middle hepatic vein, hug the back of the middle hepatic vein, and aim for the deep edge of the left hepatic vein. This maneuver must be done gently and without forcing the clamp; do not create a hole in the middle hepatic vein or inferior vena cava. Keep in mind that the left and middle hepatic veins have a common trunk in 85–90 %. If it is not easy to open the window deep to the middle hepatic vein and left hepatic vein, divide them later as the parenchymal transection is completed.
- Pass an umbilical tape through this window and divide the common trunk of the middle

hepatic vein and left hepatic vein with a vascular stapler.

- Ultrasound to confirm the transection plane on the anterior surface; stay close to the demarcated line. Protect the middle hepatic vein as it passes tangentially from the left to the right lobe.
- Along the line of demarcation in the liver, Bovie approximately 1 cm into the liver parenchyma, and then switch to a LigaSure device. Continue parenchymal division with the LigaSure device until segment V/VIII middle hepatic vein branches are encountered.
- Pringle maneuver around the porta hepatis.
- Complete the parenchymal slice with vascular stapler (pretunnel with a large Kelly clamp). As the slice is deepened, gradually carry the transection down to exit just anterior to the caudate at the level of ligamentum venosum.
- Check the resection margin for surgical bleeding; figure-of-eight suture for bleeding or use a TissueLink device such as the Aquamantys.
- Release the Pringle maneuver; secure hemostasis on the cut edge with a saline-cooled radiofrequency sealant device.
- Ultrasound to confirm patent right portal vein and right hepatic vein.
- Inject saline via the cystic duct stump; oversew bile leaks.
- Consider a contrast cholangiogram to confirm the patency of the proximal right hepatic duct and the distal common bile duct.
- Place a closed suction drain in the left subphrenic space.

The right posterior duct comes off the left hepatic duct in 20 % of cases and the right anterior duct comes off the left hepatic duct in 5 % of cases. Thus, it is critical to divide the left hepatic duct at the base of the umbilical fissure and not more centrally in the hilum as it bifurcates. If the left hepatic duct were divided as it appears to bifurcate from the right hepatic duct, either the right posterior or right anterior duct would be transected approximately 20 % of the time. As the parenchymal transection then reaches the left side of the gallbladder fossa, the transection plane turns vertical to run parallel to Cantlie's line. The left lobe of the liver will be demarcated (unless the patient has been profoundly hypotensive) at this point (after the vascular inflow has been divided), which guides the transection plane on the anterior surface.

Left Lateral Segmentectomy [14]

- Open the gastrohepatic ligament flush with the undersurface of the left lateral section and the caudate lobe.
- Doubly ligate and divide a replaced or accessory left hepatic artery if present.
- Clamp the round ligament and pull it anteriorly as a handle to expose the left hilum.
- Divide existing parenchymal bridge between segments III and IVB.
- Dissect down from the end of the round ligament, until the segment III pedicle is encountered.
- Incise the peritoneal reflection on the left side of the round ligament as it inserts into the umbilical fissure. Segment III and II pedicles can then be encircled and divided separately with a vascular stapler. When encircling the segment II pedicle, avoid injury to the caudate inflow vessels coming off the left portal vein.
- Divide the liver parenchyma, staying flush on the left side of the falciform ligament with cautery or LigaSure device.
- Divide the left hepatic vein within the liver parenchyma with a vascular stapler as the parenchymal transection is completed.

If the patient is unstable, the left lateral segment can be removed quickly with sequential firing of a crushing stapler. Score the liver parenchyma to the patient's left side of the falciform ligament; stay to the left side of the hilar structures inferiorly and to the left side of the left hepatic vein superiorly. Use a Kelly clamp to make sequential tunnels into the liver parenchyma followed by division of the parenchyma with the stapler. The hepatic inflow and outflow structures are taken within the liver, usually with a vascular stapler. A Pringle maneuver usually is not required for a left lateral resection.

Unlikely to be necessary for trauma, other formal resections include the *right trisectionectomy* (extended right hepatectomy) and the *left trisectionectomy* (extended left hepatectomy). A right trisectionectomy includes resection of segments IV–VIII, i.e., all liver tissue to the right of the falciform ligament.

Right Trisectionectomy [30]

- The initial steps of the operation are as for right hepatectomy, including ligation of the portal triad and the right hepatic vein.
- Devascularization of segment IV
- Dissect the umbilical ligament to identify vascular pedicles to segments II, III, and IV, which run within the fissure. Usually the lower portion of the fissure is obscured by liver tissue between the segments.
- Divide this bridge of liver tissue between the segments with diathermy. The vascular pedicles to segment IV will be exposed within the umbilical fissure.
- Transect the liver tissue just to the right of the falciform ligament, resecting segment IV, from anterior to posterior toward right hepatic vein (already divided).
- Divide the middle hepatic vein as it is approached at the end of the transection.

Left Trisectionectomy

- A left trisectionectomy involves resection of segments II–V and VIII; segment I is sometimes resected as well. The operation is a left hepatectomy plus right anterior sectionectomy. The right hepatic vein must be preserved as the sole drainage in the remnant liver.
- Both lobes of the liver are fully mobilized.
- Ligate the portal triad to the left lobe.
- Expose the left hepatic vein and suprahepatic inferior vena cava.
- Ligate the left and middle hepatic veins.
- Define the plane of resection in the right lobe. The plane is horizontal, lateral to the gallbladder fossa, and anterior to the right hepatic vein in the right scissura.
- Ligate the portal pedicle to the right anterior segment.
- Parenchymal resection is from caudal to cephalad. Pringle maneuver may be needed.

Advances in understanding hepatic anatomy, operative technique and devices, and anesthesia management including maintenance of low CVP during parenchyma resection have made elective liver resection a procedure with low operative mortality. It is critical that the surgeon has a deep understanding of hepatic anatomy. Intraoperative ultrasound is an essential tool to identify and protect vascular structures during resection.

Video Captions

Video 2 Right hepatic lobe rotation (MOV 42120 kb)

Video 3 Right hepatic lobe rotation (3-D animation) (MOV 33079 kb)

References

1. Badger SA, Barclay R, Campbell P, et al. Management of liver trauma. World J Surg. 2009;33:2522–37.
2. Piper GL, Peitzman AB. Current management of hepatic trauma. Surg Clin North Am. 2010;90: 775–85.
3. Buckman RF, Miraliakbari R, Badellino MM. Juxtahepatic venous injuries: a critical review of reported management strategies. J Trauma. 2000;48:978–84.
4. Beal SA. Fatal hepatic hemorrhage: an unsolved problem in the management of complex hepatic injuries. J Trauma. 1990;30:163–9.
5. Polanco P, Leon S, Pinea J, et al. Hepatic resection in the management of complex injury to the liver. J Trauma. 2008;65:1264–70.
6. Liau KH, Blumgart LH, DeMatteo RP. Segment-oriented approach to liver resection. Surg Clin North Am. 2004;84:543–61.
7. Skandalakis JE, Gray SW, Skandalakis LJ, et al. Surgical anatomy of the liver and extrahepatic structures. Contemp Surg. 1987;30:26.
8. Skandalakis JE, Skandalakis LJ, Skandalakis PN, et al. Hepatic surgical anatomy. Surg Clin North Am. 2004;84:413–35.
9. Abdel-Misih SRZ, Bloomston M. Liver anatomy. Surg Clin North Am. 2010;90:643–53.
10. Mehran R, Schneider R, Franchebois P. The minor hepatic veins: anatomy and classification. Clin Anat. 2000;13:416–21.
11. Peitzman AB, Marsh JW. Advanced operative techniques in the management of complex liver injury. J Trauma. 2012;73:765–70.
12. Aragon RJ, Solomon NL. Techniques of hepatic resection. J Gastrointest Oncol. 2012;3:28–40.

13. DeMatteo RP, Fong Y, Jarnagin WR, et al. Recent advances in hepatic resection. Semin Surg Oncol. 2000;19:200–7.
14. Geller DA, Goss JA, Tsung A. Liver. In: Brunicardi F, Andersen D, Billiar TR, Dunn D, Hunter J, Matthews J, Pollock RE, editors. Schwartz's principles of surgery. New York: McGraw Hill; 2011. p. 1126–8.
15. Gurusamy KS, Pamecha V, Sharma D, et al. Techniques for liver parenchymal transection in liver resection. Cochrane Database Syst Rev. 2009;(1): CD006880, p. 1–38.
16. Gurusamy KS, Sheth H, Kumar Y, et al. Methods of vascular occlusion for elective liver resections. Cochrane Database Syst Rev. 2009;(1):CD007632, p. 1–47.
17. Heriot AG, Karanjia ND. A review of techniques for liver resection. Ann R Coll Surg Engl. 2002;84:371–80.
18. Lin N-C, Nitta H, Wayabayashi G. Laparoscopic major hepatectomy: a systematic review of the literature and comparison of t3 techniques. Ann Surg. 2013;257:205–13.
19. Nguyen KT, Gamblin TC. World review of laparoscopic liver resection-2804 patients. Ann Surg. 2009;250:831–41.
20. Poon RTP. Current techniques of liver resection. HPB (oxford). 2007;9:166–73.
21. Romano F, Garancini M, Uggeri F, et al. The aim of technology during liver resection-A strategy to minimize blood loss during liver surgery. Intech, open science.2013:167–205.http://dx.doi.org/10.5772/54301.
22. Smyrniotis V, Arkadopoulos N, Kostopanagiotou G, et al. Sharp liver transection versus clamp crushing technique in liver resections: a prospective study. Surgery. 2005;137:306–11.
23. Strong RA, Lynch SV, Wall DR, et al. Anatomic resection for severe liver trauma. Surgery. 1998;123: 251–7.
24. Tsugawa K, Koyanagi N, Hashizume M, et al. Anatomic resection for severe blunt liver injury in 100 patients: significant differences between young and elderly. World J Surg. 2002;26:544–9.
25. Balaa FK, Gamblin TC, Tsung A, et al. Right hepatic lobectomy using the staple technique in 101 patients. J Gastroenterol. 2008;12:338–43.
26. Fong Y, Blumgart LH. Useful stapling techniques in liver surgery. J Am Coll Surg. 1997;185:93–100.
27. Schemmer P, Friess H, Hinz U, et al. Stapler hepatectomy is a safe dissection technique: analysis of 300 patients. World J Surg. 2006;30:419–30.
28. Schemmer P, Bruns H, Weitz J, et al. Liver resection using vascular stapler: a review. HPB (oxford). 2008;10:249–52.
29. Figueras J, Lopez-Ben S, Lladó L, et al. Hilar dissection versus the "glissonean" approach and stapling of the pedicle for major hepatectomies: a prospective, randomized trial. Ann Surg. 2003;238(1):111–9.
30. Cho CS, Park J, Fong Y. Hepatic resection. In: ACS surgery: principles and practice. Available at http://206.47.151.137/bcdecker/pdfs/acs/part07_ch07.pdf.2007.
31. Lau W-Y, Lai ECH, Lau SHY. Methods of vascular control technique during liver resection: a comprehensive review. Hepatobiliary Pancreat Dis Int. 2010;9:473–81.
32. Torzilliu G, Procopio F, Donadon M, et al. Safety of intermittent Pringle maneuver cumulative time exceeding 120 min in liver resection. Ann Surg. 2012;255:270–80.
33. Rahbari NN, Koch M, Schmidt T, et al. Met-analysis of the clamp-crushing technique for transection of the parenchyma in elective hepatic resection: back to where we started? Ann Surg Oncol. 2009;16:630–9.
34. Abdalla EK, Noun R, Belghiti J. Hepatic vascular occlusion: which technique? Surg Clin North Am. 2004;84:563–85.
35. Smyrniotis V, Arkadopoulos N, Theodoraki K, et al. Association between biliary complications and technique of hilar division (extrahepatic vs. intrahepatic) in major liver resections. World J Surg Oncol. 2006;4:19–26.

Vascular Injuries of Porta Hepatis

8

Jordan A. Weinberg and Timothy C. Fabian

Introduction

Vascular injuries of the porta hepatis possess the unfavorable combination of being both rare and life threatening. Reported experience from different institutions is similar with respect to the fact that they comprise small case series over relatively long intervals of time, reflecting the infrequency with which one encounters these injuries [1–5]. Associated mortality rates have been reported between 40 and 70 %, and death is most commonly a result of exsanguination. A potentially lethal injury that is seldom encountered should give the trauma surgeon pause, and the importance of having a preestablished management strategy in mind must be emphasized. In this chapter, we will provide an overview of the relevant anatomy and physiology, techniques for hemorrhage control and operative exposure, and a strategy for the definitive management of portal vein and hepatic artery injuries.

J.A. Weinberg, MD (✉)
Department of Surgery,
University of Tennessee Health Science Center,
910 Madison Avenue, 2nd Floor Trauma Division,
Memphis, TN 38163, USA
e-mail: jaw@uthsc.edu

T.C. Fabian, MD
Department of Surgery,
University of Tennessee Health Science Center,
910 Madison Avenue, Suite 203, Memphis,
TN 38163, USA
e-mail: tfabian@uthsc.edu

Anatomy and Physiology of the Portal Vein and Hepatic Artery

The free edge of the hepatoduodenal ligament envelops the portal triad – i.e., the common bile duct, portal vein, and hepatic artery. The typical anatomic relation of these structures is demonstrated in Fig. 8.1. The portal vein originates from the confluence of the superior mesenteric and splenic veins, immediately posterior to the pancreatic neck. In the hepatoduodenal ligament, prior to forming the right and left portal vein branches at the porta hepatis, the portal vein lies between and slightly posterior to the other structures, with the common bile duct lateral and the hepatic artery medial to the vein, as demonstrated in Fig. 8.1. The common hepatic artery arises from the celiac axis and becomes the proper hepatic artery distal to the origin of the gastroduodenal artery. The proper hepatic artery typically divides into the right and left hepatic arteries at the porta hepatis, with the right hepatic artery passing posterior to the common bile duct in most individuals (Fig. 8.1). Roughly 15 % of individuals will have an accessory or replaced right hepatic artery, originating from the superior mesenteric artery and coursing posterior-lateral to the common bile duct within

Electronic supplementary material Supplementary material is available in the online version of this chapter at 10.1007/978-1-4939-1200-1_8. Videos can also be accessed at http://www.springerimages.com/videos/978-1-4939-1199-8.

R.R. Ivatury (ed.), *Operative Techniques for Severe Liver Injury*,
DOI 10.1007/978-1-4939-1200-1_8, © Springer Science+Business Media New York 2015

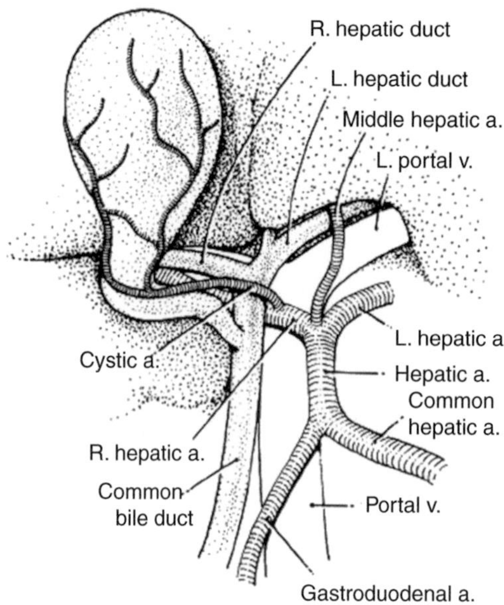

Fig. 8.1 Anatomy of the portal triad

the hepatoduodenal ligament. In the trauma setting, the surgeon should anticipate the possibility of this variant anatomy being present within a hematoma of the hepatoduodenal ligament.

The liver is a particularly unique solid organ, receiving a dual blood supply from the portal vein and the hepatic artery. The liver receives approximately 75 % of its inflow circulation from the portal vein and 25 % from the hepatic artery. The relatively oxygen-rich arterial inflow results in a division of the oxygen supply to the liver between the portal vein and hepatic artery that is roughly even. This unique situation affords the surgeon the option of ligation of an injured vessel, provided that the other vessel remains patent.

Vascular Control and Exposure of Injuries

Hematoma in the hepatoduodenal ligament strongly suggests the presence of injury to the portal vein, the hepatic artery, or both and warrants caution as disruption of the hematoma prior to adequate vascular control or exposure may result in rapid bleeding. On encountering a stable hematoma, it is wise to ensure that vascular

clamps, suture, vessel loops, and embolectomy catheters for the purpose of intravascular balloon occlusion are all at the ready. It will be the rare occasion where the anatomy allows for placement of vascular clamps across the hepatoduodenal ligament, both superior (i.e., high on the porta as close to the liver as possible) and inferior (low on the porta just above the duodenum) to the hematoma. If this so-called double Pringle maneuver can be performed, the hematoma may then be opened and the vessel injury may be identified. More often than not, however, the hematoma is too extensive and/or the hepatoduodenal ligament is too short to allow for the placement of two clamps. In this more typical scenario, we recommend proceeding with exposure as facilitated by the Kocher maneuver described below, being prepared to rapidly compress any active bleeding that becomes apparent during mobilization. Occasionally, active bleeding, rather than stable hematoma, will be initially encountered and should be immediately controlled with the application of direct digital pressure. The surgeon's left hand pinches the site of bleeding with index finger in the foramen of Winslow and thumb anterior (Fig. 8.2). The right hand is then free for dissection of the tissues above and below the pinched off area of bleeding.

Exposure of the portal vein and hepatic artery is facilitated by anterior reflection of the pancreaticoduodenal complex, known as the Kocher maneuver. Medial mobilization of the right colon is often necessary to gain the required exposure to perform the Kocher maneuver. A complete Kocher maneuver allows for the surgeon or assistant to place gentle traction on the portal triad by holding the duodenum and head of the pancreas between the fingers and thumb of the left hand and pulling inferiorly, facilitating the anterior exposure of the structures in the hepatoduodenal ligament and optimally creating space to place a clamp across the hepatoduodenal ligament for proximal control. The Kocher maneuver also allows for exposure of the lateral aspect of the portal vein (Fig. 8.3). As demonstrated in Fig. 8.3, the common bile duct obscures a portion of the portal vein. Should that portion of the vein need to be fully exposed, it is

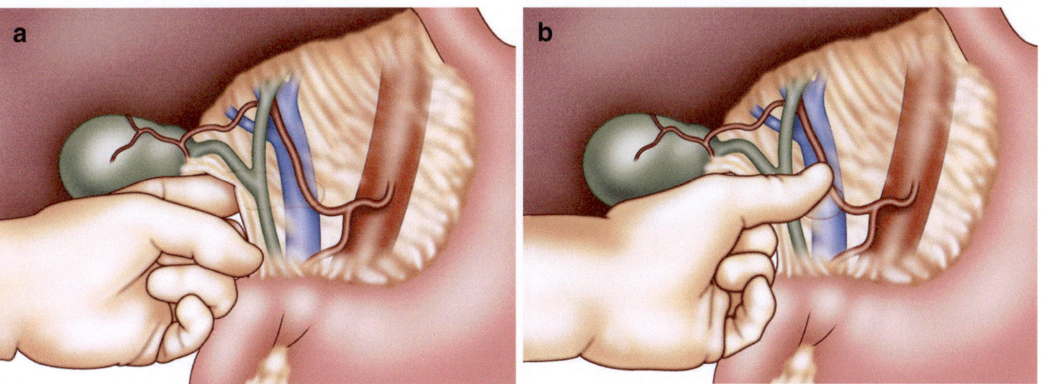

Fig. 8.2 (**a**) The surgeon's left index finger is positioned in the foramen of Winslow. (**b**) The site of bleeding is then compressed between the index finger and thumb..

Fig. 8.3 Exposure gained following anterior reflection of the pancreaticoduodenal complex (Kocher maneuver) (Reproduced with permission from Ivatury [8])

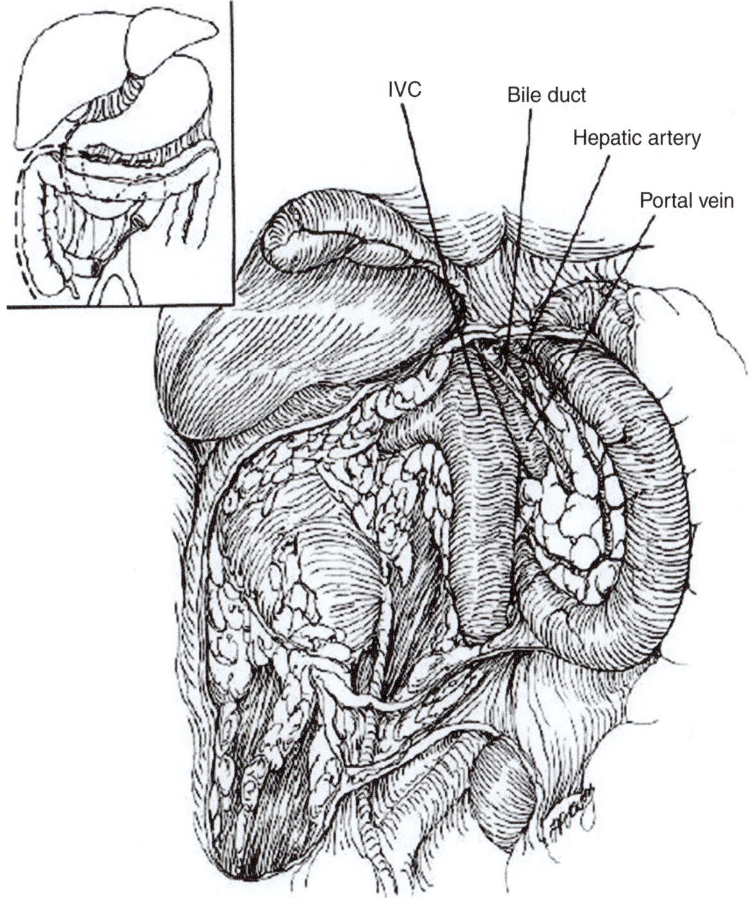

useful to divide the cystic duct and then reflect the common bile duct medially (if the cystic duct is divided, cholecystectomy should be performed prior to completion of the operation). Figure 8.3 also demonstrates the close proximity of the portal vein to the vena cava. Associated injury to the vena cava and/or adjacent aorta should be anticipated when a portal injury is encountered,

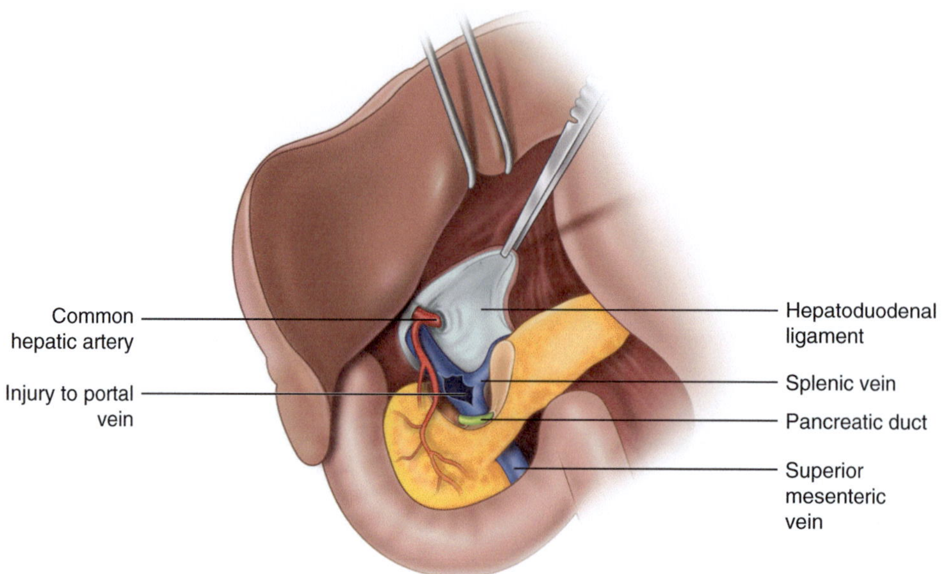

Fig. 8.4 Injury to the portal vein at the confluence of the superior mesenteric vein and splenic vein

and should be addressed once identified, leaving the portal injury temporarily controlled by a clamp or assistant's fingers for the time being.

Retropancreatic injuries of the portal vein or portal vein confluence provide an additional challenge regarding vascular control and exposure, given that the pancreas significantly limits access to the venous structures immediately posterior. Active bleeding necessitates direct anterior pressure on the point of bleeding, while working to expose the injured vessel. As demonstrated in Fig. 8.3, the Kocher maneuver exposes a large portion of the retropancreatic portal vein and allows for vascular control by way of digital compression with fingers behind and thumb on top of the pancreatic body. Division of the pancreatic neck has been advocated as an additional maneuver to expose the retropancreatic venous confluence of the superior mesenteric vein and splenic vein. Should the neck of the pancreas itself be uninjured, however, it is unlikely that the exposure gained by transecting the neck will be worth the time taken to divide the pancreas, and also risks iatrogenic venous injury in a field distorted by retroperitoneal hematoma. Often, however, retropancreatic venous injuries will be associated with a pancreatic neck injury, particularly in the context of a gunshot wound or similar penetrating injury (Fig. 8.4). In such a scenario, it is useful to convert the pancreatic neck injury to a complete transection (followed by distal pancreatectomy), thereby providing both exposure of the retropancreatic venous injury and definitive management of the wound of the pancreas.

Management of Portal Vein Injury

Once the injury has been exposed, vascular control is applied immediately proximal and distal to the area of injury to set up the field for definitive management. Should the injury be located in the midportion of the hepatoduodenal ligament, control of the vein with vascular clamps is relatively straightforward. Longitudinal injuries involving the anterior aspect of the vein, typically as a result of a stab wound, lend themselves to control of the wound with the placement of Judd-Allis clamps in side-biting fashion (Fig. 8.5). When the injury, however, extends to the liver hilum or posterior to the pancreas, clamp placement may be limited by lack of space. In such a case, intraluminal control with embolectomy balloon catheters is recommended.

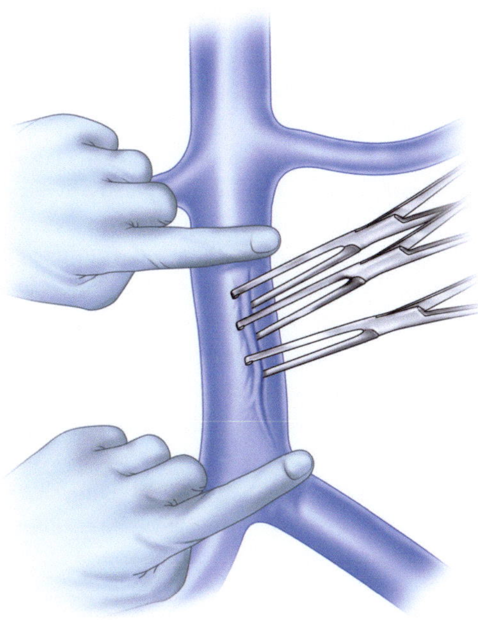

Fig. 8.5 Control of a longitudinal venous injury with Judd-Allis clamps

Definitive repair is then dictated by the extent of injury. Wounds amenable to lateral venorrhaphy should be closed with a running suture (typically 5-0 polypropylene). For wounds of greater complexity, we recommend that ligation of the portal vein at the site of injury be strongly considered. It was heretofore believed that ligation of the portal vein was incompatible with survival, but the work of Child demonstrated that this was not, in fact, the case [6]. Although occlusion of the portal vein will result in acute portal venous hypertension, this will in fact resolve over days to weeks as collateral flow develops.

Experience has demonstrated that portal vein ligation can be a lifesaving treatment, particularly when it is performed early in the decision-making process, rather than as a bailout maneuver following the failure of attempted complex repair with a graft or otherwise. It will be the rare occasion when a completely transected portal vein can be simply put back together with a primary anastomosis. The large majority of portal vein injuries that require more than lateral suture repair will require a graft to return directional flow. These injuries, however, are usually associated with multiple vascular and other injuries that need to be addressed. Consequently, the patient is unlikely to have the physiologic reserve necessary to sustain the time and blood loss required for a complex repair of the portal vein. Clinical experience has demonstrated that such patients have a higher likelihood of survival when the portal vein is ligated, and ligated early in the course of management, thus saving time and ongoing blood loss [1]. In the rare scenario of an isolated portal vein injury that lends itself to end-to-end repair, it may be reasonable to pursue repair rather than ligation, but as stated above, such a case will be rarely encountered.

When faced, however, with injury to both the portal vein and hepatic artery, ligation of both vessels will result in complete inflow occlusion of the liver and is not compatible with survival. In such a case, we recommend that the hepatic artery be managed with ligation (if it is beyond simple primary repair) and the portal vein be repaired, typically with saphenous vein or polytetrafluoroethylene graft. The secondary option would be to ligate the vein and repair (rather than ligate) the artery, should one find that the portal vein injury be excessively destructive.

Management of Hepatic Artery Injury

Following identification of an injury to the hepatic artery, vascular control immediately proximal and distal to the injured artery should be obtained, utilizing either vascular clamps or vessel loops with a Potts technique. Definitive management of the majority of hepatic artery injuries should be ligation. Hepatic artery ligation is generally well tolerated, and injury to the hepatic artery is often associated with other major injuries, whereby the time taken to repair the artery would be better applied to the management of the associated injuries. Following ligation of the common hepatic artery, the gastroduodenal artery can provide collateral flow to the proper hepatic artery. Nonetheless, the proper hepatic artery itself is not truly an "end artery," as flow develops via translobar and subcapsular hepatic collaterals within

24 h of ligation, as demonstrated in an innovative in vivo study by Mays and May [7]. The gallbladder, however, is at risk of irreversible ischemia should the hepatic artery be ligated, particularly proximal to the cystic artery, but also more distally, including selective ligation of the left or right hepatic artery (gallbladder ischemia is more commonly associated with right-sided ligation but has been reported to have occurred after left-sided ligation as well). Following ligation of the hepatic artery or its main branches, cholecystectomy should be performed.

Hepatic necrosis has been reported to occur following hepatic arterial ligation in the setting of hemorrhagic shock, but it is the consensus that such a complication is unlikely. Associated injury to the portal vein, however, increases the risk of irreversible hepatic ischemia. As stated above, injury to both inflow vessels to the liver mandates repair of one of them. Restoration of inflow via portal vein repair is favored, but in the case of a minor arterial injury and massive vein injury, it may be advisable to repair the artery and ligate the vein.

Postoperative Management

Acute occlusion of the portal vein results in significant pooling of circulating blood volume in the splanchnic circulation at the expense of the peripheral circulation. This results in the combination of massive bowel edema and systemic hypotension. Therefore, diligent attention to maintenance of cardiac preload by volume resuscitation is paramount and is best guided with invasive monitoring such as a pulmonary artery catheter.

As a result of venous outflow obstruction of the portal circulation and subsequent bowel edema, there is risk for the development of bowel ischemia. The traditional teaching was to perform a "second-look" laparotomy at 24 h to inspect the bowel for this complication. In contemporary practice, however, these cases are almost always managed with an open abdomen approach. To prevent the development of abdominal compartment syndrome secondary to bowel edema, the abdomen is left open at the completion of operation, utilizing some form of temporary abdominal closure. As the bowel edema may be extreme in these particular cases, we favor the use of a sterile x-ray cassette cover (or similar clear plastic sheet) sewn circumferentially to the skin edge to allow for maximum amount of space for bowel expansion and visual inspection of the visceral block. Over time (typically by 72 h), the portal venous hypertension resolves as collaterals develop, and the development of chronic portal venous hypertension is highly unlikely. While it is possible that delayed primary closure of the fascia may be achievable with subsequent trips to the operating room, it is likely that a planned ventral hernia strategy will be necessary given the typical severity of bowel edema, whereby the fascial gap is bridged with an absorbable mesh with subsequent skin grafting and eventual abdominal wall reconstruction.

Video Captions

Video 6   Pringle maneuver (MP4 14015 kb)
Video 8   Finger fracture of the liver (MP4 22289 kb)

References

1. Stone HH, Fabian TC, Turkleson ML. Wounds of the portal venous system. World J Surg. 1982;6(3):335–41.
2. Jurkovich GJ, Hoyt DB, Moore FA, et al. Portal triad injuries. J Trauma. 1995;39(3):426–34.
3. Busuttil RW, Kitahama A, Cerise E, McFadden M, Lo R, Longmire Jr WP. Management of blunt and penetrating injuries to the porta hepatis. Ann Surg. 1980;191(5):641–8.
4. Ivatury RR, Nallathambi M, Lankin DH, Wapnir I, Rohman M, Stahl WM. Portal vein injuries. Noninvasive follow-up of venorrhaphy. Ann Surg. 1987;206(6):733–7.
5. Pearl J, Chao A, Kennedy S, Paul B, Rhee P. Traumatic injuries to the portal vein: case study. J Trauma. 2004; 56(4):779–82.
6. Child CG, Milnes RF, Holswade GR, Gore AL. Sudden and complete occlusion of the portal vein in the Macaca mulatta monkey. Ann Surg. 1950;68: 155–75.
7. Mays 2nd ET, Mays ET. Are hepatic arteries end-arteries? J Anat. 1983;137(Pt 4):637–44.
8. Ivatury RR. Basic operative techniques in trauma and emergency surgery. In: Britt LD, Peitzman A, Barie P, Jurkovich G, editors. Acute care surgery. Philadelphia: Lippincott Williams & Wilkins; 2012.

L.D. Britt

General Concepts

Blunt trauma contributes over 75 % of mechanisms of injuries for most of the trauma centers in the United States. The liver, the largest solid organ in the body, is one of the most frequently injured abdominal organs by either blunt or penetrating mechanisms. Fortunately, the majority of hepatic injuries are not severe and require no surgical repair. These are low-grade injuries (see Table 5.1, page 48). Suspicion of liver injury is predicated on several factors: clinical suspicion derived from the mechanics of the crash and the hemodynamic state of the patient in the field and upon arrival at the hospital, along with findings obtained during abdominal examination obtained in the hospital (Fig. 9.1). High-energy crashes involving application of force to the upper abdomen or to the right thoracoabdominal area should arouse immediate suspicion of a possible hepatic injury. Hemodynamic lability, although not an exclusive feature of liver injury, mandates evaluation to exclude it as the source of the hemorrhage. Tenderness in the right upper quadrant, in the absence of other signs, can be suggestive of subcapsular hematoma requiring attention and further evaluation. Unfortunately, the physical examination is not perfect and has a false-positive rate of approximately 50 % and a false-negative rate of 40 %.

The additional methods available to evaluate the abdomen include focused abdominal sonography for trauma (FAST), computed tomography, and diagnostic peritoneal lavage. FAST has become a highly reliable test used when seeking to determine whether there is blood in the abdomen in a patient who is hemodynamically labile. In the stable patient in whom liver injury is suspected, the use of computed tomography has become widespread. Several classification schemes have been described for liver injuries. There are inconsistencies in the terminology, but a grading scheme proposed by the American Association for the Surgery of Trauma (AAST) is now in wide use (see Table 5.1, page 48).

These diagnostic adjuncts are not intended to replace clinical judgment and examination by the surgeon. Whatever method is used for abdominal evaluation should be readily available, and the surgeon should be proficient in its use and interpretation.

Penetrating abdominal injury presents a more straightforward situation for the evaluating surgeon. What must be remembered is the anatomic position of the liver, under the costal margin, especially as this relates to thoracoabdominal injuries. Hemodynamic lability mandates explor-

L.D. Britt, MD, MPH
Department of Surgery, Eastern Virginia Medical School, 825 Fairfax Avenue, Norfolk,
VA 23507, USA
e-mail: brittld@evms.edu

Electronic supplementary material Supplementary material is available in the online version of this chapter at 10.1007/978-1-4939-1200-1_9. Videos can also be accessed at http://www.springerimages.com/videos/978-1-4939-1199-8.

R.R. Ivatury (ed.), *Operative Techniques for Severe Liver Injury*,
DOI 10.1007/978-1-4939-1200-1_9, © Springer Science+Business Media New York 2015

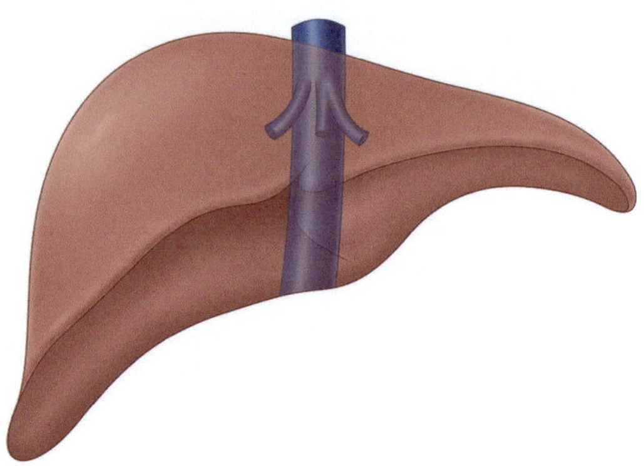

Fig. 9.1 Juxtahepatic (or retrohepatic) vena cava is in direct contact with the posterior aspect of the liver

atory celiotomy, irrespective of the mechanism of injury (stab versus gunshot wound).

Approach to the Injured Liver

With hepatic injuries, the paramount decision is to determine if an intervention is needed to control hemorrhage. Hemodynamic instability mandates expeditious operative management or angiography/embolization (if the patient can be stabilized with volume resuscitation) in order to make transportation to the radiographic suite less risky for the patient. The hemodynamically stable patient may be evaluated by any of the methods noted earlier. Minor grade I or II injuries frequently require no operative intervention. When diagnosing by CT scan, the surgeon must be cognizant of the magnitude and anatomy of the liver injury. Contusion contained within the liver capsule or minor laceration, such as in grade I or II injuries, may be observed. These diagnoses together constitute most liver injury cases, accounting for 60 or 70 %. Grade III injuries (deeper, larger wounds with more tissue destruction) occur in approximately 25 % of cases. Grade IV and V injuries, involving large amounts of tissue destruction, have an incidence of 7 and 3 %, respectively, and are highly lethal. It should be emphasized that evidence of blood in the peritoneal pericolic gutters, in the pelvis, or tracking along the periportal triads [1] is suggestive of a more significant injury than the liver anatomy

may indicate and mandates exploration. Also, the concomitant existence of hollow viscous injury occurs in 5 and 20 % of major hepatic injuries.

In addition, it is important to realize that massive parenchymal injuries can occur with surprisingly little bleeding and that minor lacerations may bleed profusely. An understanding of the tissue architecture of the liver is a prerequisite to successful management. Most blunt lacerations may occur along segmental fissures, because the vascular and biliary duct structures are moderately shear resistant. This explains why a large stellate or "bear claw" laceration may be seen, with little or no intraperitoneal blood in a hemodynamically stable patient. This can be managed nonoperatively with observation and repeated CT scan. Nonoperative treatment of the stable patient sustaining a blunt liver injury is the management approach of choice today [2–7].

Conversely, the deceleration forces are responsible for a shear effect that can result in avulsion of the hepatic veins from the vena cava or major branches of the portal venous or hepatic venous systems. Hemorrhage is devastating, difficult to control, and responsible for the high mortality rate seen with such injuries.

Penetrating injuries present their own set of difficulties; missile tracts may bleed profusely. The same elasticity that can protect the vascular structures from shear forces has little if any effect when confronted with a missile.

Intraoperative Decisions: General Principles

Once the decision to operate has been made, the surgeon needs to proceed in an orderly fashion, to a fully equipped operative theater, including the capabilities of invasive monitoring. Before opening the abdomen, the surgeons must ensure that there is optimal venous access. Large-bore central access is essential. The prudent, historic dictum is that access should be from the upper torso in the event there is a retrohepatic caval injury. The blood bank must be notified of the potential for massive transfusion of packed cells and blood components to treat the often associated coagulopathy. The development of blood salvage systems has greatly improved the care of these patients; shed blood from the operative field can be washed and reinfused, provided there is no evidence of gastrointestinal contamination. Infusion systems are available that allow rapid delivery of large volumes of warmed fluid to help minimize hypothermia and hypovolemia. Hypothermia is a common cause of coagulopathy and must be aggressively defended against. Invasive monitoring capabilities are essential in the management of these critically injured patients.

Optimal surgical exposure is essential and starts with performing a midline vertical incision for expedient entry into the abdominal cavity. The incision should extend from the xiphoid process to the symphysis pubis. Such an approach allows, if necessary, relatively easy extension into the thorax through either a median sternotomy or a lateral thoracotomy.

Performing a celiotomy could potentially decompress the tamponade, thereby necessitating expeditious vascular control. The need to perform an emergency thoracotomy for vascular control of the aorta before opening the abdomen is rarely indicated. Such control of the bleeding can usually be obtained with the assistant's manual compression of the liver.

Once the abdomen is open, a rapid assessment of the injury is made and priority management begun. All clot is evacuated, and the four quadrants are packed to control bleeding. A sequential examination is then carried out with priority given to control of blood loss followed by control of any enteric content spillage.

The general approach to the liver injury requires adequate visualization of the anatomic features of the injury. This may require mobilization of the liver along the falciform and triangular ligaments. Full mobilization of the liver allows delivery onto the abdominal wall that can often facilitate suture repair of a hepatic wound in a difficult area. When mobilizing the liver, care must be taken that the hepatic veins are not injured. The coronary ligaments are in close proximity to hepatic veins. Also, the surgeon must be cautious during the mobilization of the liver that venous return through the vena cava is not obstructed for a prolonged period. Hemorrhage control during mobilization can often be done by the assistant's applying direct pressure with laparotomy packs, compressing the liver between the hands.

As noted previously, most of the injuries encountered are grade I or II and require little more than simple suture repair. Grades III, IV, and V injuries require an organized approach for successful control of hemorrhage, which includes manual compression, direct ligation, or clipping of lacerated vessels, along with sophisticated techniques for more complex wounds.

Vascular occlusion of the portal triad (performing the Pringle maneuver) is a useful method of controlling hepatic arterial and portal venous inflow to the liver. A noncrushing or vascular clamp can be applied to the porta hepatis and safely left in place for approximately 45 min, although the specific duration threshold is not known for the hemodynamically labile patient. Also, an umbilical tape placed around the porta hepatis structures can be used for such control. If this maneuver markedly reduces the liver's bleeding, the parenchymal injury can be assessed and a method of repair decided on. However, if hemorrhage persists, then an intrahepatic portal vein injury or a major hepatic vein injury must be suspected.

Proceeding with hepatotomy for localization and control of hemorrhage requires fastidious cooperation between the surgeon and the first assistant. With the depth of the hepatic wound exposed, it is usually the first assistant who controls the bleeding. The finger-fracture technique for hepatotomy, with the first assistant compressing the liver, is very effective. The operating surgeon using the fingertips or the handle of a scalpel to separate the liver parenchyma and the assistant using a multiple loaded clip applier, made popular for laparoscopic cholecystectomy, ligate severed vessels. Nonabsorbable suture ligation can also be performed to control vessels as each is encountered. Knowledge of the anatomy of the liver (along with reported anatomic variants) is a prerequisite to this approach. The confluence of the left and middle hepatic veins must be kept in

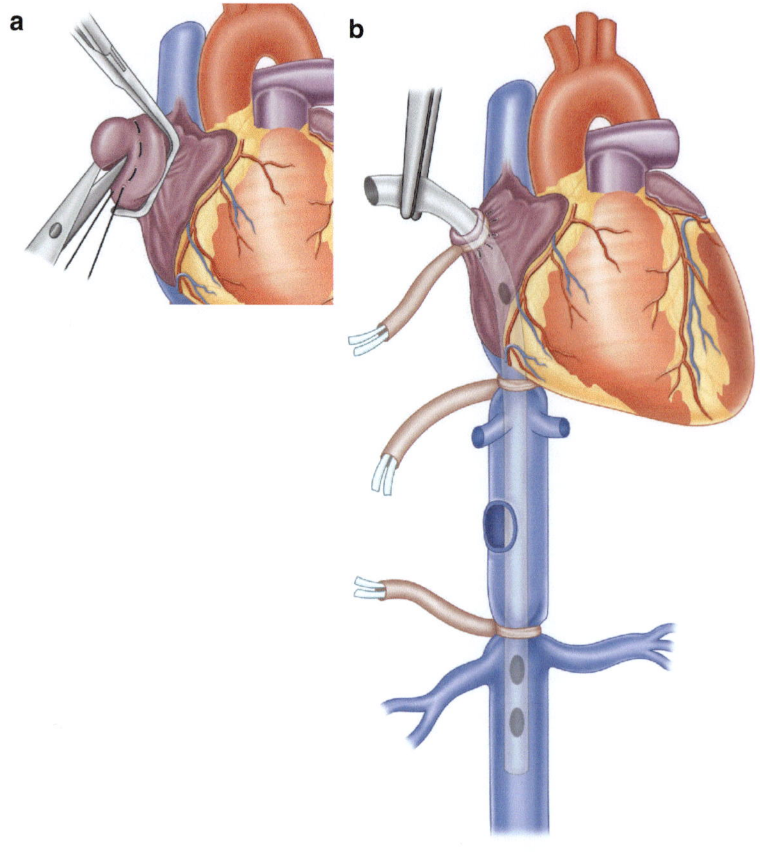

Fig. 9.2 After obtaining the necessary exposure (thoracotomy, mediasternotomy), an opening—along with 2-0 Prolene purse-string suture—is created in the right atrial appendage (**a**) to provide the access needed for insertion of the atriocaval shunt (**b**) which is usually a No. 36 chest tube. An extra hole needs to be made at the level of the right atrium. With the chest tube holes being outside of umbilical tape occlusion, blood is directed from the lower half of the body and the kidney through the atriocaval shunt

mind to avoid overzealous ligation (Fig. 9.2). Likewise, the position of the inferior vena cava and the hepatic veins to the caudate lobe should be noted to avoid unnecessary injury that may complicate the surgical management. The placement of random deep sutures is fraught with difficulty. Failure of the abovementioned maneuvers to control hepatic bleeding means that the surgeon either has not adequately identified the source or is dealing with coagulopathic bleeding (or both).

Although specific ligation of the hepatic artery or portal vein branch supplying a specific portion of the liver is rarely needed, the suspected branch should be isolated, and its occlusion should control hemorrhage while the Pringle maneuver is released. If such is the case, then the identified branch should be ligated.

Liver injury, infrequently, follows the anatomic lines of demarcation delineating the right and left lobes, much less the segments. Anatomic resection, a once popular approach, has poor outcome with high mortality rates. This technique has been, essentially, abandoned. Resectional debridement of devitalized liver is not formal lobectomy but rather a completion of the injury to remove nonviable hepatic tissue and to facilitate vascular control. This usually entails a degree of finger fracture through uninjured liver, which allows visualization of the bleeding raw surface and more direct control. Application of specific liver clamps, such as the Lin clamp, designed to aid in lobectomy, is difficult because of positioning of the injury laceration and maneuvering around the clamp.

Being able to perform a tractotomy of a missile wound should be in a surgeon's armamentarium when dealing with penetrating hepatic injury. In addition, a variety of methods designed for tamponade of the bleeding missile tract have been described, using various materials. Bluett et al. [8] described a tamponade device with multiple Penrose drains dragged through the liver tract. However, it is more preferable to open the liver and suture or clip-control the bleeding site directly, if possible.

Once the bleeding has been controlled, the large, raw surface of the liver can be problematic, as persistent oozing of bile or blood continues. A viable omental patch sutured to the liver bed is an excellent homeostatic agent and internal drain. Stone and Lamb [9] popularized the omental pack in their initial report. Fabian and Stone [10] reported 90 % successful hemostatic control with this procedure. For large, raw liver surfaces resulting from debridement or tractotomy, the omental patch held in place with several liver sutures is an excellent hemostatic agent. Also, utilization of the argon beam coagulator is another option in addressing bleeding of raw liver surfaces. The argon gas removes the blood from the hepatic tissue and ionizing energy is transmitted. A maximum of 110 °C is achieved and an eschar is formed.

An alternative to surgical repair of the injured liver is a mesh wrap intended to provide compression, to control bleeding, and to close parenchymal defects. Delaney et al. [11] reported success in six liver injuries controlled in this manner. Brunet et al. [12] reported 35 liver injuries wrapped for control. Sequential CT examination of the patients demonstrated progressive restoration of normal liver architecture.

The premise underlying much of the preceding discussion is that liver bleeding can be controlled. However, even when advanced techniques of liver control are used, hemorrhage control can be precarious, at best. A critical error that can be made when dealing with major liver injury is to continue operative intervention in the face of a hypothermic (less than 32 °C), acidotic patient who has developed coagulopathy. Although the specific time to make a decision to pack the liver and restore normothermia and coagulation factors is not always clear, the operating surgeon should always have a low threshold to incorporate packing and prepare the patient to be expeditiously transferred to the intensive care unit for aggressive resuscitation and monitoring. Once a patient has required a 10-U transfusion, packing

should be seriously considered. Garrison et al. [13], in a review in which they tried to predict the need for packing in severe abdominal injuries, noted that patients with severe injuries, hypothermia, refractory hypertension, coagulopathy, and acidosis need early packing. It needs to be emphasized that large-vessel bleeding must be controlled before packing can be effective.

Perihepatic packing was popularized during World War II. The high incidence of complications, plus the advent of more sophisticated techniques for control of liver bleeding, led to the demise of packing until its revival in the 1970s. Feliciano et al. [14] noted the major indications for perihepatic packing to be the postrepair coagulopathy that developed or an extensive subcapsular hematoma or capsular avulsion. They reported 57 % survival rate in their series. Carmona et al. [15] reported similar success with perihepatic packing to control bleeding when other methods failed. Perihepatic packing is broadly embraced today. It is also a valuable adjunct to resectional debridement and tractotomy. Walt [16] has enumerated several guidelines regarding liver packing. The use of a folded, disposable plastic drape is helpful. It is placed against the liver and the packs placed on it, preventing the laparotomy pads from adhering to the liver and possibly minimizing the recurrent bleeding upon removal of the packs. Gauze packs are then placed in order to compress the liver. The packs should be placed at both the superior and inferior surfaces of the liver. The packing should be tight enough to control the bleeding but not so tight that it unnecessarily compresses the renal vessels and possibly the inferior vena cava, resulting in intra-abdominal hypertension. Patients who have undergone packing will require continued sedation with mechanical ventilation until pack removal, because of the interference of optimal diaphragmatic movement. Abdominal wall closure is rapid and is performed by towel clips or by running nylon suture in the skin. Utilization of silo-like closures with sterile towels and plastic drapes should be used to minimize fluid loss and to maintain abdominal pressure. In addition, there should always be a high index of suspicion for the development of intra-abdominal compartment syndrome.

Pack removal can be planned when the patient has regained normothermia and coagulation parameters have been normalized. This usually occurs within 24–72 h. Packs are then removed during a second operation, and the surgical team again must be prepared to manage bleeding. Repacking at the second operation might be indicated. The complication rate of packing is appreciable. Ivatury et al. [17] noted an increased incidence of sepsis in a group of patients subjected to liver packing. An additional benefit of liver packing is that it may allow transport of a critically ill patient from one center to a definitive treatment center where the liver injury can be treated. Clark et al. [18] emphasized this point in the context of a trauma system, with a number of smaller, more rural hospitals transporting seriously injured patients to the tertiary center for definitive care.

Juxtahepatic Venous Injuries

The lethality of juxtahepatic venous injuries in blunt hepatic trauma and the management challenges of definitively addressing such injuries have been well chronicled [19–23]. Fortunately, such liver wounds are seen infrequently. However, the downside is that very few acute care surgeons are familiar with and comfortable operating in this specific setting. Depending on the specific series, the mortality ranges from 50 to 80 %, with massive hemorrhage being the overwhelming cause of death.

The deadly nature of this injury is a result of the difficulty in expeditiously getting access to the injury site. The retrohepatic vena cava and major hepatic veins are within the depth of the least mobile area of the liver—making expose and direct control of bleeding very challenging. Attempting to rotate the liver in an effort to access the injury can actually extend the wound and cause increased bleeding. Also, such a misguided effort could result in a fatal air embolus.

Detailed knowledge of the pertinent anatomy is imperative for any surgeon attempting an operative management strategy. The juxtahepatic vena cava, which is within the "bare area" of the liver, extends for approximately 7 cm and is bordered by the phrenic veins and right adrenal vein—cephalad and caudad, respectively. Approximately three centimeters above the most superior aspect of the retrohepatic vena cava, the inferior vena cava enters the right atrium. The retrohepatic cava is an extraparenchymal structure. The three major hepatic veins, along with its tributaries, enter directly into the anterior aspect of the retrohepatic vena cava. This anatomy is relatively constant, with major anomalies being uncommon. While the course of the extraparenchymal hepatic veins is short, the intraparenchymal veins have a long course. Substantial blunt trauma can lacerate/avulse either or both.

Probably because of its highly lethal nature, juxtahepatic venous injuries are infrequently managed. Surrounding structures can provide a tamponade effect and contain juxtahepatic venous hemorrhage. Such structures include the liver, the diaphragm, and the suspensory ligaments of the liver. Adequate containment of hemorrhage by these structures might allow an attempt at expectant or nonoperative management. However, if these supporting structures are disrupted, substantial bleeding will ensue. As a consequence, overly aggressive or injudicious hepatic mobilization can result in uncontrollable hemorrhage.

Juxtahepatic injuries, which can be caused by blunt or penetrating injuries, are often classified as type A or B, with the former being hepatic venous wounds that are intraparenchymal and the latter being extraparenchymal venous wounds. Both type A and B injuries can occur together. In addition, there can be associated injuries to the portal vein and its tributaries, which occur more frequently with type A wounds. Fortunately, the extraparenchymal hepatic venous or the associated retrohepatic caval injuries are infrequent. Penetrating wounds to this anatomic region or the sheer forces from blunt injury are the predominant mechanisms of injury. Irrespective of the reported series on the management of juxtahepatic venous injuries, the mortality rates are overwhelmingly high.

There are, basically, three operative approaches in the management of juxtahepatic venous injuries: (1) direct repair of the venous wound(s), (2) surgical resection, and (3) pressure application (containment/tamponade measures) with reinforcement of the natural containment structures that have been disrupted. While there have been several reports of the specific strategy and efficacy of operative exposure and direct repair of juxtahepatic venous injuries, the success is sporadic and overall outcomes dismal [19–23]. In 1966, Feldman [19] was credited with reporting the first successful application of direct suture repair of a juxtahepatic venous injury. Schrock introduced, in 1968, the concept of vascular isolation with the utilization of an atriocaval shunt (Fig. 9.2) [23]. However, the majority of surgeons have abandoned atriocaval shunting because of the challenges related to the technique and the overall dismal outcomes. The paramount or overarching principle in establishing vascular isolation is obtaining proximal and distal control of all vessels to totally isolate the liver. Heaney maneuver advocates a more expedient approach to achieve vascular isolation (Fig. 9.3) to surgically address juxtahepatic venous injuries and other complex liver wounds. At all times, it is imperative that the patient is optimally resuscitated and closely monitored. Another alternative, with respect to achieving vascular isolation in an effort to access retrohepatic wounds, is the establishment of a venovenous bypass (Fig. 9.4). This approach necessitates cannulation of the femoral vein and the axillary vein in the upper arm. The cannulas are connected by a heparin-coated tubing, with a flow assisted by a centrifugal pump. Both supra- and intrahepatic clamps are required for the venovenous bypass. Along with inexperience in the above techniques, major blood loss with associated coagulopathy precludes successful utilization of any of the shunting interventions. Operative hepatic resection, in an effort to access these retrohepatic wounds, is associated with a high mortality rate and should not be attempted.

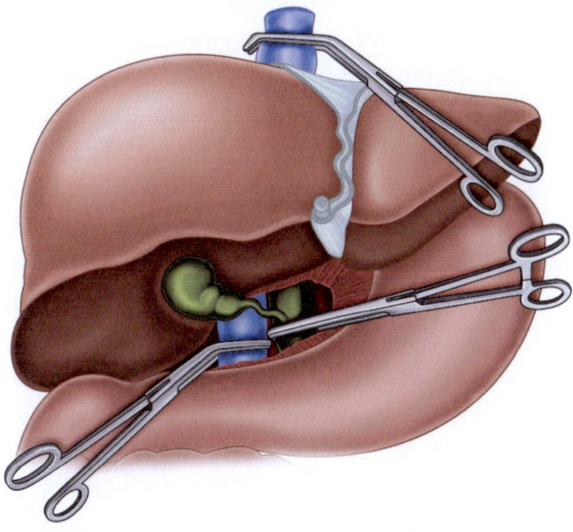

Fig. 9.3 The Heaney maneuver. Vascular isolation of the injured liver by applying vascular clamps to the suprahepatic and infra-hepatic inferior vena cava, in addition to a Pringle maneuver

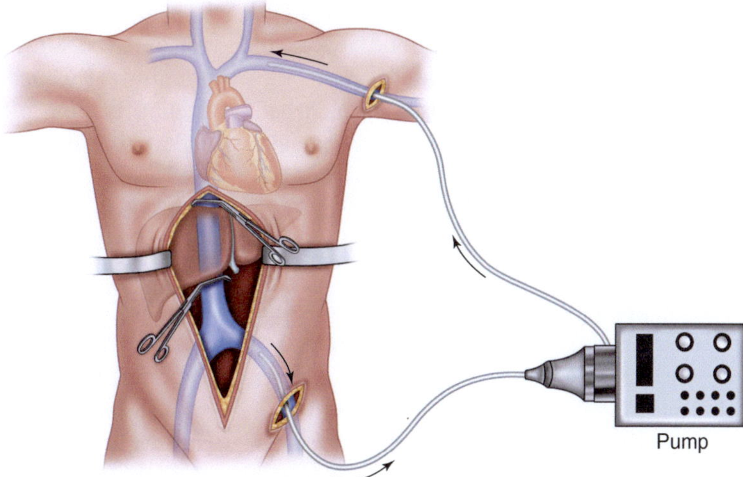

Fig. 9.4 The venovenous bypass requires cannulation of both the femoral vein and the axillary vein. A heparin-coated tubing connects the two cannulas. Flow is assisted by a centrifugal pump

Because of the inherent and overwhelming risks of surgical management of these complex injuries, tamponade with containment followed by angiography and possible embolization has become a viable option (when possible) in the management of juxtahepatic venous injuries. Such an approach often requires temporarily leaving the abdomen open. Although omentum has been proposed to create the tamponade effect, gauze packing is more expedient and effective. Pachter et al. described a "nonshunting approach" which consists of four components: (1) manual compression and aggressive fluid resuscitation; (2) prolonged portal triad occlusion (mean occlusion time, 46 min); (3) rapid and extensive finger fracture for vascular control, almost always through normal hepatic parenchyma to the site of injury; and (4) wide mobilization of the hepatic attachments with medial rotation of the liver to provide access to both the retrohepatic cava and the hepatic vein [24]. In their series, six of the nine "nonshunted" patients survived.

Porta Hepatis

Injuries to the porta hepatis are rare, usually complex, and highly lethal. Review of the recent literature showed three large series that cumulatively report 180 patients treated between 1965 and 1994 [25–27]. These injuries are usually penetrating, occurring in 50–100 % of the populations reported. Isolated injuries to the portal structures occur and are far more survivable than are multiple injuries. Overwhelming hemorrhage is the usual cause of death in all reported series.

The porta hepatis is composed of the hepatic artery, extrahepatic bile duct system, and the portal vein. The proximity of these structures to other major structures, and their relatively difficult exposure, explains their high lethality. In the multi-institutional survey compiled by the Western Trauma Association and reported by Jurkovich et al. [27], an overall 51 % mortality rate was recorded. When broken down, the mortality rate in single-structure injuries is still 45 %, whereas the mortality rate in multiple-structure injuries rises to 80 %. This is in line with results in other reports in the literature.

Portal Vein

Injuries to the portal vein are responsible for most deaths ascribed to portal structures. Once identified and the bleeding controlled, the question of repair versus ligation must be addressed. Ligation of the portal vein can be tolerated, in that there will be decompression of the portal hypertension by collateral vessels. Unfortunately, in patients subjected to ligation of the portal vein, the mortality rate is as high as 90 %. This is in disagreement with survival rates of 50–80 % reported previously by Pachter et al. [28] and Stone et al. [29]. Patients treated by ligation of the portal vein have greater circumferential disruption of the vein and overwhelming hemorrhage, and ligation is used as a rapid method of bleeding control. Repair of the portal vein is used with lesser degrees of injury—in circumferential injury less than 25 %—and is reported to have increased survivability. Many of the deaths occur because of massive hemorrhage before a repair can be accomplished. When confronted with a portal venous injury, repair is preferable to ligation, although ligation is an acceptable option. Second-look laparotomy to check for bowel viability has been advocated when the portal vein has been ligated.

Hepatic Artery

The liver receives a dual blood supply from the hepatic artery and the portal vein, allowing ligation of the hepatic artery without absolutely compromising hepatic blood supply. Lobar artery ligation is well tolerated, but overall mortality rate remains in excess of 40 %.

Extrahepatic Biliary Ducts

Bile duct injuries are uncommon, even in this relatively uncommon injury cluster. Partial circumferential disruption can be treated by primary repair as well as demonstrated from the experience with iatrogenic bile duct injury at the time of cholecystectomy. Complex or complete disruption of the ductal tree is best managed by biliary-enteric anastomosis. End-to-end anastomosis has an excessive stenosis rate. Adequate drainage of the area is essential, because bile leaks can occur. On rare occasion, stenting and external drainage have been used in an unstable patient, with biliary reconstruction accomplished at a later date [30].

The key to the diagnosis of bile duct injury is suspicion that the injury has occurred. Evidence of bile staining and the presence of a duodenal injury should prompt investigation that is best done by an intraoperative cholangiogram. Small injuries may be missed at initial exploration. Endoscopic retrograde cholangiopancreatogram with stenting may provide diagnostic therapeutic answers if a patient develops a biloma subsequent to a missed injury.

Video Captions

Video 3	Right hepatic lobe rotation (3-D animation) (MP4 33079 kb)
Video 4	Left hepatic lobe rotation (MP4 53192 kb)
Video 5	Left hepatic lobe rotation (3-D animation) (MP4 30377 kb)
Video 6	Pringle maneuver (MP4 14015 kb)
Video 7	Liver suture (MP4 39685 kb)
Video 9	Hepatic vascular exclusion (MP4 22289 kb)
Video 15	Case 02 A 30-year-old man was a victim of 3 gunshot wounds: he was hemodynamically stable (MP4 94193 kb)

References

1. Yokota J, Sugimoto T. Clinical significance of periportal tracking on computed tomographic scan in patients with blunt liver trauma. Am J Surg. 1994;68:247–50.
2. Karp MP, Cooney DR, Pros GA, et al. The nonoperative management of pediatric hepatic trauma. J Pediatr Surg. 1983;18:512–8.
3. Oldham KT, Guice KS, Ryckman F, et al. Blunt liver injury in childhood: evolution of therapy and current perspective. Surgery. 1986;100:542–9.
4. Bond SJ, Eichelberger MR, Gotschall CS, et al. Nonoperative management of blunt hepatic and splenic injury in children. Ann Surg. 1996;223:286–9.
5. Meredith JW, Young JS, Bowling J, et al. Nonoperative management of blunt hepatic trauma: the exception or the rule? J Trauma. 1994;36:529–34.
6. Pachter HL, Knudson MN, Esrig B, et al. Status on nonoperative management of blunt hepatic injuries in 1995: a multi center experience with 404 patients. J Trauma. 1996;40:31–8.
7. Smith RS. Nonoperative management of hepatic trauma. Mil Med. 1991;156:472–4.
8. Bluett MK, Woltering E, Adkins RB. Management of penetrating hepatic injury: a review of 102 consecutive patients. Am Surg. 1984;50:132–42.
9. Stone HH, Lamb JM. Use of pedicle omentum as an autogenous pack for control of hemorrhage in major injuries of the liver. Surg Gynecol Obstet. 1975;141:92–4.
10. Fabian TC, Stone HH. Arrest of severe liver hemorrhage by omental pack. South Med J. 1980;73:1487–90.
11. Delaney HM, Ivatury RR, Blau SA, et al. Use of biodegradable (PGA) fabric for repair of solid organ injury: a combined institution experience. Injury. 1993;24:585–9.
12. Brunet C, Sielezneff I, Thomas P, et al. Treatment of hepatic trauma with perihepatic mesh: 35 cases. J Trauma. 1994;37:200–4.
13. Garrison JR, Richardson JD, Hilakos AS, et al. Predicting the need to pack early for severe intra-abdominal hemorrhage. J Trauma. 1996;40:923–9.
14. Feliciano DV, Mattox KL, Burch JM, et al. Packing for control of hepatic hemorrhage. J Trauma. 1986;26:738–42.
15. Carmona RH, Peck DZ, Lim RC. The role of packing and planned reoperation in severe hepatic trauma. J Trauma. 1984;24:779–84.
16. Walt AJ. The diagnosis and treatment of hepatic trauma. In: Najarian JS, Delaney JP, editors. Trauma and critical care surgery. Chicago: Year Book Medical Publisher; 1987. p. 127–36.
17. Ivatury RR, Nallathambi M, Gunduz Y, et al. Liver packing for uncontrolled hemorrhage: a reappraisal. J Trauma. 1986;26:744–53.
18. Clark DE, Cobean RA, Radke FR, et al. Management of major hepatic trauma involving interhospital transfer. Am Surg. 1994;60:881–5.
19. Feldman EA. Injury to the hepatic vein. Am J Surg. 1966;111:244–6.
20. Waltuck TL, Crow RW, Humphrey LJ, et al. Avulsion injuries of the vena cava following blunt abdominal trauma. Ann Surg. 1970;171:67–72.
21. Yellin AE, Chaffee CB, Donovan AJ. Vascular isolation in treatment of juxtahepatic venous injuries. Arch Surg. 1971;102:566–73.
22. Bricker DL, Morton JR, Okies JE, et al. Surgical management of injuries to the vena cava: changing patterns of injury and newer techniques of repair. J Trauma. 1971;11:725–35.
23. Schrock T, Blaisdell W, Matthewson C Jr. Management of blunt trauma to the liver and hepatic veins. Arch Surg. 1968;96:698–704.
24. Coppa GF. The management of juxtahepatic venous injuries without an atriocaval shunt: preliminary clinical observations. Surgery 1986;99:569–75.
25. Busuttil RW, Kitahama A, Cerise E, et al. Management of blunt and penetrating injuries to the porta hepatis. Ann Surg. 1980;191(5):641–8.

26. Sheldon GF, Lim RC, Yee ES, et al. Management of injuries to the porta hepatis. Ann Surg. 1985; 202:539–45.
27. Jurkovich GJ, Hoyt DB, Moore FA, et al. Portal triad injuries. J Trauma. 1995;39:426–34.
28. Pachter H, Drager S, Godfrey N, et al. Traumatic injuries to the portal vein. The role of acute ligation. Ann Surg. 1979;189:383–5.
29. Stone HH, Fabian T, Turkelson M. Wounds of the portal venous system. World J Surg. 1982;6:335–41.
30. Ivatury RR, Rohman M, Nallathambi M, et al. The morbidity of injuries of the extrahepatic biliary system. J Trauma. 1985;25:967–73.

Juxtahepatic Venous Injuries: Emergency Measures, Definitive Control, and Atriocaval Shunts

Donald D. Trunkey and K. Shad Pharaon

Introduction

The liver is one of the most frequently injured organs in abdominal trauma due to its anterior location in the abdominal cavity and fragile parenchyma. Prior to World War II, the mortality from liver injuries that were diagnosed and addressed in the field was very high. After World War II, a better working knowledge of the anatomy of the liver, popularized by Couinaud, and subsequent liver transplantation furthered our understanding of the organ. Even with these surgical, until about twenty years ago, many liver injuries still resulted in lethal outcomes. The operations were time consuming and prone to significant blood loss. Recent advancements in imaging studies, angiography, embolization, damage control surgery, and enhanced critical care have shifted the paradigm for the management of liver injuries. Most grade I and II liver injuries do not require surgery. Some grade III injuries (approximately 40 %) may require surgery depending on the amount of blood loss or if there are operative lesions such as extravasation of blood or aneurysm seen on CT. Eighty percent of grade IV and V injures will require surgical intervention. Many liver injuries can be treated nonoperatively, and those that do require operation can be treated with packing. The survival of these patients has greatly improved. Rarely, however, a retrohepatic injury occurs which remains a devastating and lethal injury. These injuries do require an emergent operation, despite the high risks of significant blood loss and time-consuming exposure. Unfortunately, after many years of research and exploring new techniques, this injury and operation are still associated with high mortality. This chapter explains the sequence and methods of care of liver injuries.

D.D. Trunkey, MD (✉)
Section of Trauma and Critical Care, Department of Surgery, Oregon Health and Science University, 3181 SW Sam Jackson Park Rd., Portland, OR 97239, USA
e-mail: trunkeyd@ohsu.edu

K.S. Pharaon, MD
Division of Trauma, Critical Care, and Acute Care Surgery, Department of Surgery, Oregon Health and Science University, Portland, OR USA

Division of Trauma and Acute Care Surgery, Surgical Critical Care, PeaceHealth Southwest Medical Center, Vancouver, WA 98664, USA
e-mail: pharaon@ohsu.edu,
spharaon@peacehealth.org

Stable

The critical decision that a surgeon must determine on all trauma patients, particularly ones with suspected liver injuries, is if the patient is stable or unstable. A stable patient should get a CT scan of their abdomen and pelvis with IV

Electronic supplementary material Supplementary material is available in the online version of this chapter at 10.1007/978-1-4939-1200-1_10. Videos can also be accessed at http://www.springerimages.com/videos/978-1-4939-1199-8.

contrast. CT scan is the standard imaging study for hemodynamically stable patients following blunt trauma. A grading of liver injuries I through VI has been described. However, the main indication of the operative approach is hemodynamic instability, not the grading of the injury. If on CT scan the patient has a liver injury, but has no extravasation of contrast and no other reason to go to the operating room theater, the patient should be monitored in an ICU setting with serial hematocrits. If on CT scan there is extravasation of contrast, and the patient remains stable, the injury can still be treated nonoperatively with angiography and embolization with help from interventional radiology.

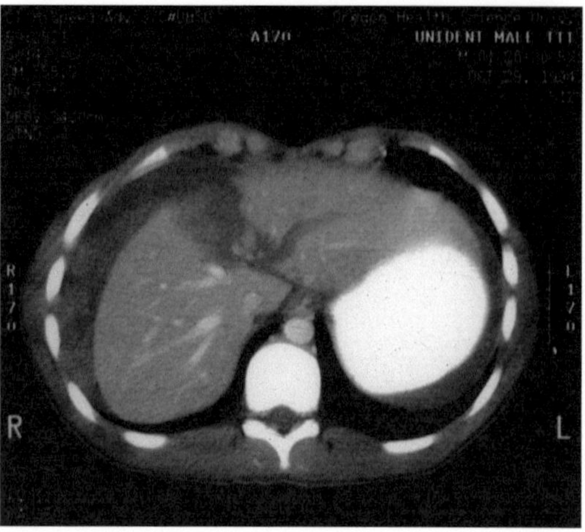

Fig. 10.1 CT scan of a 17-year-old boy with near traumatic liver resection. In this case, you may need to complete the liver resection on the initial operation

Unstable

If the patient is unstable, he or she should be taken to the operating room within 15 min. The main objective is to quickly identify the source of bleeding, be ready to expose the injury, repair it, and get out of the operating room quickly. The massive transfusion protocol should be initiated and the operating room warmed up. The patient is prepped and draped from midnek to midthighs anteriorly and from tabletop to tabletop laterally. Enter the abdomen through a midline incision extending from the xiphoid to the pubis. Evacuate as much clot as possible and then pack all four quadrants. The anesthesiologist should replace volume as needed. Remove the lower packs first and check for associated injuries, particularly those that can cause fecal contamination. Then, remove the packs in the left upper quadrant. If the spleen is bleeding, do not spend time trying to repair it. Eliminate the bleeding source by performing a splenectomy. Last, remove the right upper quadrant packs. If there is bleeding from the right upper quadrant, the critical sequence of events is to determine if the bleeding is coming from the top of or from behind the liver.

Blood coming from on top of the liver should be initially managed with direct pressure on the liver fracture or the missile tract. Some require direct suture ligation with absorbable suture on a large curved needle. Blood on top of the liver can also be managed with adjuncts such as Gelfoam®, Surgicel®, thrombin, fibrin glue, or omental packing. On occasion, a resection is performed if a portion of the liver is nonviable or has significant disruption (Figs. 10.1 and 10.2). If these maneuvers do not stop the bleeding, perform a Pringle maneuver by initially inserting your index finger into the foramen of Winslow and your thumb through the avascular portion of the gastrohepatic ligament. A Penrose or non-crushing vascular clamp can then be used to get control of the portal circulation. If the bleeding stops with the Pringle maneuver, the injury is within the portal system and can be repaired primarily or it may be due to a hepatic artery injury. If the hepatic artery is transected, it can be ligated (Figs. 10.3, 10.4 and 10.7).

A failure of a Pringle maneuver to slow the bleeding likely indicates an injury behind the liver, to the retrohepatic inferior vena cava or a hepatic vein. Be sure to check for a replaced right hepatic artery. Immediately push back and up on the liver, against the spine and diaphragm, to stop the hemorrhage temporarily, followed by prompt perihepatic packing. If hemorrhage is not controlled after a Pringle maneuver and perihepatic packing, there are a few ways to obtain definitive control of the blood supply to the liver—the

Heaney maneuver, venovenous bypass, and atriocaval shunting. There have been case reports of interventional radiologists temporarily occluding the inferior vena cava above and below the injury, with catheters, by accessing the femoral vein and internal jugular vein. Rarely, a hepatectomy for trauma has been performed with subsequent transplantation (Fig. 10.2).

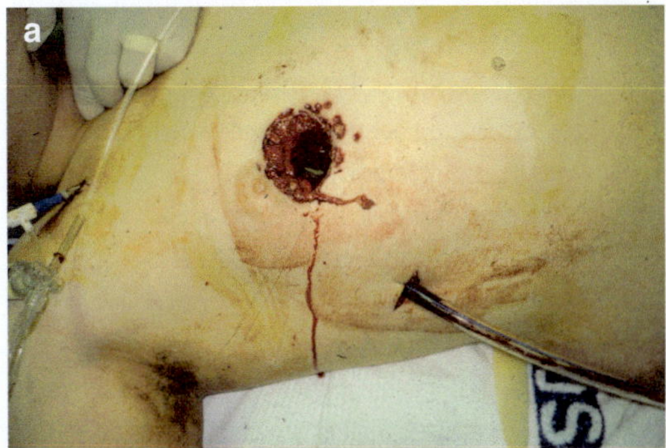

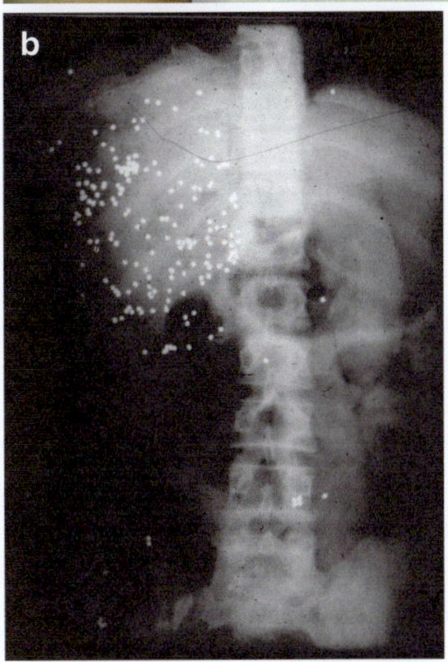

Fig. 10.2 (**a**) 14-year-old boy with shotgun injury just below the right nipple. On laparotomy, the blast injury nearly resected his liver and had the appearance of currant jelly. (**b**) Plain film of a 14-year-old boy accidentally shot by his brother at close range while hunting. The entrance wound was at the inferior border of the right nipple. He was transported to the nearest emergency room, where he was given eight units of blood and transported by helicopter to the level I trauma center 50 miles away. The highest blood pressure was 80 mmHg. He was taken immediately to the operating room where a right lobectomy was performed. The wadding from the shotgun shell was found in the middle of the right lobe

Juxtahepatic Venous Injury

The Heaney maneuver is performed by clamping both the suprahepatic and infrahepatic inferior vena cava while simultaneously applying the Pringle maneuver (Fig. 10.3). During the Heaney maneuver, clamping of the inferior vena cava can lead to cardiac arrest because of the sudden decrease in cardiac preload. It is crucial that central pressures are monitored and that fluid replacement is adequate. The aorta should not be clamped. Doing so will result in worsening acidosis. Once you have control of the inferior vena cava and portal vein, there is less than one hour to repair the injury. Begin by taking down the falciform and right triangular ligament as well as freeing the liver posteriorly from the diaphragm. Occasionally, the right hepatic artery may arise from the superior mesenteric artery (replaced right hepatic). The right hepatic lobe is freed up from the diaphragm and rotated medially away from the diaphragm, exposing the small hepatic veins from segment one communicating directly into the inferior vena cava.

Each of these small veins should be ligated. In extreme deceleration injuries, the small veins are avulsed from the anterior surface of the inferior vena cava creating a linear laceration (Fig. 10.4).

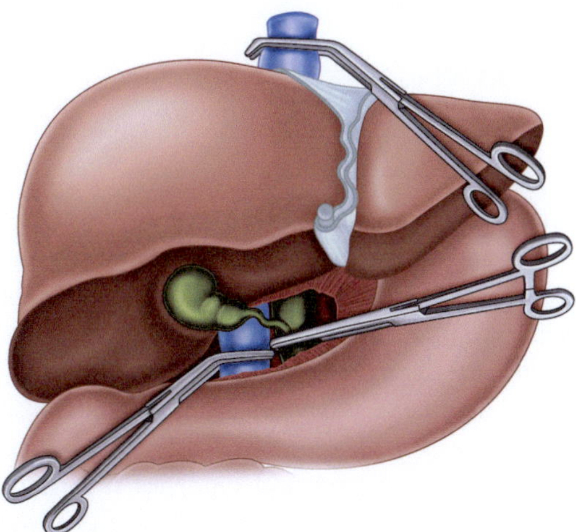

Fig. 10.3 The Heaney maneuver. Vascular isolation of the injured liver by applying vascular clamps to the suprahepatic and infra-hepatic inferior vena cava, in addition to a Pringle maneuver

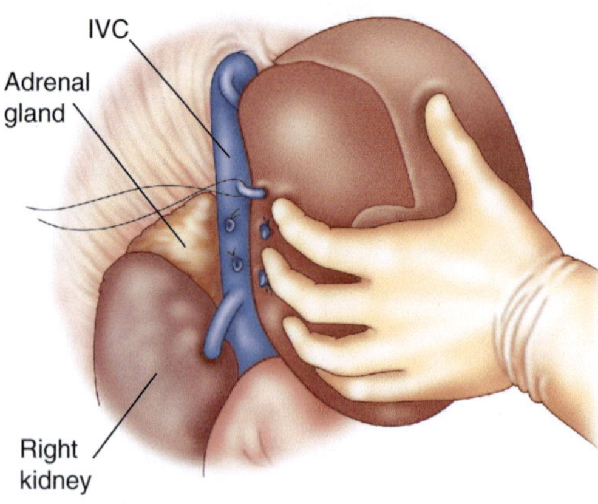

Fig. 10.4 Retrohepatic inferior vena cava

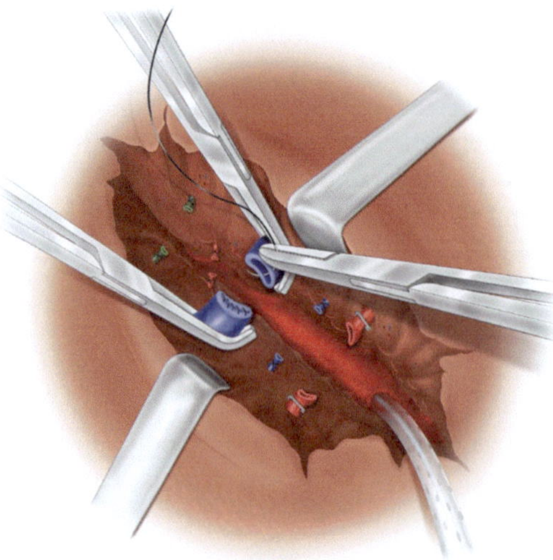

Fig. 10.5 Clamping of right hepatic vein (Reproduced with permission from Ivatury)

If the right hepatic vein is avulsed from the inferior vena cava, place a clamp on the hepatic vein and ligate it (Fig. 10.5). If there is a hole in the inferior vena cava, you can repair this with 4-0 Prolene, taking care to minimize reducing the lumen.

An injury to the left hepatic vein should also be considered. The left lobe is mobilized by division of the falciform and coronary ligaments. Medially rotate the left lobe of the liver. You should keep in mind that the left hepatic artery may arise from the left gastric artery (replaced left hepatic). If the left hepatic vein is avulsed from the inferior vena cava, a Satinsky clamp in

some injuries can be placed and oversewn. Alternatively, the forefinger can be placed in the hole of the inferior vena cava and a running suture of 5-0 Prolene is advanced as the surgeon's finger is withdrawn from the laceration. Once the repair is complete, release the clamps from the portal vein and inferior vena cava. If there is control of bleeding, it may be prudent to place a few packs around the repair. The abdomen should be left open with a temporary abdominal closure system such as ABThera™. The patient will be brought to the intensive care for rewarming and resuscitation. This can usually be achieved in three to six hours. The patient is returned to the operating room for another look, pack removal, and closure of the abdomen if possible. Although the Heaney technique involves occlusion of inferior vena cava with no bypass or shunting of blood, it is the preferred method of retrohepatic injury repair. It is the easiest of the three techniques to perform, does not involve additional equipment or teams, and provides the patient with the best chance of survival.

A second method of hepatic vascular isolation is venovenous bypass using a centrifugal pump that was initially described by Starzl (Fig. 10.6). The following explanation is an advanced maneuver and should only be attempted by an experienced liver or trauma surgeon. In addition to having the necessary equipment including the circulating pump, a perfusion team should be immediately available. While the patient is being prepped and draped for surgery, two simultaneous cutdowns are performed. One is over the left saphenofemoral junction and an 18 F Argyle tube is inserted into the saphenous vein, which extends into the inferior vena cava. The other cutdown is performed over the left axillary vein and an 18 F Argyle tube is inserted which extends into the subclavian vein. A vascular clamp is placed across the portal triad to control bleeding from the viscera. The right triangular ligament is taken down (Fig. 10.7). Massive bleeding will be encountered from behind the liver. Venovenous bypass is achieved by attaching the Argyle tubes to the centrifugal pump and circulating blood from the catheter in the saphenous vein through the pump and returning it through the catheter in the axillary vein. Concomitant total hepatic

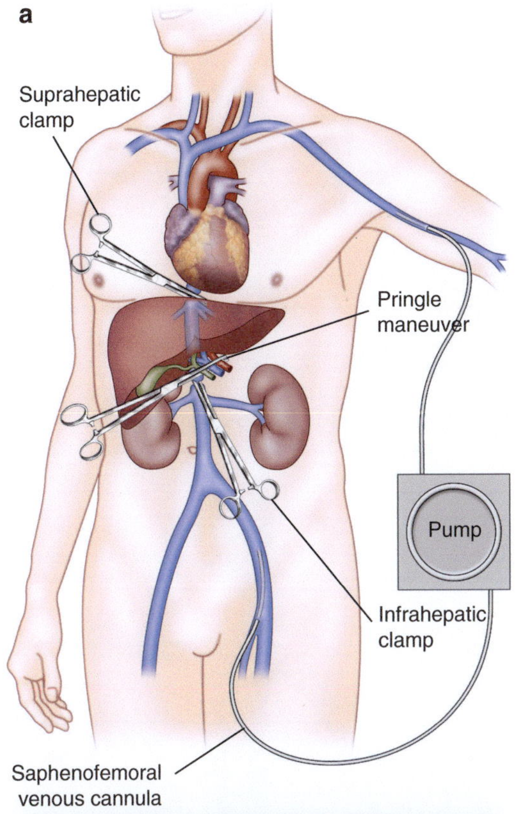

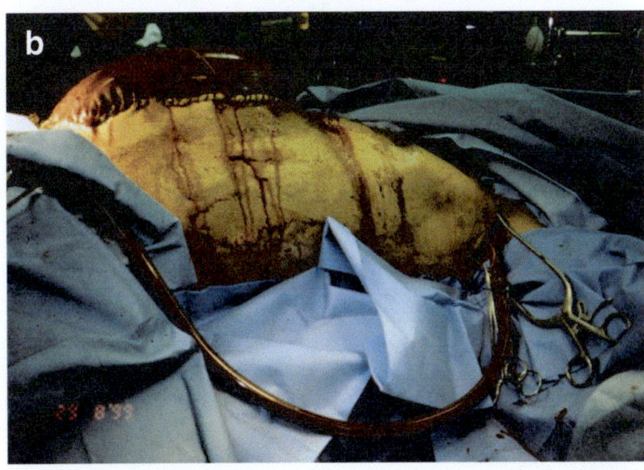

Fig. 10.6 (**a**) Venovenous bypass. (**b**) Venovenous bypass setup from left groin to left axilla. In this patient, we achieved 1,200 cc of flow without a pump

isolation is achieved by clamping or placing Rummel tourniquets around the inferior vena cava just above the renal veins and on the suprahepatic inferior vena cava. In some injuries, it is possible to clamp the suprahepatic inferior vena cava below the diaphragm. Another approach is to perform a sternotomy and clamp or place a Rummel tourniquet above the diaphragm. If the right or left hepatic

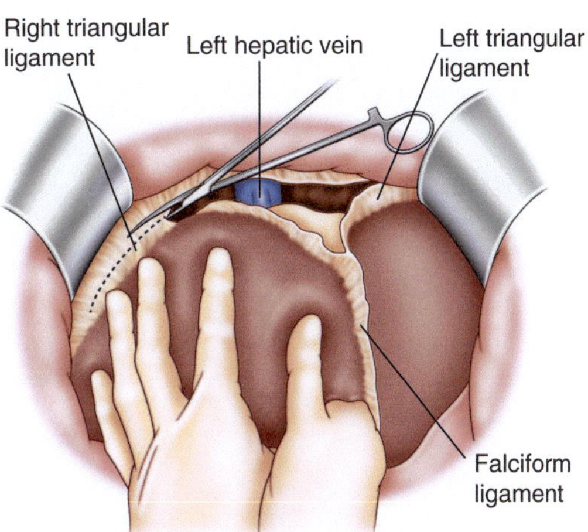

Fig. 10.7 Mobilization of liver

veins are avulsed from the inferior vena cava, place clamps on the vessels and ligate them. A hole in the inferior vena cava can be repaired with a 4-0 Prolene. Venovenous bypass has the advantage of creating a bloodless field while still returning blood to the heart. This method does not require sternotomy or thoracotomy unless it is necessary to control the inferior vena cava above the diaphragm. Another advantage is the ability of using the circuit to rewarm the patient. The disadvantage is that it is a moderately complex procedure that must happen quickly. While in theory the operation makes sense, the practicality of all the necessary parts coming together makes it difficult. Quick recognition of the retrohepatic injury, a readily available perfusion team and equipment, facile venous cutdown, mobilization of the liver, and placement of catheters are all complex time-consuming tasks that must be done quickly and correctly in order to achieve success with this maneuver (Fig. 10.5).

The third way to obtain definitive control of blood to the liver is by atriocaval shunting. Atriocaval shunting was reported by Schrock et al. in 1968 and was the mainstay of treatment for complex liver injuries for many years. Most surgeons have now abandoned this technique. For historical purposes, we will explain how it was set up (Fig. 10.8). The patient requires sternotomy and laparotomy to expose the heart and intra-abdominal vena cava. A thoracoabdominal incision is contraindicated since it is difficult to access

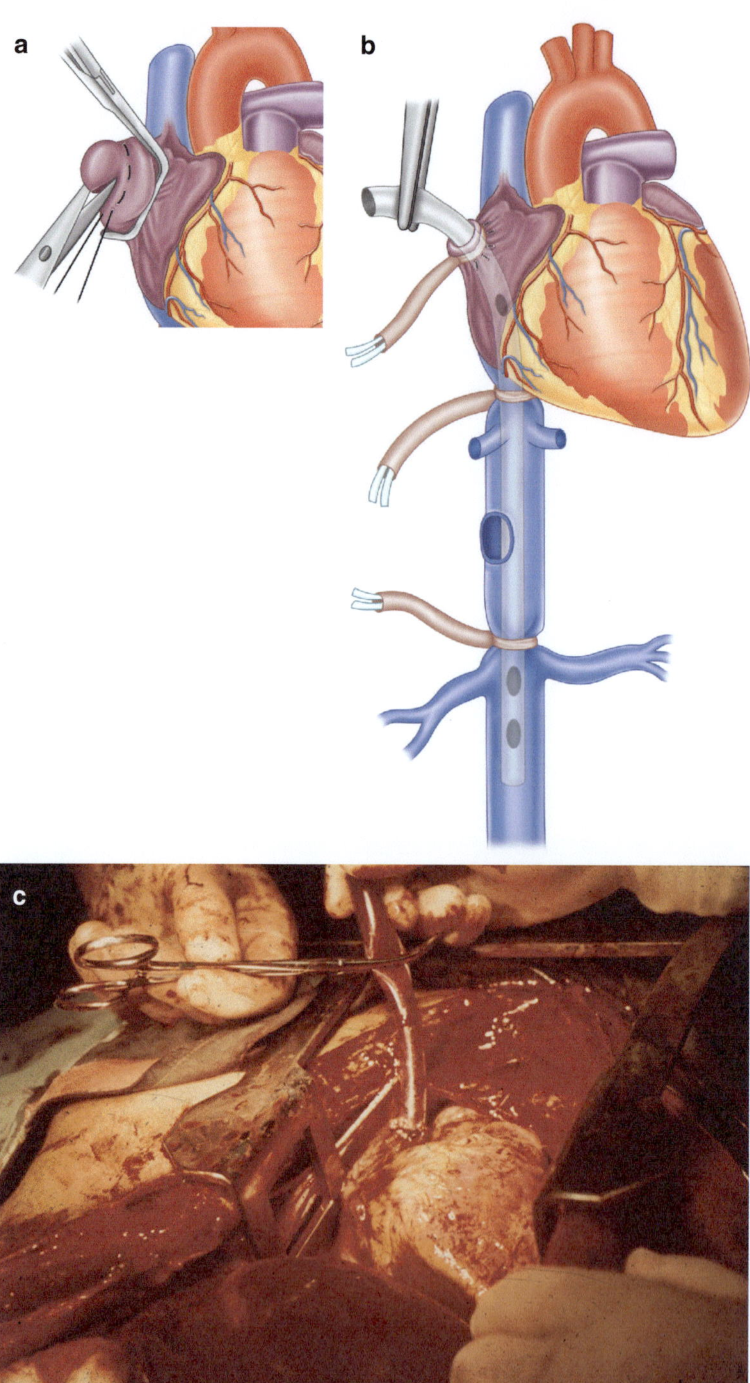

Fig. 10.8 (**a**) Schrock shunt. (**b**, **c**) Schrock shunt entering right atrial appendage

the right atrium and the inferior vena cava inside the pericardium. A purse-string suture is placed in the right atrial appendage using a 3-0 Prolene. Control of the supradiaphragmatic inferior vena cava is obtained inside the pericardium with a Rummel tourniquet. Another Rummel tourniquet is fashioned around the suprarenal inferior vena cava. A 36 F chest tube or 9 mm endotracheal tube with strategically placed side holes is inserted through the right atrial appendage down the vena cava to the level of the renal veins. Two teams of experienced surgeons working simultaneously are required, one in the chest and one in the abdomen. The surgeon working in the abdomen directs the shunt in the inferior vena cava past the area of injury and positions it so that the distal portion of the shunt is just below the renal veins and the proximal side holes are at the level of the right atrium. The side holes allow flow from the renal veins and lower extremities to flow through the lumen of the shunt into the right atrium. Tourniquets are tightened preventing back bleeding and to ensure that blood flows only through the shunt. The advantage of this operation is the creation of a bloodless field for the repair to be completed while returning blood to the heart through a shunt. However, there are also numerous barriers to its success. Care must be taken to insert the shunt correctly as there are a number of ways to incorrectly position the shunt that can cause exacerbation of the bleeding. It requires sternotomy and laparotomy. Two cavities simultaneously open subjects the patient to hypothermia. There are few technical maneuvers in surgery as dramatic or desperate as the use of the atriocaval shunt. The death rate from atriocaval shunting is extraordinarily high. It is often used after other attempts at control of bleeding have failed. At San Francisco General Hospital, there were seven survivors out of 18 patients (Figs. 10.1, 10.6 and 10.8).

The emergence of interventional vascular techniques has had a profound impact on many groups of patients, including trauma patients. There have been case reports of the placement of catheters to control bleeding from retrohepatic and juxtahepatic vena cava injuries. The catheters can be introduced using fluoroscopic guidance and positioned precisely for maximal hemostasis and minimal additional tissue trauma. Primary repair of the original injury then can be undertaken in the standard fashion. This requires the recognition in the operating room of the injury, movement of the patient to the interventional radiology suite, and then moving the patient back to the operating room for repair. However, the practicality of moving the patient so many times is time consuming. If, however, you have the ability to operate and perform endovascular procedures in the same room, this option becomes more attractive.

Other structures can simultaneously be injured. While injuries to the extrahepatic biliary tree are usually associated with penetrating trauma, blunt trauma can cause stretch or avulsion injuries. Injuries to the extrahepatic biliary tree are usually associated with penetrating trauma; however, blunt trauma can cause stretch or avulsion injuries. In the unstable patient, temporary biliary drainage can be accomplished by placing catheters into the right and left hepatic ducts or the common duct, which are then brought out of the abdomen laterally. Delayed reconstruction of the biliary systems can be accomplished after the patient recovers from other injuries.

There are many pitfalls in grade IV and V liver injuries that can lead to the patient's demise. The most common pitfall is failure to recognize the lethal triad of acidosis, hypothermia, and coagulopathy. This emphasizes the role of the anesthesiologist who must monitor the patient for these three problems. The anesthesiologist may also capitalize on having a hematologist come to the operating room to expedite the procurement of blood and help with hemotherapy. The military has shown that a 1:1:1 ratio of packed cells, fresh frozen plasma, and platelets is the optimal ratio of component treatment. The military has also shown that fresh warm blood is the best resuscitation in these severely injured patients. This has been confirmed in San Francisco and Houston. Thromboelastography is a useful adjunct in assessing a patient's clotting abnormalities. Heating the operating room is essential. As earlier noted, venous injuries lend themselves to control by packing, returning the patient to the ICU and, over a three-hour period, reversing the acidosis, hypothermia, and coagulopathy. Some patients may benefit from pooled plasma protein, tranexamic acid, and occasionally factor 7. This is planned based on the coagulation studies during the initial operation. If one chooses to use the atriocaval shunt, it must be instituted very early in the operative management. It should not be used after the patient has developed acidosis, hypothermia, and coagulopathy. Failures of the Schrock shunt at San Francisco General Hospital were due to using it very late in the course of the initial surgery.

In summary, juxtahepatic venous injuries, including those to the retrohepatic vena cava or major hepatic veins, represent the most difficult and lethal form of liver trauma. The mortality of such injuries is very high. The reason for the high mortality is due to the difficulty in achieving hemorrhage control in this surgically inaccessible area. Consequently, several therapeutic options have been designed. Many early treatments of liver injury that were abandoned, have again become safe, popular treatment modalities. Hepatic packing was initially abandoned due to its high associated complications in the early twentieth century, but we now know that some liver trauma can be treated nonoperatively. Most patients with liver injury that do require an operation can be managed with hepatic packing alone, particularly if the bleeding is due to injury to the veins. It is the uncommon patient that has a liver injury, is hemodynamically unstable, requires an operation, and fails hepatic packing and a Pringle maneuver. These juxtahepatic venous injuries represent the biggest challenge to trauma surgeons. On occasion, advanced techniques are needed. Although several techniques have been described, we feel that only the Heaney maneuver for total vascular isolation of the liver should be used. Mobilization of the liver and occlusion of the portal triad and suprahepatic and infrahepatic vena cava takes skill and must be done expeditiously. Exposing the retrohepatic inferior vena cava will sometimes reveal that the hepatic veins have been avulsed from the cava. Ligating them and getting out of the operating room quickly are the patient's only hope for survival. Any treatment strategy used to manage juxtahepatic and retrohepatic inferior vena cava injuries must rapidly control hemorrhage. Plan on returning to the operating room in a few hours after rewarming and resuscitation in the intensive care. And lastly, multidisciplinary management with early angioembolization and/or temporary caval occlusion may improve patient outcomes.

Take-Home Points
- Nonoperative therapy of liver injuries has become an acceptable approach to management of hemodynamically stable patients without associated injury requiring laparotomy
- Surgical intervention is based on unstable hemodynamics, not the grade of the liver injury
- Grades III, IV, and V usually will require an intervention
- As a general rule, occlusion of the portal triad is safe for about 60 min
- When portal triad occlusion does not control the hemorrhage, assume that bleeding is coming from behind the liver.
- Heaney maneuver, venovenous bypass, and atriocaval shunt are three methods of temporarily controlling the hemorrhage from behind the liver. We prefer Heaney.
- Newer techniques involving interventional radiology may prove to be an additional tool in the surgeon's armamentarium.

Video Captions

Video 6   Pringle maneuver (MP4 14015 kb)
Video 9   Hepatic vascular exclusion (MP4 99239 kb)
Video 12   Atriocaval shunt (MP4 256971 kb)

Suggested Readings

Burch JM, Feliciano DV, Mattox KL. The atriocaval shunt: facts and fiction. Ann Surg. 1988;207(5):555–68.

Krige JE, Worthley CS, Terblanche J. Severe juxtahepatic venous injury: survival after prolonged hepatic vascular isolation without shunting. HPB Surg. 1990;3(1):39–43.

Pringle JH. Notes on the arrest of hepatic hemorrhage due to trauma. Ann Surg. 1908;48:541.

Richardson JD, Franklin GA, Lukan JK. Evolution in the management of hepatic trauma: a 25-year perspective. Ann Surg. 2000;232:324–30.

Rogers FB, Reese J, Shackford SR, Osler TM. The use of venovenous bypass and total vascular isolation of the liver in the surgical management of juxtahepatic venous injuries in blunt hepatic trauma. J Trauma. 1997;43(3):530–3.

Schrock T, Blaisdell FW, Mathewson Jr C. Management of blunt trauma to the liver and hepatic veins. Arch Surg. 1968;96:698–704.

Strong RW. The management of blunt liver injuries. Aust N Z J Surg. 1999;69(8):609–16.

Trunkey D, Shires T, McClelland R. Management of liver trauma in 811 consecutive patients. Ann Surg. 1974;179:722–8.

Ivatury RR. Basic operative techniques in trauma and emergency surgery. In: Britt LD, Peitzman A, Barie P, Jurkovich G, editors. Acute care surgery. Philadelphia: Lippincott Williams & Wilkins; 2012.

Rao R. Ivatury

In patients with missile wounds of the liver that traverse the entire thickness of the lobes, the so-called transfixing wounds, control of the hemorrhage by extensive tractotomy, and debridement-resection may not be the optimal approach, given the presence of extensive associated injuries and/or coagulopathy. In such situations, lesser procedures are available for hemorrhage control.

Omental pack. A graft of viable omentum with an intact vascular supply can be mobilized to fill in this dead space and control the venous bleeding [1, 2]. This living tissue not only acts as a pack to control bleeding but also may serve as a rich source of macrophages to help minimize the risk of subsequent sepsis. The omental graft is pulled through the tract and hemostasis is ensured (Fig. 11.1; Video 11). The most important requisite for success is the vascularity of the omentum [3, 4].

Penrose pack. Described by Bluett et al. [4], it involves using a pack of Penrose drains as a tamponading plug inside the long, penetrating tract. A long Kelly clamp is passed through the missile tract. A pack made of a collection of 0.5″ or 1″ Penrose drains is pulled back through the tract and left in the laceration (Figs. 11.2 and 11.3). The Penrose pack serves to exert gentle pressure on the surrounding hepatic parenchyma and controls the bleeding. The drains, brought to the

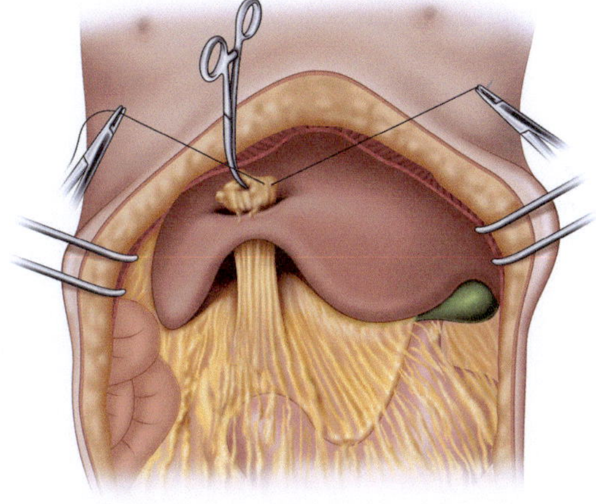

Fig. 11.1 Omental pack. A graft of viable omentum is pulled through the penetrating tract in the liver

exterior through the flank, also serve to drain the laceration. The drains may be "shortened" gradually over the next few days to allow the tract to collapse behind the receding drains. This technique facilitates hemostasis and helps to avoid a tractotomy or major resection in difficult circumstances.

Balloon tamponade. As reported by Morimoto et al. [5], this therapeutic modality has shown to be effective and less traumatic than hepatotomy. Several methods are available for balloon

R.R. Ivatury, MD, MS, FACS
Department of Surgery, Virginia Commonwealth University, 3010 Newquay Lane,
Richmond, VA 23236, USA
e-mail: raoivatury@gmail.com

Electronic supplementary material Supplementary material is available in the online version of this chapter at 10.1007/978-1-4939-1200-1_11. Videos can also be accessed at http://www.springerimages.com/videos/978-1-4939-1199-8.

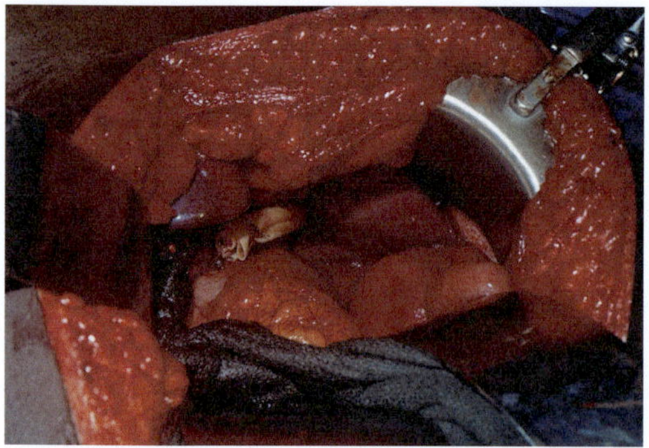

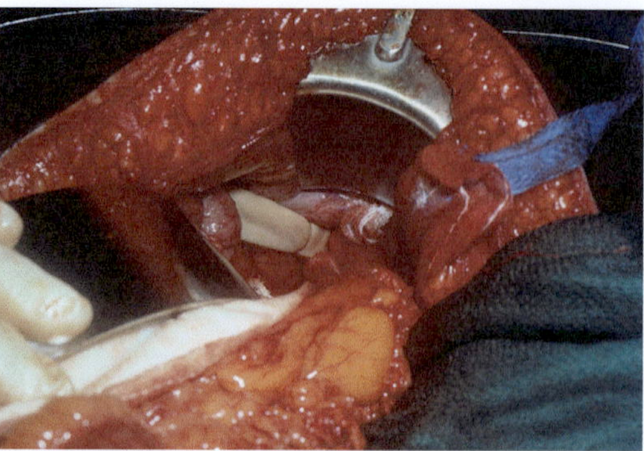

Fig. 11.2 Penrose pack through a bi-lobar transfixing gunshot wound of the liver

Fig. 11.3 The pack is pulled through the other surface of the liver and exteriorized as a drain

Fig. 11.4 Sengstaken-Blakemore tube. The esophageal balloon may be used for balloon tamponade of transfixing gunshot wounds of the liver. The tube is exteriorized through the abdominal wall and can also function as a drain

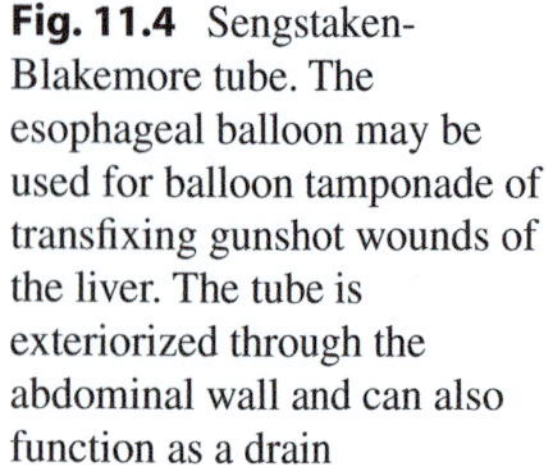

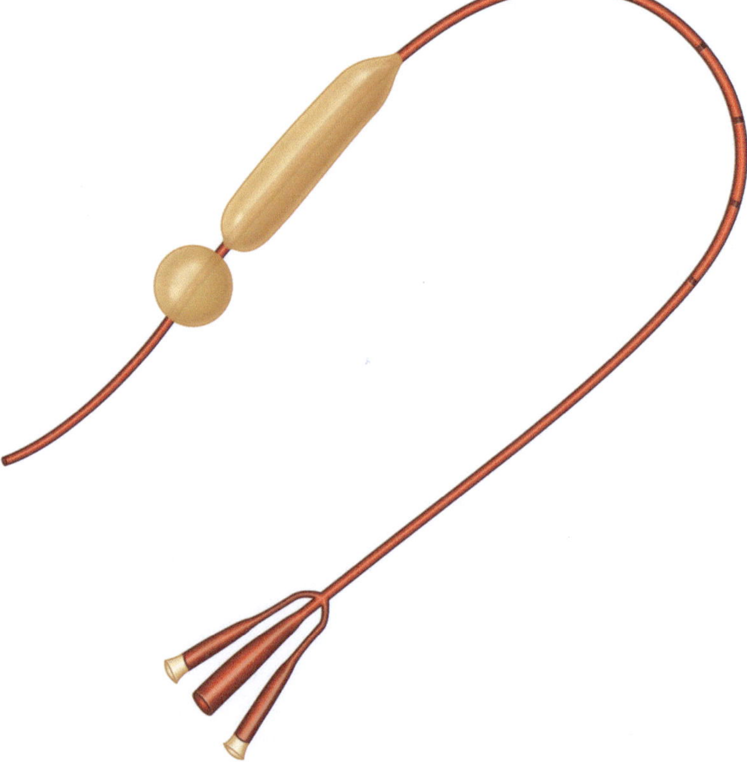

tamponade. We have achieved intrahepatic balloon tamponade of missile tracts by using a sterilized Sengstaken-Blakemore tube (S-B tube). This tube, traditionally used for esophageal variceal bleeding, has a gastric balloon, a long esophageal balloon, and a lumen for drainage (Fig. 11.4). The sterilized tube is introduced into the long bi-lobar intrahepatic tract through a suitable point in the abdominal wall that is aligned to the tract, such that the esophageal balloon lies in the tract. It is then inflated with saline, enough to tamponade the tract and control bleeding. The balloon may be deflated over the next few days gradually as hemostasis is secured. Morimoto et al. [5] used a similar technique of balloon tamponade. The balloon can be "manufactured" in the operating room

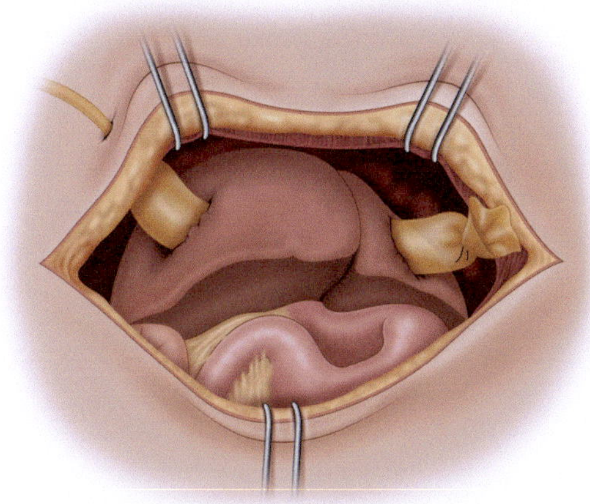

Fig. 11.5 Intrahepatic balloon tamponade. The inflated balloon seen entering and exiting from the penetrating tract within the liver

using a tube and a Penrose drain. The balloon consists of two drains arranged coaxially, an internal tubular one (no. 14 or 16 Levine tube or a red rubber catheter) and an external, laminar one of the Penrose type. The Penrose drain is firmly tied to the tubular one at the ends and the tube is occluded with a ligature at its distal end. The balloon portion should be longer than the intrahepatic tract by about 6 cm. The device is then introduced into the tract, leaving about 2–3 cm protruding from either end of the tract (Fig. 11.5). Video 13 illustrates the technique. The balloon is then inflated with saline enough to lie snugly in the tract and procuring hemostasis by gentle compression on the liver parenchyma. Some authors instill some radiopaque contrast material into the saline in the balloon, so it can be studied radiologically. The end of the tube is brought out to the exterior and serves as a drain. This usually controls bleeding and the balloon can be deflated gradually over the next week or so and eventually removed. Several successful series using the technique were published by Smaniotto et al. [6], Branco et al. [7], and others [8]. Poggetti et al. [9] succinctly described the procedure of intraoperative manufacturing of the balloon device and quoted their experience with more than 35 patients without failures or "breakthrough" bleeding. The advantages of using a tamponading balloon are the easy preparation of the device and the

efficiency in obtaining hemostasis, with no need for major or more aggressive surgical procedures. In fact, Poggetti et al. [9] commented that they believed that many of the major injuries involved hepatic veins, and this technique may also control hepatic venous bleeding. While intrahepatic abscesses have been noted as a complication in a small number of cases, a direct cause and result to balloon compression has not been established.

In summary, several easily applicable alternatives to major hepatic resection are available in the trauma surgeon's armamentarium. They can be highly successful in carefully selected patients with complex, bi-lobar transfixing lesions of the liver.

Video Captions

Video 11   Digital compression (MP4 16750 kb)
Video 13   Intraparenchymal balloon tamponade (MP4 92292 kb)

References

1. Stone HH, Lamb JM. Use of pedicled omentum as an autogenous pack for control of hemorrhage in major injuries of the liver. Surg Gynecol Obstet. 1975;141: 92–4.
2. Fabian TC, Stone HH. Arrest of severe liver hemorrhage by an omental pack. South Med J. 1980;73: 1487–90.
3. Pachter HL, Spencer FC. The management of complex hepatic trauma. Controversies in surgery II. Philadelphia: WB Suanders; 1983.
4. Bluett MK, Woltering E, Adkins RB. Management of penetrating hepatic injury. A review of 102 consecutive patients. Am Surg. 1984;50:132–42.
5. Morimoto RY, Birolini D, Junqueira Jr AR, et al. Balloon tamponade for transfixing lesions of the liver. Surg Gynecol Obstet. 1987;164(1):87–8.
6. Smaniotto B, Von Bahten L, Filho D, et al. Hepatic trauma: analysis of the treatment with intrahepatic balloon in a university hospital of Curitiba. Rev Col Bras Cir. 2009;36(3):217–22, Rio de Janeiro.
7. Branco PD, Poggetti R, Bernini CO, et al. Balão de tamponamento em ferimentos transfixantes do fígado: resultados imediatos. Rev Hosp Clin Fac Med Sao Paulo. 1988;43(1):20–5.
8. Fávero S, Corsi P, Coimbra R, et al. Treatment of transfixing hepatic lesions with a hydrostatic balloon. Sao Paulo Med J. 1994;112(4):629–34, São Paulo.
9. Poggetti RS, Moore EE, Moore FA, et al. Balloon tamponade for bilobar transfixing hepatic gunshot wounds. J Trauma. 1992;33:694.

Liver Packing

12

David V. Feliciano

Introduction

With a blood supply of 1,500 ml/min, the greatest priority in patients with hepatic trauma is control of hemorrhage. Simple techniques such as temporary pressure, topical hemostatic agents, use of the electrocautery or argon beam coagulator, or suture will stop bleeding in approximately 90 % of patients with penetrating wounds and 60 % of patients with blunt trauma [1]. More advanced techniques described elsewhere in this text will control hemorrhage in most of the remaining patients. There are several subsets of patients, however, in whom the surgeon will need to use the technique of "liver packing" for hepatic hemostasis. While very useful, liver packing is a trade-off for the trauma surgeon in that there is now a foreign body in the abdomen and the need for a reoperation for removal.

History

Packing to control hemorrhage from the liver is not a new technique. In the 1890s and early 1900s, hepatic lacerations were filled with gauze and sutures placed over this to create a tampon

D.V. Feliciano, MD
Division of General Surgery, Department of Surgery,
Indiana University Medical Center,
545 Barnhill Drive, EH 509, Indianapolis,
IN 46202, USA
e-mail: davfelic@iupui.edu

[2–5]. Carl Beck of Chicago used rolled-up iodoform packing to obtain hemostasis after resection of a massive hepatic angioma during this same period [6]. Intrahepatic packing for trauma remained a common form of operative management though perihepatic packing was employed for the first time in civilian life in the late 1920s. In 1936, Krieg from Detroit Receiving Hospital stated that "the hepatic wound was treated by packing in forty-one cases and by suture in 15 cases. It is of interest to note that in the majority of cases the gauze was not inserted into the wound with enough pressure to control hemorrhage and frequently it was merely placed against the wound, yet in no case was there alarming bleeding after the patient returned to the ward" [7]. Intrahepatic packing was performed in selected American casualties during World War II but was eventually condemned by former military and civilian authorities [8, 9]. In 1947, J.D. Martin Jr. of Atlanta stated that "hemorrhage is controlled in most instances by packing. The possibility of infection is increased by this procedure and after removal, secondary hemorrhage may occur and necessitate repacking. A liver which has been too tightly packed may develop pressure necrosis" [10].

Packing of some type continued to be used in civilian centers in the "more massive hepatic injuries where there was a loss of hepatic substance" [11]. Despite the recognized need for occasional packing, there was continuing concern "because of necrosis and infection around the packing and hemorrhage after its removal"

R.R. Ivatury (ed.), *Operative Techniques for Severe Liver Injury*,
DOI 10.1007/978-1-4939-1200-1_12, © Springer Science+Business Media New York 2015

[12]. In A. J. Walt's oft-quoted lecture to the Royal College of Surgeons of England in 1969, he stated that "there is virtually no place in modern surgery for gauze packing of the liver as sepsis and recurrent bleeding are almost inevitable sequelae" [13].

It is of interest that C.E. Lucas and A.M. Ledgerwood from Walt's department at Wayne State University subsequently helped along with others to revive the technique of perihepatic packing [14, 15]. In 1976, they described three patients in a series of 637 with hepatic injuries who survived following the insertion of perihepatic packs [14]. Subsequently, Calne et al. at the University of Cambridge reported on four patients transferred to their hospital in England after perihepatic packing had been inserted at other hospitals [16].

In 1980, the group from Ben Taub General Hospital/Baylor College of Medicine reported on ten patients with major hepatic trauma and secondary intraoperative hypothermia, acidosis, and coagulopathies [17]. After using standard techniques of hepatic hemostasis, perihepatic packs were inserted. Nine of ten patients survived, and there were no instances of rebleeding following removal of the packs. A large number of papers on perihepatic packing followed over the next decade, and all but one were supportive of the technique including two large clinical reviews [18–26].

Over the past 25 years, further descriptions of indications, newer operative techniques, and the risks of perihepatic packing have been published.

Indications

As perihepatic packing is the prototypical and one of the original techniques of "damage control laparotomy," it is used in a highly selected group of injured patients undergoing laparotomy [27, 28].

In the era before "damage control resuscitation" (limit crystalloids; administer packed red blood cells: fresh frozen plasma; platelets as "1:1:1") and even at present, the most common indication for insertion of perihepatic packing is an *intraoperative coagulopathy* associated with hypothermia and acidosis. When a coagulopathy does occur during operation on an AAST grade IV–V injury, commonly used advanced techniques of hemostasis such as resectional debridement or hepatotomy with selective vascular ligation may be ineffective. This is primarily because further hepatic parenchyma including numerous small vessels is exposed utilizing these approaches. Options at this point include topical application of oxidized regenerated cellulose, microfibrillar collagen hemostat, or commercially available fibrin glue. With the cellulose or collagen products, temporary intraoperative perihepatic packing is used to add a tamponade effect to the hemostatic effect of the topical agent. When these options are ineffective, the use of the electrocautery or argon beam coagulator is appropriate. As per the technique utilized by elective hepatic surgeons in the days before advanced power sources such as the CUSA (Cavitron Ultrasonic Surgical Aspirator, Integra LifeSciences, Plainsboro, NJ) device or the Aquamantys (Medtronic, Minneapolis, MN), the electrocautery is increased to 80 J to coagulate the oozing areas mentioned above. Should hepatic oozing continue and the patient remains hypothermic and acidotic from the hemorrhage-induced shock state, perihepatic packing is inserted.

A second major indication for the insertion of perihepatic packing is the presence of a *large subcapsular hematoma* of the liver. Such hematomas often have a laceration under them, so formal operative management mandates opening of the elevated hepatic capsule, evacuation of the hematoma, repair of the laceration, and reclosure of the capsule versus application of a synthetic capsule (absorbable mesh). In patients with multiple intra-abdominal injuries and extensive bilobar or expanding hematomas, this combination of procedures may be too time-consuming. The goals of inserting perihepatic packing with this clinical scenario are tamponade of hemorrhage from the underlying laceration and prevention of expansion and possible rupture of the subcapsular hematoma [20].

A third major indication for the insertion of perihepatic packing is the presence of a *hepatic injury in the setting of multiple other intra-abdominal injuries.* When multiple resections or repairs of other organs will be necessary in the patient with profound hypovolemic shock, the insertion of perihepatic packing around the hepatic injury is appropriate. Such a maneuver saves time during a "damage control laparotomy" and will allow for earlier transfer of the patient to the intensive care unit for rewarming and resuscitation [27, 28]. Perihepatic packing that does not control the hemorrhage from the hepatic injury, however, is inappropriate.

A fourth major indication for the insertion of perihepatic packing is the *presence of a major hepatic injury (grade IV or V) and an inexperienced surgical team and/or patient in a hospital with limited resources* (i.e., *no blood bank, no intensive* care unit, *no interventional radiology*). Tight perihepatic packing, even if it subsequently causes an abdominal compartment syndrome, is appropriate till a more experienced surgeon is available or the patient is transferred to a trauma center or to next higher echelon of military care [29].

A fifth major indication for the insertion of perihepatic packing is a *slowly enlarging, non-pulsatile, unruptured retrohepatic hematoma* [30]. The risk of this "conservative" approach is that some of these hematomas may cover a right renal injury rather than an injury to a hepatic vein or retrohepatic vena cava. Therefore, hemorrhage could be controlled by treatment of the right renal injury without the need for perihepatic packing. In other patients in whom the hematoma is obviously retrohepatic, perihepatic packing is inserted to avoid the complex, low-yield techniques traditionally used for venous injuries in this location (direct lateral approach, hepatic vascular isolation, transhepatic direct approach, and insertion of an atriocaval shunt) [31, 32].

Timing of Packing

In addition to the choice of appropriate patients who will benefit from the technique of perihepatic packing, the proper timing of insertion must be decided upon, as well.

A patient with a solitary major hepatic injury (AAST Hepatic Organ Injury Scales IV–V) should have a Pringle maneuver placed, division of the ligaments of the injured lobe, and advanced techniques of hepatic hemostasis performed. If hepatic hemostasis is difficult to attain or if attempts are prolonged (>30 min), the surgeon should decide as to whether nonmechanical (coagulopathy) vs. mechanical bleeding is present. The absence of mechanical bleeding, the presence of diffuse oozing, the presence of other components of the "lethal triad" (hypothermia, metabolic acidosis), and a total body "exchange transfusion" ($\geq$10 units packed red blood cells) should prompt perihepatic packing. It should be noted that some authors in the past have stated that perihepatic packing should be inserted immediately upon visualization of a major blunt hepatic injury [30]. If hemorrhage from the liver is controlled, the surgeon is encouraged to leave the pack in place rather than get into the "pack and peek" technique criticized by Beal in 1990 [30].

When a patient undergoing an emergency or urgent laparotomy is noted to have a hepatic subcapsular hematoma in isolation or in the presence of other intra-abdominal injuries, the extent is quickly marked with a marker pen. Perihepatic packing is immediately placed if anatomically feasible, and the time is recorded. In the patient with an isolated subcapsular hematoma, the packs are removed 15 min later. A hematoma that has not expanded and does not do so over 15 more minutes of intraoperative observation does not need further packing. Expansion of the hematoma after removal of the packs is managed with repeat packing and closure of the skin of the incision or application of a Pringle maneuver, capsulotomy, and hepatic repair as needed. The same sequence would be used in the hemodynamically stable patient with multiple injuries after these have been treated.

In patients with multiple intra-abdominal injuries that are causing bleeding, immediate perihepatic packing of an AAST grade III or less hepatic injury is appropriate. Should some hemorrhage from the liver continue to occur, a carefully timed Pringle maneuver (15–30 min) is performed as

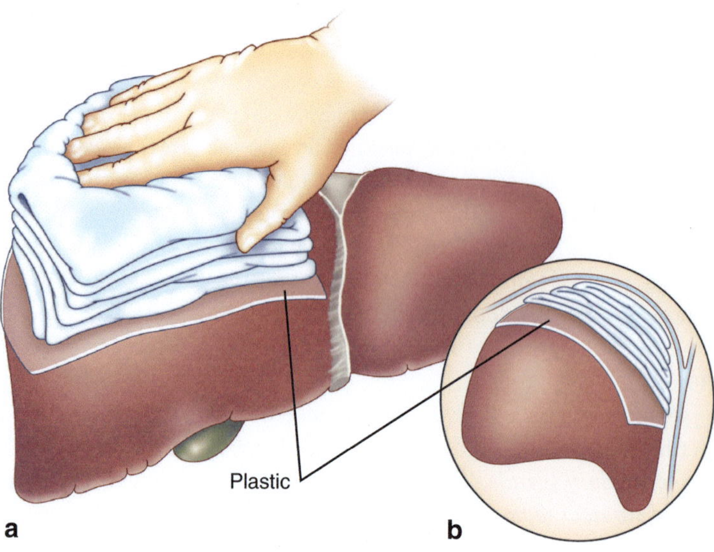

Fig. 12.1 A folded plastic drape is placed between the surface of the liver and the folded dry laparotomy pads used as perihepatic packing (**a**) anterior view (**b**) saggital view (Adapted from Feliciano et al. [20]. Used with permission)

other severe injuries are treated. As a bleeding grade IV or V hepatic injury is less likely to respond to perihepatic packing, only temporary intraoperative packing is used until direct hepatic hemostasis is attempted.

A patient with a major hepatic injury being treated by an inexperienced surgeon or in a hospital with limited resources *or* one with a slowly enlarging unruptured retrohepatic hematoma is treated with immediate insertion of perihepatic packing. "Pack and peek" is avoided, once again, if the packing has controlled hepatic hemorrhage or the expansion of the retrohepatic hematoma. Patients in the former group are transferred once stabilized as previously noted. In the latter group, a reoperation for removal of the packs and inspection of the hematoma is planned within 24–72 h.

Technique of Perihepatic Packing

Depending on the indication, hepatic packing for tamponade will be placed directly on the injured liver, on the area of repair, or on the lobe overlying a retrohepatic hematoma. When first revivified in the 1970s and early 1980s, little thought was given to the technique of perihepatic packing other than to accomplish tamponade of venous bleeding and capillary oozing. Once complications related to the insertion of perihepatic packing (rather than intrahepatic packing) were

recognized in the early series, a number of refinements in packing were described [20, 33]. These have continued through the present era [34].

With packing onto an injured lobe directly or onto sites of hepatic sutures, there is a tendency for the packs to dry out if bleeding is rapidly controlled. Much as with intrahepatic packing used in the past, this can result in adherence of the packs to the injured liver at the time of pack removal. Therefore, bleeding may recur when the packs and adherent clot are removed. For this reason, it is worthwhile to insert some type of plastic barrier between the injured or repaired liver and the packs [20] (Fig. 12.1). This technique was first described by William S. Halsted in the early 1900s when treating patients needing packing for "cavities after sequestrectomy" in the extremities [35]. A readily available piece of plastic is the nonadherent part of one of the skin covers commonly used in the operating room. This material is thin, lightweight, can be cut to size to cover the injured liver only, and is easily removed at the time the packs are removed.

Perihepatic packing placed directly over the liver anterior to the suprarenal and retrohepatic inferior vena cava can lead to compression of these structures. This compression can potentially collapse the renal veins and contribute to an abdominal compartment syndrome or be a direct cause of acute kidney injury. The risk of this secondary insult is surely increased in patients with recent hemorrhage and hypovolemic shock. In almost all patients with injuries crossing hepatic segments V, VIII, and IV, every effort should be made to place perihepatic packs either laterally or medially and direct posterior pressure in an oblique fashion. Avoiding direct posterior compression at a pressure greater than 30 mmHg in this location should prevent collapse of the renal veins [36].

Perihepatic compression from packs is lost in patients in whom the abdomen is left open under a silo or vacuum suction device. For this reason, it is appropriate to towel clip the skin edges of the upper 1/3 of the midline abdominal incision in patients in whom the rest of the abdomen will remain open. This will maintain the tamponading effect of the perihepatic packs in such patients and, if performed properly, should still avoid causing an abdominal compartment syndrome.

Other Techniques

In 1994, McHenry et al. [33] described an approach to packing that combined the use of intrahepatic omental packs and current perihepatic approaches [37]. After selective intrahepatic ligation of major vessels and segmental bile ducts, a mobilized piece of viable omentum is placed into the hepatic defect. This is covered with a nonadherent plastic drape, and perihepatic packs are placed anterior and posterior to the liver (Fig. 12.2). At the time of reoperation, the perihepatic gauze packs and plastic drape are removed. The omentum is left in place in the hepatic defect without suturing, perihepatic drains are inserted, and the midline incision is closed.

Another variation of the old technique of intrahepatic packing was reported by Ong et al. [38] in 2007. In a patient on anticoagulants who sustained a gunshot wound from the "dome of the right lobe" to the inferior surface of "segment IV", a large "tunnel" was left in the liver. Because of ongoing hemorrhage, a plastic bowel bag was inserted through the "tunnel" in the liver. Three laparotomy pads were then placed into the bag creating intrahepatic tamponade (Fig. 12.3). At the time of relaparotomy, the laparotomy pads were removed from the intrahepatic bag. Bleeding

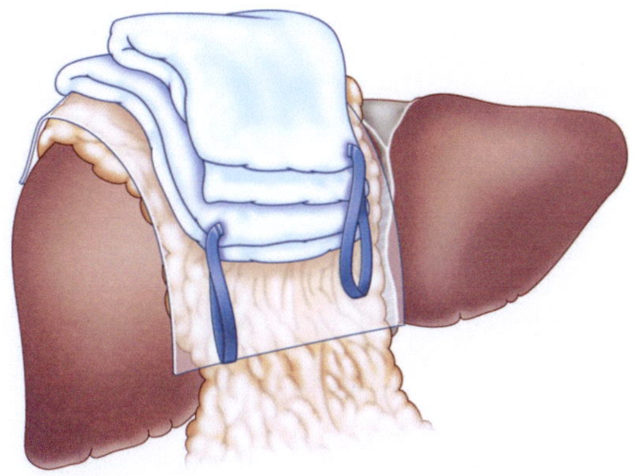

Fig. 12.2 Intrahepatic omental packing is covered with a plastic drape and laparotomy pads are placed above this for compression (Adapted from McHenry et al. [33], Copyright 1994, with permission from Elsevier)

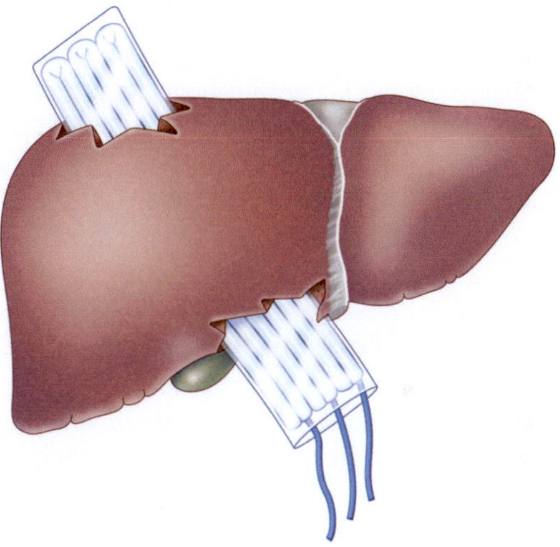

Fig. 12.3 Intrahepatic plastic bag filled with laparotomy pads (Adapted from Ong et al. [38])

did not recur over a period of 20 min, and the plastic bag was removed.

A "refinement in the technique of perihepatic packing" has been described by Baldoni et al. [34] from Bologna, Italy, in recent years. The right lobe of the injured liver is completely mobilized by division of the right triangular and anterior right coronary ligaments. Laparotomy pads are then packed around the posterior paracaval surface (without compressing the retrohepatic inferior vena cava [36]); the lateral right lobe, anterior to the lobe; and posteroinferior to the lobe. The authors' comparison of results in

Table 12.1 Comparison of the results in two groups of patients treated with the old and "refined" perihepatic packing

	Old technique 1996–2004	"Refined" technique 2005–2008	p
# Patients	23	12	–
Grade IV/V	16/7	9/3	.260
Base deficit on arrival	–10.7	–8	.200
Liver-related complications	41.7 %	18.2 %	0.97
Intra-abdominal sepsis	41.7 %	9.1 %	0.076
Death within 24 h	52.2 %	8.3 %	0.01
Overall survival	30.4 %	75 %	0.015

Modified from Baldoni et al. [34], Copyright 2011, with permission from Elsevier

patients with grades IV–V injury using an older technique of packing in 23 patients from 1996 to 2004 versus the "refined" technique described above in 12 patients from 2005 to 2008 is in Table 12.1. The authors have continued to analyze their results with this newer approach [39].

Removal of Perihepatic Packing

In the past, there was a technique of bringing long gauze perihepatic packing out of a hole in the lateral abdominal wall at the first operation. The intent was to allow for subsequent removal of the packing without a relaparotomy. This technique has been slowly abandoned over the past 35 years as rebleeding was common, missed injuries could not be searched for, and the abdomen could not be irrigated.

The need for a relaparotomy, however, has its own "side effects." It mandates a return trip to the operating room, a second general anesthetic, and a further manipulation of the injured liver and edematous midgut, and it may cause a "second hit" phenomenon [40]. Therefore, the timing of a relaparotomy would appear to be a critical decision for the trauma surgeon. Unfortunately, little scientific evidence exists to support any postsurgery day as being ideal for all patients.

In the 1981 review of ten patients by Feliciano et al. [17], perihepatic packing was removed from 8 h to 10 days (mean 5.2 days). The patient with the longest delay till pack removal developed severe respiratory failure and anuric renal failure after the first trauma laparotomy. A second review of 49 patients from the same group in 1986 described the timing of removal as being based on the patient's condition: "Patients without evidence of further bleeding are returned to the operating room for pack removal when the cardiovascular system is stable, coagulopathies have been corrected, and only the respiratory system is being supported" [20]. The authors noted that the timing of pack removal depended on the timing of insertion of the packing, as well. In 22 patients who survived after perihepatic packing was inserted at the first trauma laparotomy, removal of the packing was performed at a mean of 3.3 days. The six patients who survived after perihepatic packing was inserted at a reoperation (continuing hemorrhage; ruptured subcapsular hematoma) had removal of the packing performed at a mean of 5.5 days. Of interest, later postoperative intra-abdominal fluid collections, hematomas, or abscesses occurred in 9 of the 47 patients (18.4 %) surviving the first trauma laparotomy in this review. Five of the ten drained collections in these nine patients were purulent for a 10.2 % incidence of perihepatic abscess.

Another approach was used by Carmona et al. [19] in the early 1980s. In a review of 17 patients who underwent temporary perihepatic packing: "The average time between the first and second operation was 17 h (range of 10–28 h) to remove the packs and reexplore the liver." No rationale for such early removal of the packing was presented in the manuscript.

In the later review of patients with perihepatic packing by Krige et al. [41] from Cape Town, South Africa, the authors noted that "six of the 16 survivors in this series developed sepsis and one patient died of septicaemia; five of these seven patients had an associated bowel or biliary injury." The authors recommended that patients with isolated hepatic injuries have removal of packing at 48 h "after correction of coagulation and metabolic abnormalities…in the liver injuries with gross bowel contamination or bile leaks…packs should be retrieved at relaparotomy within 24 h."

One of the most helpful reviews with regard to timing of pack removal was by Caruso et al. [42] from the University of California, Davis, in 1999. In this interesting report, outcomes were compared between 39 patients who had perihepatic packing removed within 36 h of insertion and 24 patients who had packing removed 36–72 h after insertion. While rebleeding requiring repacking was significantly more common in the early pack removal group (early 21 % vs. late 4 %, $p<0.001$), liver-related complications (early 33 % vs. late 29 %) and mortality (early 18 % vs. late 29 %) were similar.

Similar findings were noted in the review by Nicol et al. [43] from Groote Schuur Hospital in Cape Town, South Africa, in 2007. Perihepatic packing was inserted in 17 % of all patients with hepatic injuries noted at laparotomy, and the mean duration of packing was 2.4 days. Early removal of packs at 24 h led to a higher rate of rebleeding when compared to the group of patients with removal at 48 h ($p=0.006$). As in the review by Caruso et al. [42], the total duration of perihepatic packing (1 vs. 2 vs. 3 or longer days) had no impact on postoperative liver-related complications or the development of intra-abdominal collections.

In essence, "damage control" principles apply when considering the timing of removal of perihepatic packing. Hypothermia, acidosis, and coagulopathies should be corrected, and the patients should be in the "diuretic phase" of recovery from resuscitated hemorrhagic shock. Consideration should be given to an earlier return to the operating room (48 h) in patients with extensive gastrointestinal contamination noted at the first trauma laparotomy.

Complications

Complications related to perihepatic packing are difficult to distinguish from those due to the hepatic injury itself. For example, the earliest complication that might be attributed to perihepatic packing would be *failure to control hepatic hemorrhage*. This could be due, however, to failure of the surgeon to control intrahepatic arterial hemorrhage or delaying the insertion of packs till an intraoperative coagulopathy is well established. The former is the most likely cause of persistent post-packing hemorrhage in the modern era. For this reason, immediate postoperative hepatic arteriography with therapeutic embolization is indicated whenever the surgeon is aware that hepatic hemorrhage has not been fully controlled by the perihepatic packing. In the intensive care unit, continued hepatic hemorrhage is suggested by the need for continuing transfusion of two units of packed red blood cells per hour.

It has been recognized for over 25 years that the insertion of perihepatic packing will elevate intra-abdominal pressure and may cause an *abdominal compartment syndrome* [20]. This may occur with formal musculofascial closure of the midline incision, towel clip closure of the skin of the incision only, or the application of a silo. This complication is acceptable in the short term as previously noted if tight packing will maintain hemostasis until the patient can be transferred, a senior surgeon arrives, or therapeutic embolization can be performed [29]. In the 1995 review by Meldrum et al. [44] from Denver General Hospital, cardiopulmonary data were measured in patients before and after removal of perihepatic packing. Pulmonary capillary wedge pressure and systemic vascular resistance decreased, while cardiac index and oxygen delivery increased significantly after removal of packing. In similar fashion, peak airway pressure decreased, while static compliance and PaO_2 to FiO_2 ratios increased significantly after removal. As noted previously, packing should be inserted in an oblique fashion to avoid compression of the suprarenal and retrohepatic inferior vena cava if at all possible. Should towel clip closure of the upper 1/3 of the midline incision be used to maintain hepatic tamponade as previously suggested, loose silo coverage of the remainder of the abdomen should decrease the incidence of the abdominal compartment syndrome.

Other complications related to the magnitude of the hepatic injury and the presence of perihepatic packing are intra-abdominal fluid collections, hematomas, and abscesses. In Moore's review of the management of hepatic injuries at eight level I trauma centers in 1984, the post-repair perihepatic abscess rate was 4 % when all grades of injury were included [25].

As noted above, the author's review in 1986 documented an incidence of 18.4 % of perihepatic fluid collections, hematomas, or abscesses in patients with perihepatic packing who survived beyond the first operation [20]. The actual incidence of perihepatic abscesses was 10.2 %, which falls in the range of similar complications from major elective hepatic resection or hepatic transplantation at the time [45]. In the review by Ivatury et al. [21] in 1986, five of the six survivors (83.3 %) developed intra-abdominal abscesses after removal of the packing. The incidence of "intra-abdominal sepsis" has been reported as low as 9.1 % in the recent review by Baldoni et al. [34] and the incidence of "intra-abdominal collections" as high as 44.4 % in the 2007 review by Nicol et al. [43].

Survival

The survival for patients with hepatic injuries who were treated with perihepatic packing as primary therapy or as an adjunct over the past 40 years is summarized in Table 12.2.

Table 12.2 Results with perihepatic packing of hepatic injuries

Author	Year	Total patients	Survival	Survival rate (%)
Lucas [14]	1976	3	3	100
Calne [16]	1979	4	4	100
Feliciano [17]	1981	10	9	90
Svoboda [18]	1982	12	10	83
Carmona [19]	1984	17	15	88
Feliciano [20]	1986	49	28	57
Ivatury [21]	1986	14	6	43
Baracco-Gandolfo [22]	1986	36	30	83
Krige [41]	1992	22	16	23
Caruso [42]	1999	123	47	38[a]
Richardson [46]	2000	21	13	62
Nicol [43]	2007	72	65	90[b]
Baldoni [34]	2011	12	11	92
DiSaverio [39]	2012	39	19	48[a]
Total	–	434	276	64

[a]Grade IV and V injuries only
[b]Deaths in first 24 h not included

References

1. Feliciano DV, Mattox KL, Jordan Jr GL, et al. Management of 1000 consecutive cases of hepatic trauma. Ann Surg. 1986;204:438–43.
2. Ponfick VA. Surgery of the liver. Lancet. 1890;1:881.
3. Kousnetzoff L, Penski J. Sur la resection partielle du foie. Rev Chir. 1896;16:501,954.
4. Tilton BT. Some considerations regarding wounds of the liver. Ann Surg. 1905;41:20–30.
5. Schroeder WE. The progress of liver hemostasis – reports of cases (resection, sutures, etc.). Surg Gynecol Obstet. 1906;2:52–61.
6. Beck C. Surgery of the liver. JAMA. 1902;38:1063–8.
7. Krieg EG. Hepatic trauma. Analysis of 60 cases. Arch Surg. 1936;32:907–14.
8. Madding GF. Injuries of the liver. Arch Surg. 1955; 70:748–56.
9. Madding GF. Wounds of the liver. Surg Clin North Am. 1958;38:1619–29.
10. Martin Jr JD. Wounds of the liver. Ann Surg. 1947; 125:756–67.
11. Mikesky WE, Howard JM, DeBakey ME. Injuries of the liver in 300 consecutive patients. Surg Gynecol Obstet. 1956;103:323–37.
12. Morton JR, Rays GD, Bricker DL. The treatment of liver injuries. Surg Gynecol Obstet. 1972;134:298–302.
13. Walt AJ. The surgical management of hepatic trauma and its complications. Ann R Coll Surg Engl. 1969;45:319–39.
14. Lucas CE, Ledgerwood AM. Prospective evaluation of hemostatic techniques for liver injuries. J Trauma. 1976;16:442–51.
15. Lascar R. A propos de plaies hepatiques. Le tamponnement par change a demeure. Bull Mem Soc Chirurg Paris. 1971;61:201–2.
16. Calne RY, McMaster P, Pentlow BD. The treatment of major liver trauma by primary packing with transfer of the patients for definitive treatment. Br J Surg. 1979;66:338–9.
17. Feliciano DV, Mattox KL, Jordan Jr GL. Intra-abdominal packing for control of hepatic hemorrhage: a reappraisal. J Trauma. 1981;21:285–90.
18. Svoboda JA, Peter ET, Dang CV, Parks SN, Ellyson JH. Severe liver trauma in the face of coagulopathy. A case for temporary packing and early reexploration. Am J Surg. 1982;144:717–21.
19. Carmona RH, Peck DZ, Lim Jr RC. The role of packing and planned reoperation in severe hepatic trauma. J Trauma. 1984;24:779–84.
20. Feliciano DV, Mattox KL, Burch JM, Bitondo CG, Jordan Jr GL. Packing for control of hepatic hemorrhage. J Trauma. 1986;26:738–43.
21. Ivatury RR, Nallathambi M, Gunduz Y, Constable R, Rohman M, Stahl WM. Liver packing for uncontrolled hemorrhage: a reappraisal. J Trauma. 1986; 26:744–53.
22. Baracco-Gandolfo V, Vidarte O, Baracco-Miller V, del Castillo M. Prolonged closed liver packing in

severe hepatic trauma: experience with 36 patients. J Trauma. 1986;26:754–6.

23. Saifi J, Fortune JB, Graca L, Shah DM. Benefits of intra-abdominal pack placement for the management of nonmechanical hemorrhage. Arch Surg. 1990;125:119–22.

24. Cué JI, Cryer HG, Miller FB, Richardson D, Polk Jr HC. Packing and planned reexploration for hepatic and retroperitoneal hemorrhage: critical refinements of a useful technique. J Trauma. 1990;30:1007–13.

25. Moore EE. Critical decisions in the management of hepatic trauma. Am J Surg. 1984;148:712–6.

26. Cogbill TH, Moore EE, Jurkovich GJ, Feliciano DV, Morris JA, Mucha P. Severe hepatic trauma: a multi-center experience with 1,335 liver injuries. J Trauma. 1988;28:1433–8.

27. Feliciano DV, Burch JM, Spjut-Patrinely V, Mattox KL, Jordan Jr G. Abdominal gunshot wounds: an urban trauma centers experience with 300 consecutive patients. Ann Surg. 1988;208:362–70.

28. Rotondo MF, Schwab DC, McGonigal MD, Phillips GR, Fruchterman TM, Kauder DR, et al. Damage control: an approach for improved survival in exsanguinating penetrating abdominal injury. J Trauma. 1993;35:375–82.

29. Strong RW. The management of blunt liver injuries. ANZ J Surg. 1999;69:609–16.

30. Beal SL. Fatal hepatic hemorrhage: an unresolved problem in the management of complex liver injuries. J Trauma. 1990;30:163–9.

31. Pachter HL, Spencer FC, Hofstetter SR, Liang HC, Coppa GF. The management of juxtahepatic venous injuries without an atrial-caval shunt: preliminary clinical observations. Surgery. 1986;99:569–75.

32. Burch JM, Feliciano DV, Mattox KL. The atriocaval shunt. Facts and fiction. Ann Surg. 1988;207:555–68.

33. McHenry CR, Federle GM, Malangoni MA. A refinement in the technique of perihepatic packing. Am J Surg. 1994;168:280–2.

34. Baldoni F, DiSaverio S, Antonacci N, Coniglio C, Giugni A, Montanari N, et al. Refinement in the technique of perihepatic packing: a safe and effective surgical hemostasis and multidisciplinary approach can improve the outcome in severe liver trauma. Am J Surg. 2011;201:e5–14.

35. Halsted WS. The employment of fine silk in preference to catgut and the advantages of transfixion of tissues and vessels in control of hemorrhage. Also an account of the introduction of gloves, gutta-percha tissue and silver foil. JAMA. 1913;60:1119–26.

36. Gadzijev EM, Stanisavaljevic D, Mimica Z, Wahl M, Butinar J, Tomazic A. Can we evaluate the pressure of perihepatic packing? Results of a study on dogs. Injury. 1999;30:35–41.

37. Stone HH, Lamb JM. Use of pedicled omentum as an autogenous pack for control of hemorrhage in major injuries of the liver. Surg Gynecol Obstet. 1975;141:92–4.

38. Ong AW, Kelly R, Jeremitsky E, Cortes V, McAuley CE, Rodriguez A. Liver packing: a variation of an old technique. J Trauma. 2007;63:1405–6.

39. DiSaverio S, Catena F, Filicori F, Ansaloni L, Coccolini F, Keutgen XM, et al. Predictive factors of morbidity and mortality in grade IV and V liver trauma undergoing perihepatic packing: single institution 14 years experience at European trauma centre. Injury. 2012;43:1347–54.

40. Dewar D, Moore FA, Moore EE, Balogh Z. Post injury multiple organ failure. Injury. 2009;40:912–8.

41. Krige JE, Bornman PC, Terblanche J. Therapeutic perihepatic packing in complex liver trauma. Br J Surg. 1992;79:43–6.

42. Caruso DM, Battistella FD, Owings JT, Lee SL, Samaco RC. Perihepatic packing of major liver injuries. Complications and mortality. Arch Surg. 1999;134:958–63.

43. Nicol AJ, Hommes M, Primrose R, Navsaria PH, Krige JE. Packing for control of hemorrhage in major liver trauma. World J Surg. 2007;31:569–74.

44. Meldrum DR, Moore FA, Moore EE, Haenel JB, Cosgriff N, Burch JM. Cardiopulmonary hazards of perihepatic packing for major liver injuries. Am J Surg. 1995;170:537–42.

45. Feliciano DV, Pachter HL. Hepatic trauma revisited. Curr Probl Surg. 1989;26:453–524.

46. Richardson DJ, Franklin GA, Lukan JK, Carrillo EH, Spain DA, Miller FB, et al. Evolution in the management of hepatic trauma: a 25-year perspective. Ann Surg. 2000;232:324–30.

Damage Control Laparotomy

Carlos A. Ordoñez, Mauricio Millán,
and Michael W. Parra

Introduction

Abdominal trauma is a very common pathology at a busy emergency room department and associated liver injuries occur in up to 5 % of cases. This is probably due to the organ size in relationship to the rest of the abdominal cavity, which makes it vulnerable to penetrating and blunt trauma. Approximately 40 % of all penetrating abdominal traumas that require an emergent laparotomy are secondary to uncontrollable liver bleeding. The overall mortality from penetrating liver trauma fluctuates between 10 and 15 % and is dependent on the grade of the liver injury and the number of associated injuries [1]. In 1970, the concept of liver packing was introduced as a useful tool in the control of liver hemorrhage and as an integral component of damage control surgery. Since then, the management of parenchymal liver injuries has continued to evolve. Based on our experience, we set forth to describe a comprehensive surgical approach that deals with severe penetrating liver injuries which attempts to include all validated past and present techniques.

Hepatic Trauma Grading

According to the American Association for the Surgery of Trauma (AAST), liver trauma is graded by depth of organ injury (Table 13.1). This organ injury scale has its limitations due to the fact that it is a computerized tomography (CT)-based blunt trauma organ injury scale. Ferrada et al., from the University Hospital of Cali, Colombia, published a series of 1,005 patients with penetrating liver trauma with the following reported results.

Eighty-five percent of patients had AAST-OIS liver injuries grades I, II, and III and 15 % had injuries grades IV, V, and VI. The author created a new classification that can be performed intraoperatively and permits the surgeon to take rapid and concise treatment options accordingly:

Grade I: The bleeding is minor and can be controlled by temporary liver packing, topical hemostatic agents, and/or hepatorrhaphy.

Grade II: Moderate liver bleeding that requires a Pringle maneuver and perihepatic liver packing that is left in as part of a damage control approach.

C.A. Ordoñez, MD (✉)
Division of Trauma and Acute Care Surgery, Hospital Universitario del Valle, Fundación Valle del Lili, Cra 127 # 6-120, Cra 98 # 18-49, Cali 0000, Colombia

Department of Surgery, Universidad del Valle, Cali, Colombia
e-mail: ordonezcarlosa@gmail.com

M. Millán
Division of Trauma and Acute Care Surgery, Department of Surgery, Universidad del Valle, Calle 5a # 36-08, Cali 760050, Colombia

M.W. Parra, MD
Division of Trauma Critical Care, Broward General Level I Trauma Center, 1600 S. Andrews Avenue, Fort Lauderdale, FL 33316, USA

R.R. Ivatury (ed.), *Operative Techniques for Severe Liver Injury*,
DOI 10.1007/978-1-4939-1200-1_13, © Springer Science+Business Media New York 2015

Grade III: Liver bleeding that cannot be controlled with a Pringle maneuver and perihepatic packing or rebleeds once the Pringle is released. The source of bleeding is probably secondary to hepatic veins or retrohepatic vena caval injury. Additional advance surgical maneuvers are required for hemorrhage control [2].

Table 13.1 The American Association for the Surgery of Trauma (AAST) liver injury scale (1994 revision)

Grade	Injury description	
I	Hematoma	Subcapsular, <10 % surface area
	Laceration	Capsular tear, <1 cm parenchymal depth
II	Hematoma	Subcapsular, 10–50 % surface area; intraparenchymal, <10 cm diameter
	Laceration	1–3 cm parenchymal depth, <10 cm length
III	Hematoma	Subcapsular, >50 % surface area or expanding. Ruptured subcapsular or parenchymal hematoma; intraparenchymal hematoma >10 cm or expanding
	Laceration	>3 cm parenchymal depth
IV	Laceration	Parenchymal disruption involving 25–75 % of hepatic lobe or >3 Couinaud's segments within a single lobe
V	Laceration	Parenchymal disruption involving >75 % of hepatic lobe or 1–3 Couinaud's segments within a single lobe
	Vascular	Juxtahepatic venous injuries, i.e., retrohepatic vena cava/central major hepatic veins
VI	Vascular	Hepatic avulsion

Used with permission from Moore et al. [20]

Surgical Approach

The initial surgical approach to any penetrating abdominal trauma victim who arrives in severe hypovolemic shock is to perform an immediate exploratory laparotomy that permits a full exposure of the abdominal cavity and/or retroperitoneum. We recommend a stepwise approach:

Step 1: The hemoperitoneum must be collected, quantified, and autotransfused when possible. All four quadrants of the abdominal cavity should then be packed with special attention directed toward adequately packing the liver. We do not recommend using initially any plastic protective barrier between the liver and the packs because it is our experience that this interferes with the adequate placement of the packs. Following the initial perihepatic packing, we recommend a Pringle maneuver which can remain in place in most non-cirrhotic patients for up to 60 min and up to 15 min in those who are cirrhotic. The porta hepatis cross clamping can be repeated with reperfusion intervals of 5 min [3–7] (Fig. 13.1). Immediate bowel contamination is controlled

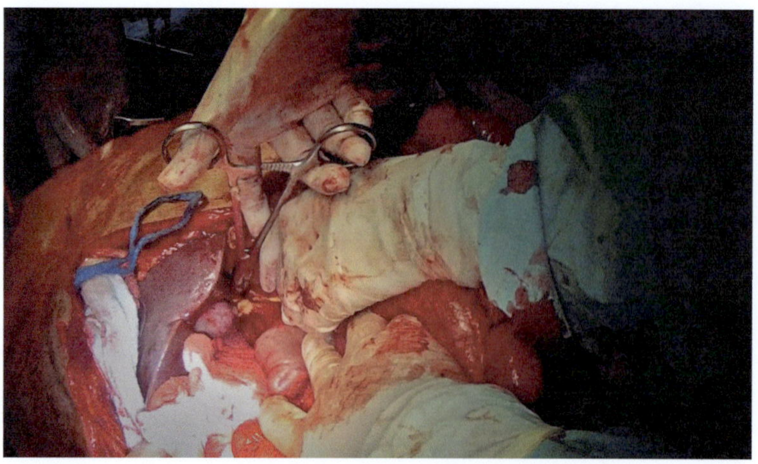

Fig. 13.1 Pringle maneuver

by quickly stapling or tying off any injured segments of small or large bowel.

Step 2: A complete quick systematic evaluation of all infra- and supra-mesocolic organs of the abdominal cavity is performed to determine the amount and extent of all associated injuries. At this point, an early determination must be made to determine the need to establish damage control resuscitation (DCR). For this purpose, we follow an explicit set of parameters that we have simplified in an easily remembered *ABCD* mnemonic. The presence of all four of the following components is necessary:

A = acidosis (base deficit > −8)

B = blood loss (hemoperitoneum > 1,500 mL)

C = cold (temperature < 35 C)

D = damage (New ISS [NISS] > 35)

At the same time, concepts of damage control surgery are simultaneously performed such as abdominal packing, aortic cross clamping, shunt placements for vascular trauma, and fecal contamination control [5].

Step 3: After having evacuated the hemoperitoneum and controlled all possible fecal contamination sources, we proceed on grading the liver injury. We use a modified penetrating liver injury scale devised by Ferrada et al., which is based on a vast experience over many years of an unfortunate Colombian drug-funded civil war:

Grade I: Upon removal of perihepatic packing, liver bleeding has stopped or requires simple techniques of hemostasis such as topical hemostatic agents and/or hepatorrhaphy and the procedure is truncated.

Grade II: The bleeding is controlled by combining a Pringle maneuver and perihepatic packing. The initial immediate liver packing upon laparotomy is removed, the extent of the liver injury is determined, a Pringle maneuver is placed resulting in a significant decrease in the bleeding, and then a definitive 8–10 packs are placed perihepatically. The definitive packing should be done as quickly as possible before the patient becomes coagulopathic. A prime principle of perihepatic packing is that the vectors of

compression created by the selective placement of the packs should result in an adequate compressive opposition of the fractured liver borders. To obtain this kind of packing, the liver needs to be completely mobilized and compressed manually by an assistant while the surgeon places the perihepatic packs. This usually requires two to four packs on each vector plane of compression. If there is a large deep laceration, then placement of intraparenchymal hemostatic agents should be done first, followed by gauze packing in a folded accordion fashion. We have learned that there are several technical mishaps regarding liver packing. The first is the issue of overpacking which can result in intra-abdominal hypertension with an associated decrease in cardiac preload and subsequent hemodynamic instability due to the decrease blood return from the compressed retrohepatic vena cava. Another common error is the other extreme of too few packs placed which results in an inefficacious compression of the liver injury and subsequent persistent bleeding. The initial damage control surgery should not be terminated until all ongoing surgical bleeding from the liver has been controlled. This can be verified by assuring that the most superficial packs remain dry and white. If this is not the case, then the packs should be removed and the liver injury reevaluated. In the case that the packs are dry, the Pringle maneuver is removed, and the condition of the packs is re-examined, if dry, then the surgery can be truncated. All of this should be done in the least time possible to avoid that the patient develops the triad of death: hypothermia, coagulopathy, and acidosis. The abdomen is washed out, temporary abdominal closure coverage is placed, and the patient is taken immediately to the intensive care unit to continue his damage control resuscitation.

Step 4: Some trauma surgeons advocate the complete mobilization of the liver at the time of the take back of the patient to visualize the injury and remove the packs (Fig. 13.2). We believe that if required, the mobilization of the liver should be done during the initial

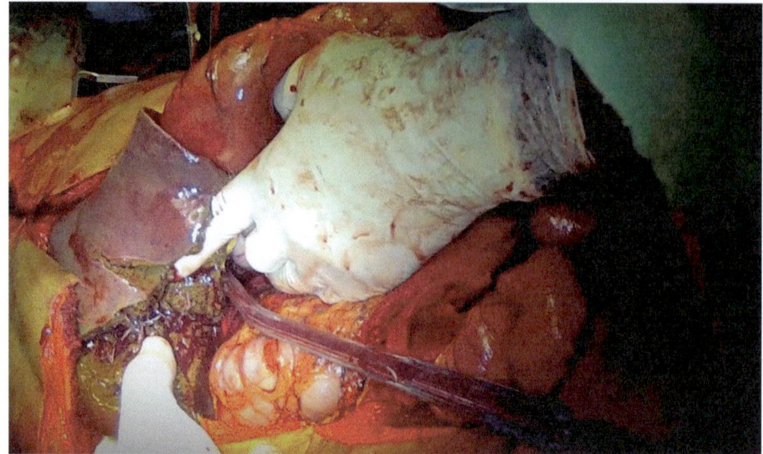

Fig. 13.2 Liver parenchymal injury exploration

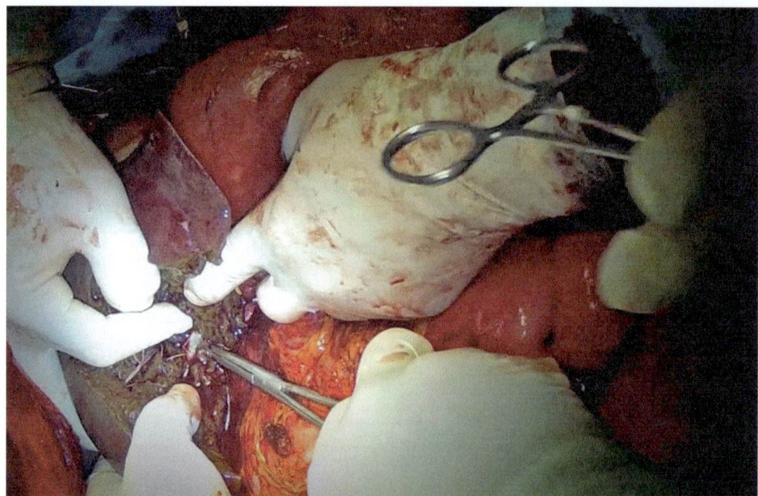

Fig. 13.3 Intraparenchymal vessel ligation

laparotomy and that performing it at any other time just increases the chances of rebleeding of an injury that had already subsided.

Some surgeons also advocate that after removal of the initial liver packing, the parenchymal injury should be reexplored leaving in discontinuity all exposed vascular or biliary duct ends. This is advocated by some with the aim of reducing the possibility of delayed complications such as the biliary fistulae. Although we agree with this concept, the timing of when and in whom it gets done is where we differ.

Another popular technique is liver injury packing with viable tissue such as the omentum. Although useful in minor liver injuries, we believe that in major parenchymal injuries of the liver with transected biliary ducts and/or vessels, the prevention of subsequent leaks and rebleeding is once again suboptimal in these cases.

Grade III: These are the liver injuries that fail initial management of a Pringle maneuver and perihepatic packing. This is confirmed by removing the Pringle and observing the liver bleed through the packs. The source of this bleeding is probably from transected suprahepatic vein(s) or from the retrohepatic vena cava.

Step 5: Re-clamp the porta hepatis immediately and reopen the liver injury to expose the bleeding vessel (Fig. 13.3). This is done with the finger fracture technique and systematically ligating or stapling all encountered biliary

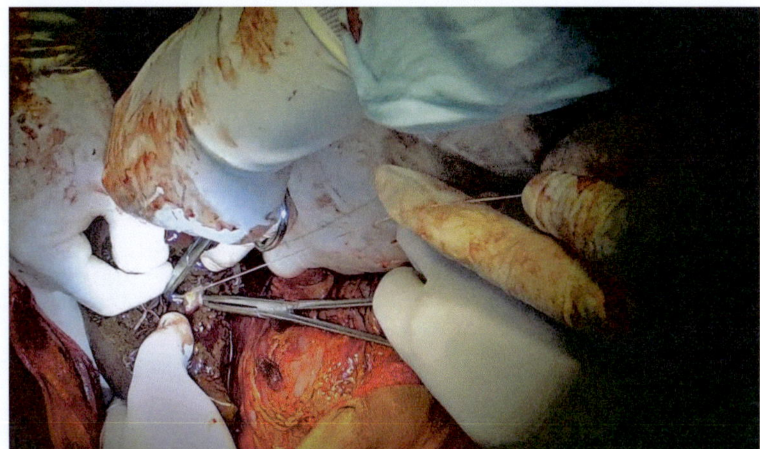

Fig. 13.4 Intraparenchymal selective vessel ligation

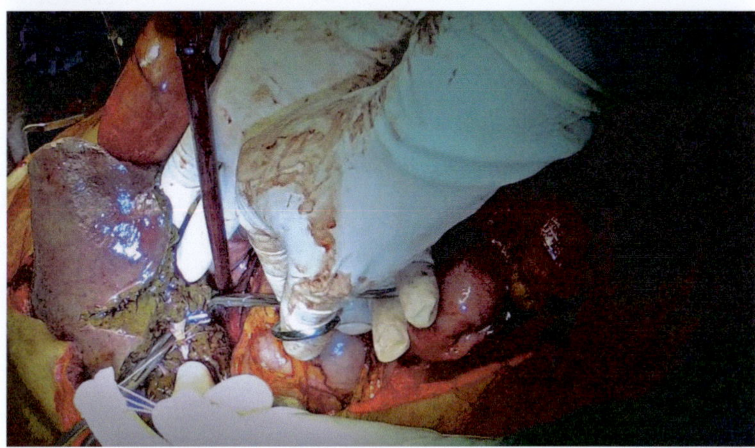

Fig. 13.5 Intraparenchymal vascular and biliary duct ligation

ducts and vasculature until the main bleeding vessel is completely exposed (Fig. 13.4). This process usually will require the joint effort of two able surgeons: one to expose and the other to tie (Fig. 13.5). Once the bleeding is controlled, then the exposed intrahepatic parenchyma is lined with hemostatic agents. If the parenchymal disruption is considerable, then we also advocate intrahepatic packing with one or two lap pads over the previously placed hemostatic agent(s), and then proceed with our conventional perihepatic packing. The Pringle maneuver is released and hemostasis of the superficial perihepatic packs is observed. If hemorrhage is controlled, then the patient undergoes temporary abdominal closure and is transferred to the ICU for further damage control resuscitation. If the

bleeding persists, then we recommend repeating step 5 and selective vessel ligation of all possible missed vascular structures.

Step 6: If hemorrhage cannot be controlled, then we recommend direct dissection of the porta hepatis and a selective ligation of the right or left hepatic artery and/or portal vein. These extreme scenarios usually lead to ischemic necrosis of the affected lobe that will most likely require a formal hepatic lobectomy. Once the bleeding is controlled, a temporary abdominal closure is performed and the patient is transferred to the ICU (Fig. 13.6).

Other techniques of hemorrhage control such as the pneumatic compression of the penetrating liver tract utilizing a Sengstaken-Blakemore or an improvised Foley catheter

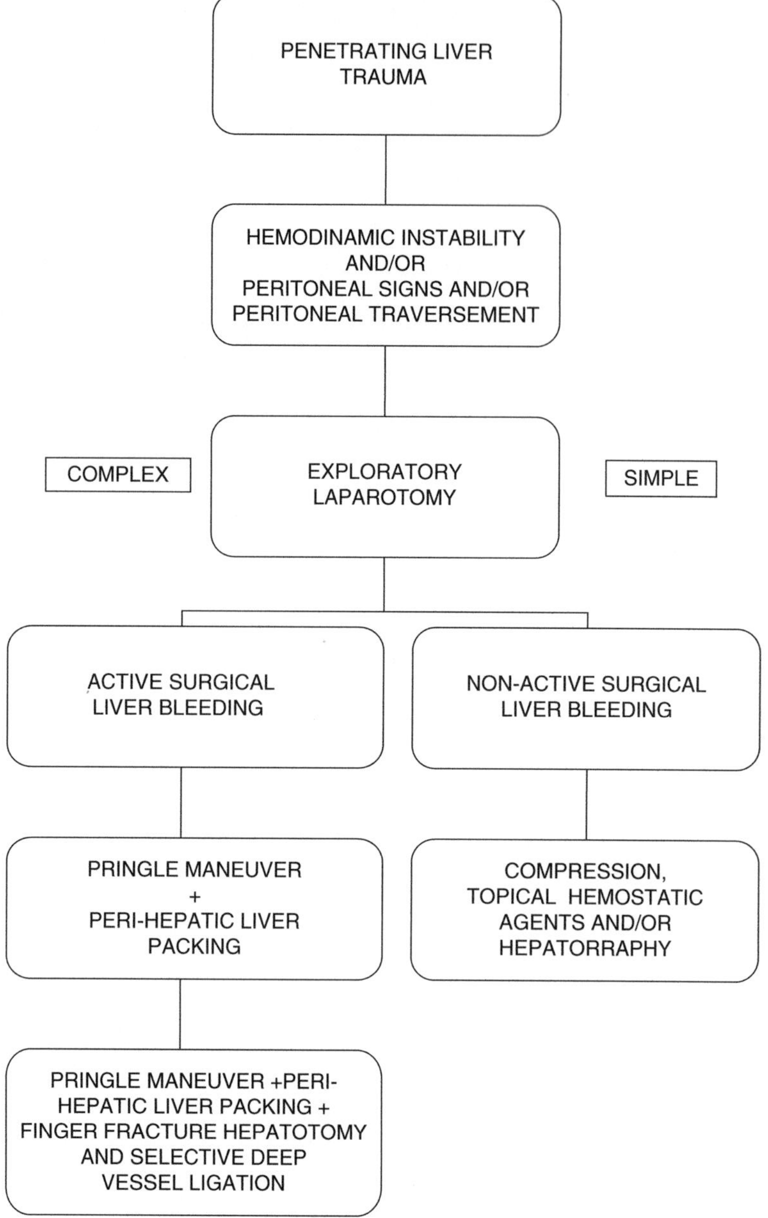

Fig. 13.6 Surgical management algorithm for severe liver trauma

with an attached condom have been advocated by some surgeons for deep transfixing liver injuries in which access seems difficult to obtain. Although this may be a viable option for many, we believe that it is more of an exceptional technique rather than the standard surgical approach to these injuries.

The actual process of unpacking should not be taken lightly by the treating surgeon. The packs are thoroughly moistened with warm crystalloid fluid and subsequently removed slowly taking great care to not evoke rebleeding. The utilization of a plastic barrier between the liver bed and the packs advocated by some surgeons has some inherent drawbacks such as the inability of the packs to promote homeostasis by direct contact and also the frequent dislodgment of the packs as they often slide out of position.

We have recently published our findings about the ideal time for abdominal pack removal in patients with damage control laparotomy which is about 2–3 days post injury. At this point in the treatment protocol, the cumulative incidence of complications with rebleeding and intra-abdominal infections is at its lowest. Abdominal packing should not be removed prior to the first postoperative day because of the increased risk of rebleeding, and if left in longer than 3 days, abdominal packing carries a significantly increased risk of infectious complications.

Injury to the retrohepatic vena cava has a well-known high mortality (65–100 %) and fortunately for the experienced trauma surgeon an overall low incidence [8–11]. This injury is commonly divided into two types:

Type A: The injury is intraparenchymal.

Type B: The injury is extraparenchymal.

These cases require an integral functioning of the trauma team especially between the trauma surgeon and the anesthesiologist who is in charge of the intraoperative damage control resuscitation. We advocate the combination of aortic cross clamping (thoracic or abdominal) followed by complete liver isolation. This is done in three steps. First, a Pringle is placed, followed by cross clamping of the infrahepatic suprarenal vena cava. The isolation is completed by cross clamping the suprahepatic vena cava which is done by opening the right diaphragm and placing the clamp supradiaphragmatic retrocardiac [12–14].

If the suprahepatic veins are injured, control of bleeding is obtained by performing a complete liver isolation followed by direct intraparenchymal ligation of the transected vessels [11].

We are currently revisiting at our institution the approach to these severe injuries and have devised a new protocol which includes the utilization of intravascular occlusion balloons (CODA®). Our inclusion criteria are all adult abdominal penetrating trauma victims who are hemodynamically unstable secondary to intra-abdominal exsanguination. The groin is incised and via a modified Seldinger technique, the femoral artery is accessed and an aortic occlusion balloon is floated up to the level of the supradiaphragmatic descending thoracic aorta.

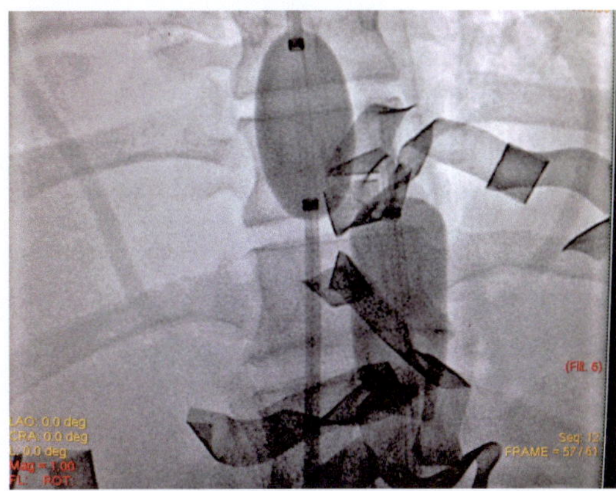

Fig. 13.7 Endovascular balloon occlusion technique

Confirmation is done by fluoroscopy visualizing the inflated balloon (intravenous contrast is utilized to inflate the balloon) in the descending thoracic aorta. For retrohepatic vena caval injuries, the femoral vein is accessed and two CODA balloons are floated, one at the level of the suprarenal infrahepatic vena cava and the second at the supradiaphragmatic vena cava (Fig. 13.7) [15–19].

References

1. Pachter HL, Feliciano DV. Complex hepatic injuries. Surg Clin North Am. 1996;76(4):763–82.
2. Ferrada R. Trauma hepatico en el hospital universitario del Valle Cali. Colomb Med. 1991;22:140–387.
3. Pringle JH. V. Notes on the arrest of hepatic hemorrhage due to trauma. Ann Surg. 1908;48(4):541–9.
4. Pachter HL, Spencer FC, Hofstetter SR, Liang HG, Coppa GF. Significant trends in the treatment of hepatic trauma. Experience with 411 injuries. Ann Surg. 1992;215(5):492–500.
5. Shaftan GW. Indications for operation in abdominal trauma. Am J Surg. 1960;99:657–64.
6. Feliciano DV, Mattox KL, Jordan GL. Intra-abdominal packing for control of hepatic hemorrhage: a reappraisal. J Trauma. 1981;21(4):285–90.
7. Anderson IB, Al Saghier M, Kneteman NM, Bigam DL. Liver trauma: management of devascularization injuries. J Trauma. 2004;57(5):1099–104.
8. Feliciano DV, Mattox KL, Burch JM, Bitondo CG, Jordan GL. Packing for control of hepatic hemorrhage. J Trauma. 1986;26(8):738–43.
9. Carmona RH, Peck DZ, Lim RC. The role of packing and planned reoperation in severe hepatic trauma. J Trauma. 1984;24(9):779–84.

10. Pachter HL. Prometheus bound: evolution in the management of hepatic trauma–from myth to reality. J Trauma Acute Care Surg. 2012;72(2):321–9.

11. Peitzman AB, Marsh JW. Advanced operative techniques in the management of complex liver injury. J Trauma Acute Care Surg. 2012;73(3):765–70.

12. Buckman RF, Miraliakbari R, Badellino MM. Juxtahepatic venous injuries: a critical review of reported management strategies. J Trauma. 2000;48(5):978–84.

13. Sankaran S, Lucas C, Walt AJ. Thoracic aortic clamping for prophylaxis against sudden cardiac arrest during laparotomy for acute massive hemoperitoneum. J Trauma. 1975;15(4):290–6.

14. Ledgerwood AM, Kazmers M, Lucas CE. The role of thoracic aortic occlusion for massive hemoperitoneum. J Trauma. 1976;16(08):610–5.

15. Millikan JS, Moore EE. Outcome of resuscitative thoracotomy and descending aortic occlusion performed in the operating room. J Trauma. 1984;24(5):387–92.

16. Wolf RK, Berry RE. Transaxillary intra-aortic balloon tamponade in trauma. J Vasc Surg. 1986;4(1): 95–7.

17. Gupta BK, Khaneja SC, Flores L, Eastlick L, Longmore W, Shaftan GW. The role of intra-aortic balloon occlusion in penetrating abdominal trauma. J Trauma. 1989;29(6):861–5.

18. Martinelli T, Thony F, Decléty P, Sengel C, Broux C, Tonetti J, et al. Intra-aortic balloon occlusion to salvage patients with life-threatening hemorrhagic shocks from pelvic fractures. J Trauma. 2010;68(4):942–8.

19. Stannard A, Eliason JL, Rasmussen TE. Resuscitative endovascular balloon occlusion of the aorta (REBOA) as an adjunct for hemorrhagic shock. J Trauma. 2011;71(6):1869–72.

20. Moore EE, Cogbill TH, Jurkovich GJ, Shackford SR, Malangoni MA, Champion HR. Organ injury scaling: spleen and liver (1994 revision). J Trauma. 1995;38:323–4.

Liver Resection and Transplantation for Trauma by Transplant Surgeons

Salvatore Gruttadauria, Duilio Pagano, and Marco Spada

Abbreviations

AAST- OIS American Association for the Surgery of Trauma-Organ Injury Scale
ISMETT Istituto Mediterraneo per i Trapianti e Terapie ad Alta Specializzazione (Mediterranean Institute for Transplantation and Advanced Specialized Therapies)
CT Computed tomography
ERCP Endoscopic retrograde cholangiopancreatography
IVC Inferior vena cava
OLT Orthotopic liver transplantation

S. Gruttadauria, MD, PhD, FACS (✉)
Department of Abdominal Surgery, IsMeTT/UPMC Italy, Mediterranean Institute for Transplantation and Advanced Specialized Therapies (IsMeTT), University of Pittsburgh Medical Center, Via Ernesto Tricomi 5, Palermo 90127, Italy
e-mail: sgruttadauria@ismett.edu

D. Pagano, MD, PhD
Department of Abdominal Surgery, IsMeTT/UPMC Italy, Mediterranean Institute for Transplantation and Advanced Specialized Therapies (IsMeTT), University of Pittsburgh Medical Center, Via Ernesto Tricomi 5, Palermo 90127, Italy
e-mail: dpagano@ismett.edu

M. Spada, MD, PhD
Department of Abdominal Surgery, IsMeTT/UPMC Italy, Mediterranean Institute for Transplantation and Advanced Specialized Therapies (IsMeTT), University of Pittsburgh Medical Center, Via Ernesto Tricomi 5, Palermo 90127, Italy

Department of Surgery, School of Medicine, University of Pittsburgh, Pittsburgh, PA, USA
e-mail: mspada@ismett.edu

Introduction

The natural tendency of choosing less or noninvasive treatment in general surgery is also followed in treating trauma injuries and has increased in recent years. Blunt and penetrating liver trauma is common and often presents significant problems in terms of diagnostics and management [1].

Current surgical management is focused mainly on packing, damage control, and early interventional radiology for angiography and embolization [2]. In our group experience, as in that of others, liver resection is, in some cases, the best possible treatment [2, 3]. Indeed, we have yet to indicate patients for OLT for this reason, though it has been used successfully in such instances by other groups [4].

The objective of this chapter is to report the most important troubleshooting areas in management of complex liver trauma and the role of transfer of these patients to tertiary referral centers for salvage resection in order to reduce morbidity and mortality.

Electronic supplementary material Supplementary material is available in the online version of this chapter at 10.1007/978-1-4939-1200-1_14. Videos can also be accessed at http://www.springerimages.com/videos/978-1-4939-1199-8.

Surgical Decision-Making and Preoperative Monitoring

An important question that skilled hepatobiliary surgeons need to clarify concerns presurgical evaluation. CT grading of hepatic injury is seldom a factor in determining the need for surgery, and most patients with higher-grade injuries that can be managed without surgical intervention are not transferred to a tertiary referral facility. However, most patients for whom nonsurgical treatment has failed are first treated in the first hospital they are admitted to.

In the planning stages of nonsurgical management of liver trauma, hemodynamic stability is a more relevant factor than grade of injury or degree of hemoperitoneum.

Experienced resuscitation teams can be helpful during initial hospitalization in achieving hemodynamic stability or rapid stabilization after initial fluid resuscitation and in correcting hypothermia, acidosis, or severe coagulopathy. Moreover, an available intensive care unit with continuous pulse and arterial blood pressure monitoring, repeated measurements of blood gas analyzer parameters, and careful clinical follow-up is mandatory.

Nonsurgical treatment is the gold standard, according to the AAST-OIS, for liver injuries grades I–III without CT detection of active bleeding. In the case of active bleeding, an angioembolization procedure can be done for grade IV injuries. Unsuccessful nonsurgical treatment, hemodynamic instability, and the presence of peritonitis on physical examination, with evidence of other abdominal injuries in diagnostic studies, constitute the principal indications for laparotomy [5, 6].

It bears emphasizing that salvage surgery is usually performed in a highly select group of patients who have undergone surgical repair and are stable enough to be transferred to a transplant referral center. It is important for the transplant surgeons at the referral center to know the following:

- What procedures did the patient undergo at the referring hospital, and how much blood did the patient receive?
- What was the patient's hemodynamic picture at the time of patient presentation?

This information is crucial in deciding if the patient *needs formal resection* [7–9]. Obviously, there is a great difference between performing a right hepatic lobectomy in a patient who is stable and performing one in a patient with severe ongoing hemorrhage.

Surgical Control of Hemorrhage and Resection Techniques

The first thing to be taken into consideration for controlling massive hemorrhage is portal triad occlusion (the Pringle maneuver), which is done by placing a nontraumatic vascular clamp across the hepatic artery, portal vein, and common bile duct at the level of the foramen of Winslow. The second is a sequential approach to total vascular exclusion/isolation of the liver, which is achieved by cross clamping both the suprahepatic and infra-hepatic IVC, with hepatic vascular control of the portal vein and hepatic artery without venous bypass. This requires active hemodynamic support carried out in agreement with the liver transplant anesthesia team.

All types of resections follow anatomic parameters, despite the extension of the resection. In semi-elective cases, when initial surgery was performed with a subcostal approach, and in patients for whom other abdominal injuries have been excluded, operations can be done with a bilateral subcostal incision, with upward midline extension.

Mobilization of the liver and skeletonization of the retrohepatic IVC with ligation of all accessory hepatic veins are usually done with *the traditional piggyback technique.*

The piggyback hepatectomy technique is paramount to decrease the theoretical risk of an iatrogenic lesion of retrohepatic vena cava margin, and it is also referred to as the "caval preservation technique" because it allows continual return of blood flow from the lower body back to the heart throughout the transplant. In transplant patients, it reduces the need for venovenous bypass by maintaining forward vena cava flow allowing decompression of the portal mesenteric system through previously established collaterals with outflow to the inferior vena cava [10].

Different techniques for hepatic resection with or without inflow occlusion have been proposed in select settings for reducing intraoperative blood loss, operative time, and improving overall surgical quality. However, there is a lack of consensus in the literature on management of liver trauma, and historical studies suggest that the gold standard technique is dependent largely on the surgeon's personal experience, as well as the kind of resection to be performed safely and quickly.

Crush clamping technique, ultrasonic dissection, vascular stapling, bipolar electrocautery, and radiofrequency can be considered equally safe and effective for transection of the liver parenchyma, so all these techniques should be available in a dedicated center for liver surgery and used according to the specific circumstances of trauma settings.

The two techniques most frequently used at our institute are liver resection using stapling devices for unstable patients and hepatic parenchyma transection for stable patients, described elsewhere [11, 12].

Hepatic parenchymal transection involves:

1. *Parenchymal tissue fragmentation and skeletonization of vascular-biliary structures with an ultrasonic dissector (Tissue-Link, Tissue Link Medical Inc, Dover, NH): the ultrasonic dissector was set at 90 % amplitude, with high tissue selection, and the irrigation rate was 5 mL/h, with suction set at maximum strength. This was applied after the liver capsule was opened using diathermy, with coagulation at 70 W. The radio-frequency setting was 75 W, and the irrigation rate was 2.5–5.0 mL/h.*
2. *Vascular hemostasis and biliostasis of the minuscule biliary ducts through a monopolar floating ball: it could be performed with using* microsurgical clips. Usually we divide the biliary duct just before the end of the parenchymal transection, using sharp instruments rather than cautery to avoid damage to the bile duct.
3. *Sectioning of fibrous and vascular-biliary structures with electrocautery: the hilar structures have to be identified and dissected with extreme care to avoid intimal damage to the hepatic artery and jeopardize the bile ducts.*
4. *Suction of organic and irrigation fluids mixed with parenchyma detritus using a pediatric* *aspirator and the integrated aspirator in the ultrasonic dissector: during this phase and parenchymal transection maneuvers, central venous pressure has to be maintained at a pressure below 5 mmHg, to minimize bleeding and therefore avoid non-autologous blood transfusion* [13, 14].

Additionally, for all procedures, we perform a presurgical setup of the Cell Saver and the Rapid Infusion System (Haemonetics Corporation, Braintree, MA). These devices are used when needed during the procedures.

We use stapling devices when we find devitalized liver parenchyma around the fracture and the Tissue-Link for major resection when the trauma is found to involve major vessels, such as hepatic veins or portal branches. We suggest to identify and confirm the plane of parenchymal transection verified with intraoperative ultrasound, near to the involved hepatic vein [15, 16].

The role of a liver transplant surgery team can be crucial not only in terms of urgent OLT, which has been used successfully in such instances [4, 17], but also in managing the potential use of extreme procedures, such as a temporary anhepatic phase using an implantation of human pericardium, or Dacron or Gore-Tex vein prosthesis, to employ back-table repair surgery or performing a complex liver resection for hepatic trauma involving the IVC [18].

Only in cases of suspected injury to the suprahepatic IVC is it a good idea to attempt a direct approach to the juxta-diaphragmatic segment of the IVC by placing the patient on an atriocaval venovenous bypass. A complete suprahepatic IVC transection can be performed by resecting the damaged section of the vessel and performing an end-to-end anastomosis with 3-0 polypropylene running sutures, using the same technique as in OLT [19].

How I Do It

In August of 2009, a 39-year-old man was hit in the abdomen by a car. He was brought to a regional hospital by an emergency rescue service of the city immediately after the accident. He was in pain, with a pulse of 145/min and a respiratory rate of 35/min.

He was resuscitated and, after stabilization, an abdominal radiograph and ultrasound were requested. Abdominal radiograph revealed no free air under the diaphragm, but the ultrasound of the abdomen showed a huge traumatic lesion of the right hemiliver, with moderate free fluid in the peritoneal cavity.

A CT scan of the abdomen was then done and also delineated liver injury, with severe grade lesions of segments IV, V, and VIII. The patient subsequently underwent right hepatic artery clipping and tube cholecystostomy and was then transferred urgently to our institute because of persistent blood outputs from the drainages. A CT scan at admission was consistent with a vast parenchymal disruption laceration involving 65 % of the right hepatic lobe, with an intraparenchymal hematoma ($60 \times 68 \times 97$ mm) and contextual air bubbles.

The hematoma was actively supplied by a segmental branch of the right hepatic arterial origin. Surgical clips were placed at the origin of the right hepatic artery, which was still patent. No other abdominal solid organ injuries were detected, with a proper appearance of the spleen, kidneys, pancreas, adrenal glands, and pelvic organs. There was a slight narrowing of the origin of the celiac trunk. On volumetric examination, the volume of the anatomic left lobe (segments I–III) was 515 cc, while the volume of the left hemiliver (I–IV) was 649 cc (Fig. 14.1).

At our institute he underwent median relaparotomy with extension to the right renal flap. We then removed roughly two liters of blood clots and found no evidence of active bleeding. Liver resection was planned by a multidisciplinary team and was aimed at excision of the gallbladder and the right lobe of the liver.

After sectioning of the falciform ligament and of the triangular ligament and right coronary, we performed a skeletonization of the retrohepatic IVC with ligature and sectioning of accessory veins. We then isolated the right hepatic vein and proceeded to isolate and section the cystic duct and cystic artery for retrograde cholecystectomy. Subsequently, we isolated the right branch of the portal vein and the right branch of the hepatic artery, which was divided between ligatures after the removal of the two metal clips from the anterior branch of the right hepatic artery.

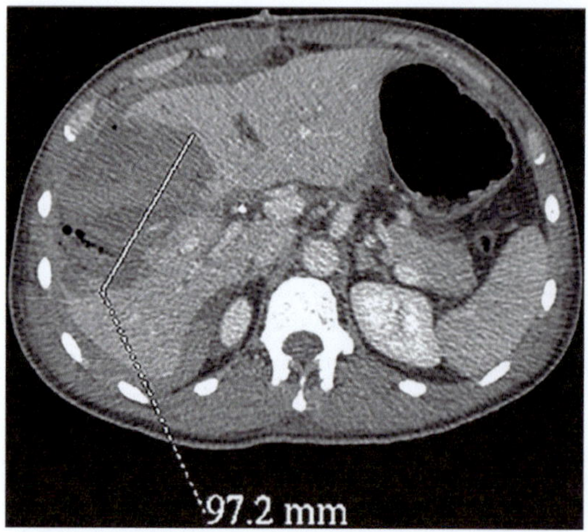

Fig. 14.1 Admission CT scan of a 39-year-old man, after hepatorrhaphy, with an extensive injury to the right liver. Right hepatic artery clipping and tube cholecystostomy were previously done at another hospital of the national health system network

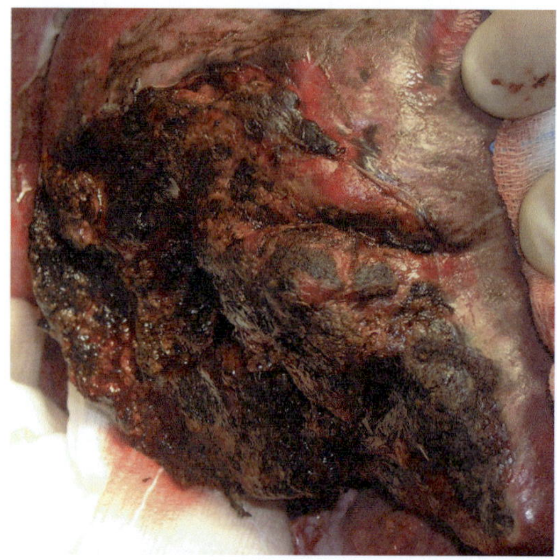

Fig. 14.2 Remnant hepatic parenchyma after right hemiliver resection. An intraoperative ultrasound was done to confirm valid flows to and from the left liver

The right branch of the portal vein and the right hepatic vein were then severed with a vascular stapler. After the intraparenchymal sectioning and cutting of the right branch of the bile duct, we proceeded to parenchymal transection with the aid of electrocautery, ultrasonic dissector, and stapler (Fig. 14.2).

One of the most relevant indications for anatomic hepatic resection in this case was the

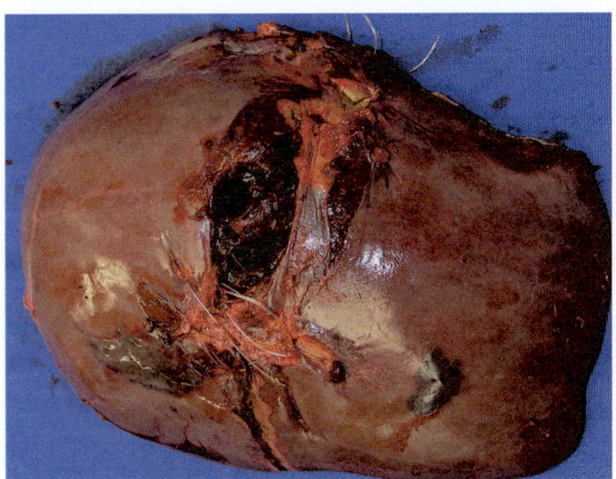

Fig. 14.3 Surgical specimen after right hepatectomy; of note is the previous surgical hepatorrhaphy for managing the liver fracture by simple suture with chromic catgut

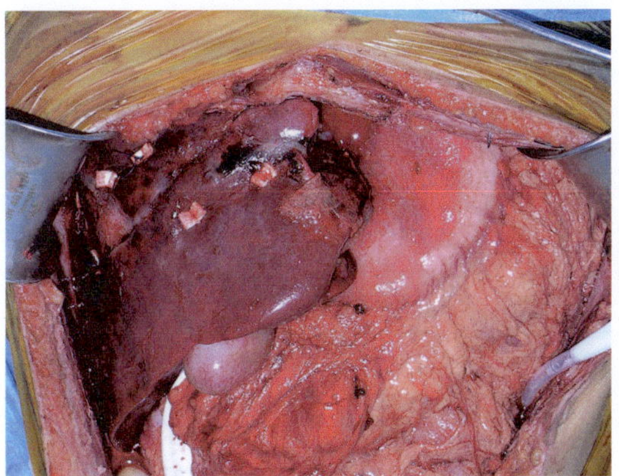

Fig. 14.4 Complex fracture of the right liver segments that was treated with hepatorrhaphy; the Teflon felts were adjuvant for supporting liver suture line fields

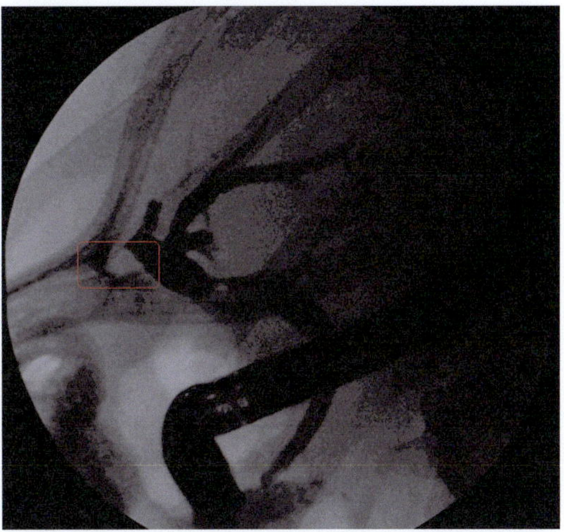

Fig. 14.5 Postoperative cholangiography confirmed mild output biliary leakage. At ERCP a metallic stent was placed (*as evidenced in the rectangle box*)

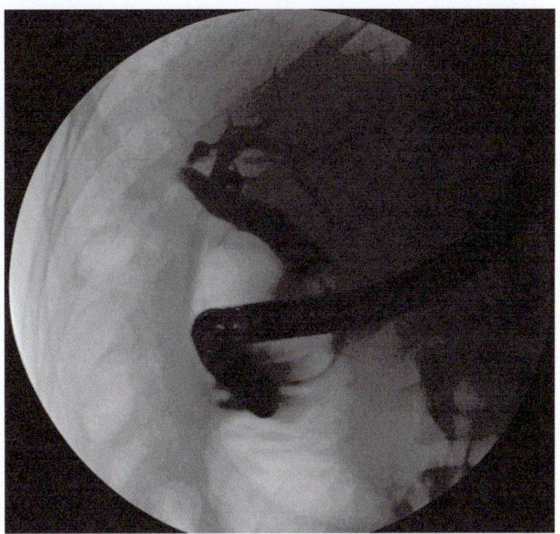

Fig. 14.6 Follow-up cholangiography, 2 months after surgery for liver injury, showing resolution of the biliary leakage

previous, inappropriate surgical treatment performed at the referring facility. Hepatorrhaphy by simple catgut suture and Spongostan application (Fig. 14.3) was less than ideal. For bailout first surgical approach, we suggest suture, supported by Teflon felt (DuPont Pharmaceuticals, Wilmington, DE), Fig. 14.4, and perihepatic packing.

An intraoperative ultrasound was performed to confirm valid blood flow to and from the left liver. Intraoperative cholangiography confirmed the patency of the left bile duct. Overall blood loss was 450 mL and operating time was 365 min. The postoperative course was complicated by mild biliary leakage, which was treated and resolved with ERCP and metallic stent placement (Fig. 14.5). The patient was discharged home on postoperative day 13. At present, he is alive and well. An uneventful ERCP and biliary stent removal was done 2 months after surgery, with no complaints (Fig. 14.6).

Conclusion

Technical skills in advanced hepatobiliary surgery, patient hemodynamic and resuscitation, diagnostic evaluations, operative indications by grade of injury, selection criteria for operative management, and criteria for the choice of operation are mandatory for indicating formal liver resection as initial or delayed management of patients with complex liver trauma.

Video Caption

Video 12 Atriocaval shunt (MP4 256971 kb)

References

1. Parks NA, Davis JW, Forman D, Demaster D. Observation for nonoperative management of blunt liver injuries: how long is long enough? J Trauma. 2011;70:626–9.
2. Li Petri S, Gruttadauria S, Pagano D, et al. Surgical management of complex liver trauma: a single liver transplant center experience. Am Surg. 2012;78(1): 20–5.
3. Piper GL, Peitzman AB. Current management of hepatic trauma. Surg Clin North Am. 2010;90: 775–85.
4. Honore C, DeRoover A, Gilson N, Detry O. Liver transplantation for hepatic trauma: discussion about a case and its management. J Emerg Trauma Shock. 2011;4:137–9.
5. Mohr AM, Lavery RF, Barone A, et al. Angiographic embolization for liver injuries: low mortality, high morbidity. J Trauma. 2003;55:1077–82.
6. Malhotra AK, Fabian TC, Croce MA, et al. Blunt hepatic injury: a paradigm shift from operative to non-operative management in the 1990s. Ann Surg. 2000;231:804–13.
7. Yildirim IO, Salihoglu Z, Bolayirli MI, et al. Prospective evaluation of the factors effective on morbidity and mortality of the patients having liver resection surgeries. Hepatogastroenterology. 2012;59(118): 1928–32.
8. van der Wilden GM, Velmahos GC, Emhoff T, et al. Successful nonoperative management of the most severe blunt liver injuries: a multicenter study of the research consortium of new England centers for trauma. Arch Surg. 2012;147(5):423–8.
9. Allard MA, Dondero F, Sommacale D, et al. Liver packing during elective surgery: an option that can be considered. World J Surg. 2011;35(11):2493–8.
10. Tzakis A, Todo S, Starzl TE. Orthotopic liver transplantation with preservation of the inferior vena cava. Ann Surg. 1989;210:649.
11. Kaneko H, Otsuka Y, Takagi S, et al. Hepatic resection using stapling devices. Am J Surg. 2004;187: 280–4.
12. Delis SG, Bakoyiannis A, Karakaxas D, et al. Hepatic parenchyma resection using stapling devices: peri-operative and long-term outcome. HPB (Oxford). 2009;11:38–44.
13. Gruttadauria S, Doria C, Vitale CH, et al. New technique in hepatic parenchymal transection for living related liver donor and liver neoplasms. HPB (Oxford). 2004;6:106–9.
14. Gruttadauria S, Doria C, Vitale CH, et al. Preliminary report on surgical technique in hepatic parenchymal transection for liver tumors in the elderly: a lesson learned from living-related liver transplantation. J Surg Oncol. 2004;88:229–33.
15. Gruttadauria S, Mandala L, Vasta F, et al. Improvements in hepatic parenchymal transection for living related liver donor. Transplant Proc. 2005;37:2589–91.
16. Polanco P, Leon S, Pineda J, et al. Hepatic resection in the management of complex injury to the liver. J Trauma. 2008;65:1264–9.
17. Gozzetti G, Mazziotti A, Frena A, et al. Il trapianto di fegato per trauma. Chirurgia. 1994;7(11):848–51.
18. Panarello G, Arcadipane A, Capitanio G, Carollo T, Burgio G, Gruttadauria S, Gridelli B. Two stage total hepatectomy as rescue therapy for primary non function. 60° SIAARTI National Congress. Bastia Umbra. 10th/13th Oct 2006
19. Marino IR, di Francesco F, Doria C, Gruttadauria S, Lauro A, Scott VL. A new technique for successful management of a complete suprahepatic caval transection. J Am Coll Surg. 2008;206(1):190–4.

Extrahepatic Biliary System

David V. Feliciano

Introduction

Injuries to the extrahepatic biliary system after abdominal trauma, especially if the gallbladder is excluded, are rare. Feliciano et al. [1] described 12 patients with injuries to the ducts over a 7-year period at a high-volume trauma center in Houston in 1985. In the 1985 review by Ivatury et al. [2] from another high-volume trauma center in the Bronx, New York, over a 10.5-year period, 13 patients with injuries to the ducts were treated. Jurkovich et al. [3] subsequently described only 26 ductal injuries at eight American level I trauma centers over a 10-year period in 1995. A later review noted an incidence of 0.37 % in 1873 patients with blunt abdominal trauma evaluated at a center in Madrid over a 20-year period [4].

In addition to being uncommon, injuries to the biliary ducts and gallbladder usually occur in patients with multiple other injuries. These are present in the abdomen in patients with penetrating trauma and systemically in patients with blunt trauma. For this reason, injuries to the ducts themselves may be missed by routine diagnostic studies and even at an emergent or urgent laparotomy [5].

Another issue complicating the management of patients with ductal injuries is that the ducts are normal size when the injury occurs. A meticulous repair is obviously needed, particularly in female patients. This is because the diameter of the normal common bile duct is only 4–5 mm and that of the right or left hepatic duct is only 2–3 mm in women. Long-term complications after repair of extrahepatic ductal injuries have been noted in many published series [2–4, 6, 7].

History

The first report of a traumatic blunt biliary ductal injury in the English language was by TM Drysdale in 1861 [8]. There were then at least five other published reports by 1900, including the oft-cited report by Battle et al. in 1894 [9, 10]. In 1972, Zollinger et al. [11] noted that there had been only 74 patients with blunt ductal injuries reported in the literature from 1921 to 1968. His report described two other patients and reviewed the operative management in three of the earlier series from 1961, 1961, and 1968 [12–14]. Reports including both penetrating and blunt etiologies and with reasonable numbers of patients since that time (injuries to the gallbladder and cystic duct excluded) have noted that only 27 % of extrahepatic ductal injuries were caused by blunt trauma from the years 1982–1995 [1–3, 6, 7].

Most reports of injuries to the extrahepatic biliary ducts have come from trauma centers in urban areas over the past 60 years [1–3, 6, 7, 15, 16]. Penetrating injuries predominate in these reviews, and most patients have a significant

D.V. Feliciano, MD
Division of General Surgery, Department of Surgery,
Indiana University Medical Center,
545 Barnhill Drive, EH 509, Indianapolis,
IN 46202, USA
e-mail: davfelic@iupui.edu

R.R. Ivatury (ed.), *Operative Techniques for Severe Liver Injury*,
DOI 10.1007/978-1-4939-1200-1_15, © Springer Science+Business Media New York 2015

number of associated intra-abdominal injuries. In reviews that have focused on injuries to one or more structures in the porta hepatis, mortality has ranged from 24 to 51% [3, 6].

Pathophysiology of Blunt Rupture

Patients who have sustained a blunt rupture or transection of the gallbladder and/or extrahepatic biliary ducts have usually received a direct blow or significant compressive force to the upper abdomen or right upper quadrant [7, 12, 17]. Several theories have been proposed to explain the mechanism of injury to only the bile duct in the porta hepatis and the consistent locations of the ductal injuries. Included among these are "blowout" of the distended duct, a shearing injury with disruption of the duct at points of anatomic fixation, the short and rigid nature of the ductal system compared with the hepatic artery and portal vein, and a direct crushing blow to the duct with or without impingement on the vertebral column [1, 2, 6, 7, 11, 12, 17, 18].

To test the "blowout" hypothesis, Fletcher et al. [12] produced intraductal pressures of 750 lb per square inch seven times in three goats. Because the gallbladder or common bile duct did not rupture, they postulated that factors responsible for ductal injury were likely to be a short wide cystic duct, a force applied to the gallbladder, and a simultaneous shearing force to the common bile duct.

Numerous authors have documented that partial avulsion or complete transection often occurs near the hilum of the liver, but the most common location of transection from blunt trauma is in the common bile duct just as it enters the pancreas [11]. Thus, much as with blunt injuries to the small intestine, shearing forces are likely to disrupt the ductal system at its points of fixation. The short and rigid nature of the ductal system presumably makes it the most likely structure to disrupt in the porta hepatis as the liver moves superiorly during the application of a shearing or compressive force [19]. Direct injury to the duct has also been noted when a macerating injury to the pancreatoduodenal complex occurs [7].

Diagnosis

Blunt Trauma

Patients with blunt injuries to the extrahepatic biliary ducts and not the gallbladder often have a delay in diagnosis. Depending on the volume of bile leakage, patients may have limited initial symptoms as sterile bile in the peritoneal cavity is reabsorbed [6, 20–23]. Even patients undergoing an abdominal CT with contrast may have a nondiagnostic study in the early post-injury period.

Patients discharged from the emergency department with a ductal injury usually return in the first 4 weeks with jaundice, biliary ascites, and inanition [11, 23]. Should further delays in diagnosis occur, death may result [8, 24]. The first diagnostic maneuver in such a patient is abdominal ultrasonography or CT to document the presence of ascites or intra-abdominal fluid collections, followed by a diagnostic peritoneal tap. With the return of bile, the point of leakage can be demonstrated by the use of technetium-99 m dimethyl iminodiacetic acid (HIDA) radionuclide scanning or by endoscopic retrograde cholangiography [25]. Scanning with HIDA or one of its analogues permits further definition of hepatic parenchymal abnormalities detected on ultrasonography or CT, while injury to the biliary tract is delineated during excretion of the tracer. Endoscopic retrograde cholangiopancreatography defines the area of ductal injury most precisely, but furnishes no information about an associated hepatic injury.

Penetrating Trauma

Patients with penetrating injuries to the gallbladder and/or extrahepatic biliary ducts almost always have other intra-abdominal injuries, especially to the liver, duodenum, pancreas, and upper abdominal vascular structures [1]. The indications for operation in these patients continue to be peritonitis, hypotension, and/or evisceration. Injuries caused by stab wounds to the biliary ducts may mimic the simpler ones caused during laparoscopic cholecystectomy – namely, partial or complete transections. When a gunshot wound is the cause, the transection and loss of tissue are similar to the most complex injuries associated with laparoscopic cholecystectomy.

Factors Affecting the Management of Gallbladder Injuries

In the patient with profound shock from multi-system trauma or multiple intra-abdominal injuries, a ruptured (blunt trauma) or perforated (penetrating trauma) gallbladder is rapidly repaired if possible. At a reoperation after the first "damage control" operation (see below), a cholecystectomy is performed.

Ruptured or perforated gallbladders in hemodynamically stable patients are managed with cholecystectomy.

Ductal Injuries Missed at Operation

Patients with either blunt or penetrating trauma have had injuries to the ductal system missed at laparotomy as previously noted [1, 3, 5, 7, 11, 14, 17, 25, 26]. In the review by Zollinger et al. [11], a mean delay of 3 weeks occurred before discovery of injuries to hepatic ducts that had been missed at a previous operation. The reasons that injuries are not detected have included hemodynamic instability and a rapid or incomplete first laparotomy with packing and silo or vacuum-assisted closure, failure to evaluate injuries near the hilum of the liver, or failure to define the source of bile staining in the hepatoduodenal ligament or retroperitoneum [5, 7, 25, 26]. In the patient with a rapid first operation for a penetrating wound near the hilum of the liver, careful inspection of the path of the knife of missile is mandatory at the time of reoperation. With the presence of bile staining at either a first or second operation, no obvious ductal injury, and a normal pancreatoduodenal complex, cholangiography through the gallbladder and compression with a bulldog clamp on the distal bile duct are indicated [5].

Factors Affecting the Choice of Operative Repair of Ductal Injuries

When the surgeon is confronted with a traumatic injury to a biliary duct, the five factors that influence management include the following:
- Hemodynamic stability of the patient
- Location and extent of the injury
- Size of the injured duct
- Tenuous blood supply of bile duct
- Presence of associated injuries in the right upper quadrant

In particular, patients with shock-induced "metabolic failure" (temperature <34 °C, pH <7.2, coagulopathy) will benefit from damage control resuscitation and operation [27–29]. In patients with injuries to the liver, pancreatoduodenal complex, or abdominal vascular structures, the lowest operative priority is the injury to the bile duct if "metabolic failure" occurs. Therefore, a temporary biliary diversion or external drainage may be all that can safely be performed at the original laparotomy.

An associated significant injury to the liver may have a major impact on the choice of repair for the injury of the bile duct. For example, if perihepatic packing is needed to control parenchymal oozing or a subcapsular hematoma above the porta hepatis of the liver, it is inappropriate to perform a delicate or complex biliary repair, such as a biliary enteric bypass, at the first operation. In similar fashion, a combined hepatic lobar and hepatic ductal injury may be better treated by resection rather than extensive attempts at repairs of both structures.

An associated significant injury to the pancreatoduodenal complex has a significant effect on the choice of ductal repair, also. For example, the patient whose condition is stable with a combined severe injury to the distal duct and head of the pancreas should have resection rather than attempted reconstruction.

The injury that is most difficult to recognize and repair is one that involves the right or left hepatic duct, particularly in a child [5, 11]. The small size of the ducts in this location eliminates many options for repair and certainly complicates the use of intraductal stents. An injury to the common hepatic or bile duct is easier to treat, although the repair used obviously depends on the magnitude and complexity of the ductal injury.

Options in Patients Who Are Hemodynamically Unstable (Table 15.1)

In patients with multiple intra-abdominal injuries, profound hypotension, and intraoperative "metabolic failure," the surgeon's goals are control of hemorrhage from major abdominal vascular structures, the mesentery, and the porta hepatis; control of oozing from the retroperitoneum, pelvis, and solid organ injuries other than the spleen by insertion of packs; removal, ligation, or stapling off of segments of the bowel containing multiple perforations; and rapid silo or vacuum-assisted coverage of the open abdomen. The injury to the bile duct is ignored in such patients because survival is unclear, and early reoperation will be necessary anyway to remove the intra-abdominal packs. These considerations are illustrated by the case report depicted in Figs. 15.1 and 15.2.

When the patient's condition is more stable but operation has been prolonged and a state of "metabolic failure" appears likely, several options short of formal repair are possible to control the leakage of bile. Included among these are insertion of a closed suction drain near the ductal injury, insertion of a red rubber tube into the proximal end of a transected hepatic or common bile duct, and insertion of a T-tube. Both the

insertion of a Jackson-Pratt drain and the creation of an end-tube hepatodochostomy or choledochostomy are best followed by early reoperation for definitive repair when the patient's condition is stable. The ideal insertion site for a T-tube is

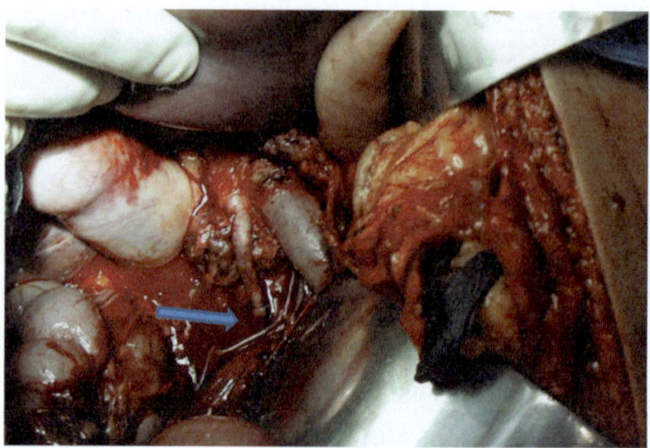

Fig. 15.1 This patient had a motor-vehicle crash and presented to the emergency department in hemodynamic instability. Laparotomy demonstrated a large amount of hemoperitoneum, grade IV crush of the right lobe of liver, crush injury of the second portion of the duodenum and the head of the pancreas, skeletonization without rupture of portal vein, and a complete avulsion injury of the common bile duct (CBD) from the duodenum (*arrow*). Hemostasis was secured by debridement-resection of liver and perihepatic packing. The common duct was ligated above and below the avulsion

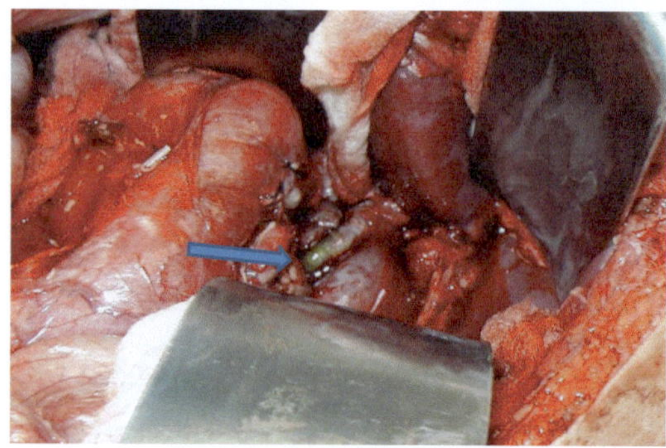

Fig. 15.2 Relaparotomy after 24 h of resuscitation showed the following: bleeding was controlled, but the lower half of the CBD had avascular necrosis (*arrow*), necessitating resection and a higher anastomosis between the common hepatic duct and the jejunum. This necrosis should be anticipated in such injuries because of the segmental blood supply of the common duct arising from the gastroduodenal artery and ascending up the duct at 3 and 9 o'clock positions

Table 15.1 Options for management in patients who are hemodynamically unstable

Reoperation mandatory
External drainage
End-tube hepatodochostomy or choledochostomy
Reoperation not always necessary
T-tube or stent with limb beneath injury

From Feliciano [9], Copyright Elsevier 1994

into a partial transection. With partial transection of a right or left hepatic duct, a small T-tube may be inserted into the common hepatic duct with a long proximal limb passing through the lacerated or partially transected area. Even without suture repair, reoperation may be avoided in such a patient, depending on the future severity of the stricture at the site of injury.

Options for Repair in Patients Who Are Hemodynamically Stable (Table 15.2)

Definitive repair or resection followed by repair is performed in a patient whose condition is stable, with the option chosen based on the extent of the ductal injury. The spectrum of ductal injuries includes avulsion of the cystic duct or clean

Table 15.2 Options for repair in patients who are hemodynamically stable

Avulsion of cystic duct or laceration
Cystic duct or gallbladder pedicle
Heineke-Mikulicz repair
Primary repair with absorbable suture
Transection without loss of tissue
End-to-end anastomosis
Choledochoduodenostomy
Roux-en-Y choledochojejunostomy
Extensive defect in the wall
Mucosal onlay patch
Serosal onlay patch
Vein patch[a]
Prosthetic patch[a]
Segmental loss of ductal tissue
Formal reconstruction
Cholecystoduodenostomy or cholecystojejunostomy (loop or Roux-en-Y)
Choledochoduodenostomy
Roux-en-Y choledochojejunostomy or hepatodochojejunostomy (hepaticojejunostomy)
Roux-en-Y hepatoportal jejunostomy
Ligation or resection
Ligation of right or left hepatic duct
Hepatic resection
Whipple procedure

From Feliciano [9], Copyright Elsevier 1994
[a]No longer recommended

laceration, transection without loss of tissue, extensive defect in the wall, or segmental loss of ductal tissue.

Avulsion of Cystic Duct or Laceration of Common Bile or Hepatic Duct

In the rare patient with avulsion of a portion of the cystic duct, the resultant defect in the side of the common bile duct can be closed using the viable cystic duct remnant or even a portion of the proximal gallbladder wall, if necessary (Fig. 15.3) [30, 31]. Many surgeons choose to insert a T-tube through a separate choledochostomy and pass the proximal limb underneath such an extensive repair.

Primary repair of a lacerated or ruptured duct can be performed in a variety of ways, but interrupted sutures of 5–0 polyglycolic acid are preferred. One option when closure of a longitudinal defect would result in narrowing of the injured duct would be to perform a Heineke-Mikulicz type of transverse repair as described by Rutledge in 1983 [31]. The use of a T-tube with a limb under a simple suture repair of a portion of the wall is controversial because the small size of the ductal system in the previously healthy individual makes insertion of the tube difficult and potentially dangerous [2, 6, 7]. In one patient of Zollinger et al. [11], small ureteral catheters were used as stents across injuries to the hepatic ducts as a #8 Fr T-tube was too large to be inserted. Technical problems associated with the insertion of T-tubes were partially responsible for the discontinuance of routine ductal drainage as an adjunct to the repair of hepatic injuries 20 years ago [32].

Transection Without Loss of Tissue

Transection of the common hepatic or common bile duct by a stab wound with little contusion to the ends is probably one of the few instances in which an end-to-end anastomosis might be considered. Dissection around the ends should be avoided because it disrupts the tenuous blood

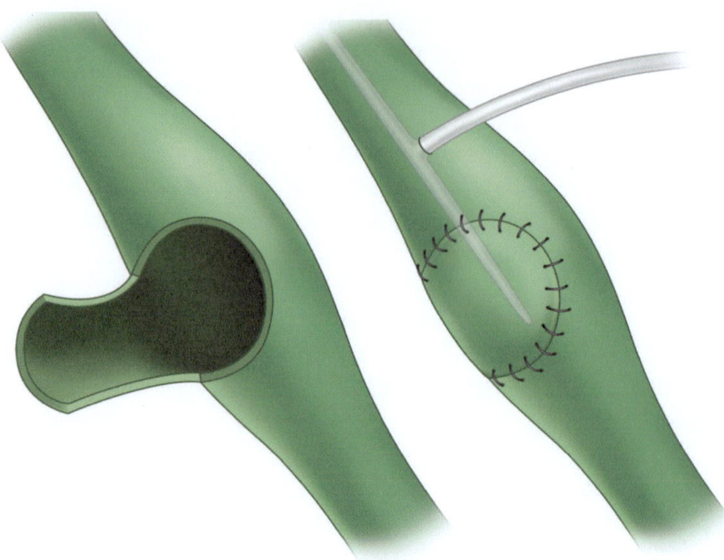

Fig. 15.3 Sandblom technique to close defect in common bile duct from cholecystocholedochal fistula can be applied to partial avulsion of cystic duct from blunt trauma (From Sandblom et al. [30], Copyright Elsevier 1975)

supply of the duct at 3 and 9 o'clock and increases the risk of a stricture at the site of repair [33]. When tension is present at the anastomosis, a stricture is inevitable. Although long-term follow-up results are lacking in many series, end-to-end anastomoses have been successful in treating traumatic transections in older series [18, 34–37]. A considerable number of reports have appeared, however, of unsuccessful end-to-end anastomoses performed for operative or traumatic transections [4, 6, 7, 38]. In a review of the literature by Ivatury et al. [2], end-to-end anastomoses for traumatic transections in 20 patients resulted in a stricture in 11 (55 %) and the need for biliary enteric bypass.

Extensive Defect in the Wall

An extensive defect in the wall (lateral defect) may result from a missile wound. Although such an injury may be managed by segmental resection of the area of injury and biliary enteric bypass, simpler and faster repairs have been suggested or used successfully in patients with either operative or traumatic injuries. Rutledge [31] originally suggested the use of a full-thickness vascularized jejunal patch in which the mucosa would be facing the lumen of the common bile duct, and this technique was subsequently used with success by another group [39]. In a similar fashion, the serosa of the mobilized duodenum, a loop of jejunum (with enteroenterostomy below), or a Roux-en-Y loop of jejunum has been used successfully to close ductal defects after longitudinal incision of strictured biliary anastomoses [39–41].These approaches would presumably be applicable, as well, to the patient who has sustained trauma with a wall defect.

An innovative approach not widely known has been the use of saphenous vein patches to close ductal defects. Originally described in 1964 [42], Rutledge [31] subsequently described its use in a patient with partial resection of the ductal wall for hepatocellular carcinoma. In 1991, Monk et al. [43] described performing a vein patch cholangioplasty in a patient who had sustained trauma with a 1 by 1 cm noncircumferential defect in the left hepatic duct. Based on the experimental studies of Belzer et al. [44] and Cushieri et al. [45] in which biliary vein patches were noted to shrink, essentially disappear, and be replaced by ingrowth of fibrous tissue, Monk et al. [43] suggested that a stent should be placed beneath the patch as it shrinks.

Prosthetic patches (knitted Teflon) have been used with success in a few patients requiring biliary reconstruction for strictures [46, 47]. Such an approach cannot be recommended in light of the success of more modern methods described for closure of traumatic wall defects.

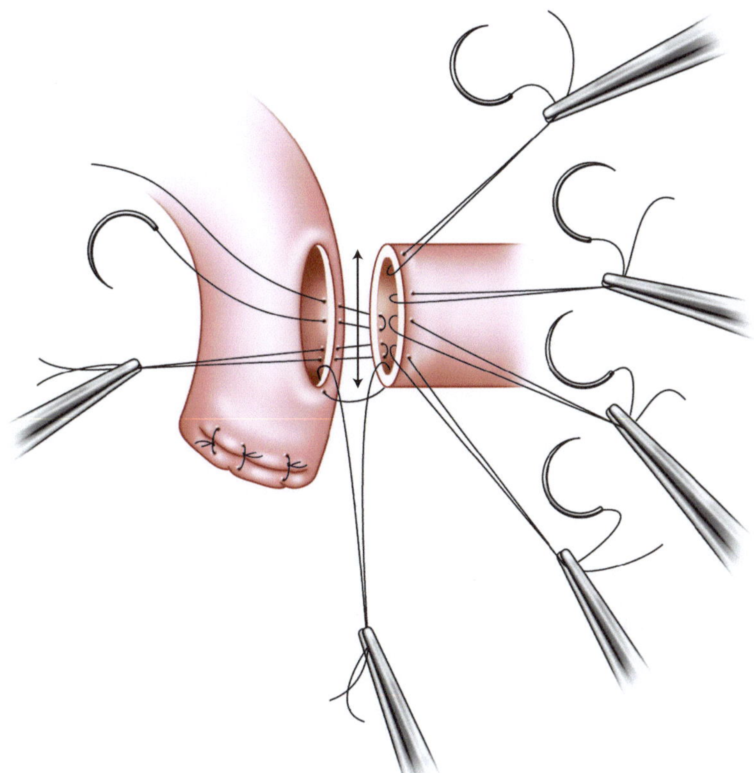

Fig. 15.4 Blumgart technique of Roux-en-Y hepaticojejunostomy after resection of ductal stricture or neoplasm can be applied to patient with significant trauma to the common bile, common hepatic, or hepatic duct. Anterior sutures are passed through biliary duct only, needles are left attached, and sutures are elevated to improve visualization as posterior row of sutures is inserted. Some surgeons place the posterior row of sutures with the knot outside the lumen (From Blumgart [53], Copyright Elsevier 1994)

Segmental Loss of Ductal Tissue

Formal Reconstruction

Segmental loss of ductal tissue results from a missile wound or a severe blunt avulsion injury requiring debridement. Ductal repairs for this group of patients are similar to those used with biliary strictures resulting from operative injuries.

With the loss of the common bile duct below the junction with the cystic duct, a normal gallbladder with a widely patent cystic duct may be used as a biliary conduit to the duodenum or jejunum. Also, it should be noted that the distal duct does not need to be identified and oversewn in such a patient [48]. This is a simple reconstruction involving only oversewing of the stump of the common bile duct at the junction with the cystic duct and an end-to-end or side-to-side cholecystoduodenostomy or cholecystojejunostomy (loop or Roux-en-Y) [31, 49]. Short-term data (<12 months) have long been available on the efficacy of cholecystojejunostomy for biliary drainage in patients with unresectable carcinoma of the head of the pancreas [50].

End-to-side choledochoduodenostomy can be used when a significant portion of the common bile duct has been injured. This option, however, has not been used in any of the large reports of biliary tract injuries in the past, presumably because of concerns about tension on the anastomosis or the potential complication of a side duodenal fistula [1, 2, 6, 7, 51].

The most popular repair when loss of ductal tissue or a significant avulsion injury has occurred in a patient whose condition is otherwise stable has been Roux-en-Y choledochojejunostomy or hepatodochojejunostomy (hepaticojejunostomy) [1, 2, 6, 7, 51]. A mobile retrocolic Roux-en-Y limb, a well-vascularized proximal bile duct, and a 1- or 2-layer anastomosis with interrupted sutures usually lead to an excellent result in the patient who has sustained trauma (Figs. 15.4 and 15.5). In the review by Ivatury et al. [2], a stricture developed in only 1 of 28 patients undergoing primary biliary enteric anastomosis for complete transection.

With avulsion of the hepatic ducts at the bifurcation, it is worthwhile to suture the right and left

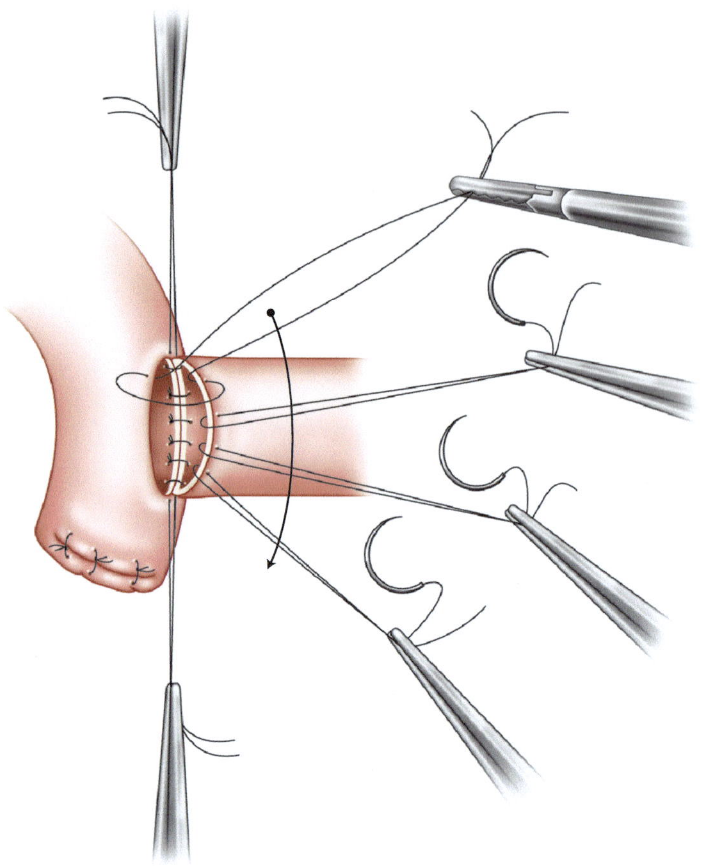

Fig. 15.5 Completion of anterior row of sutures by passing needles full thickness through jejunal in Roux limb (From Blumgart [53], Copyright Elsevier 1994)

ducts together medially before performing an end-to-side hepatodochojejunostomy [52, 53]. It may also be helpful to pass the anterior row of sutures through the common bile channel for traction before placing the sutures through the posterior row as this improves visualization [53].

Complete loss of the hepatic ducts at the surface of the liver is equivalent to the chronic E_3 or E_4 biliary strictures that Strasberg et al. [54] have described after mishaps during laparoscopic cholecystectomy. When the general surgeon is familiar with the jejunal mucosal graft-on-transhepatic stent technique described by the late Rodney Smith (Lord Smith of Marlow), this is the appropriate approach [55].

A similar injury, but one in which the stumps of the hepatic ducts cannot be identified in the hilum of the liver, is a special challenge. A Roux-en-Y hepatoportal jejunostomy similar to that used in neonates with biliary atresia is performed [56]. This approach has been used with success in Strasberg E_4 injuries with stricture after laparoscopic cholecystectomy as well [57].

Role of Stents with Formal Reconstruction

Repair of an acute injury to the extrahepatic ductal system from trauma differs significantly from repair of a chronic biliary stricture. There are no scarring and no residua from previous reconstructions, and most of the patients are young and healthy. If the stump of the resected duct(s) is bleeding freely and the Roux-en-Y choledocho- or hepatodochojejunostomy (hepaticojejunostomy) is performed without tension, there are no data that the presence of a stent will decrease postoperative leaks or strictures.

The small size of the injured ducts as previously described is the one factor that often prompts the insertion of a stent in trauma patients. The presence of a stent in a duct less than 4 mm in size may prevent narrowing during the performance of the bilioenteric anastomosis or during healing and will allow for postoperative imaging [58]. #5 or #8 Fr silastic pediatric feeding tubes, much as used by some surgeons to stent pancreatojejunostomies during Whipple procedures, make ideal biliary stents. They are soft and flexible, decrease pressure on the wall of the duct, and should minimize the incidence of arteriobiliary fistulas [59]. There are no data on the length of time that stents inserted after an acute repair should remain in place.

Role of the Local Surgeon Expert in Hepatobiliary Surgery or Hepatic Transplantation

When immediate or early repair of bile ducts injured at the time of laparoscopic cholecystectomy is performed by hepatobiliary surgeons, the results are better than when repairs are performed by "nonspecialist surgeons" [57, 59]. So, in an academic center with the availability of hepatobiliary or hepatic transplant surgeons, should the local trauma center "call for help" to care for the patient with blunt or penetrating trauma to an extrahepatic bile duct? The answer will depend on the location and magnitude of the ductal injury and the expertise of the general trauma surgeon. An injury involving the common hepatic duct or one involving the hepatic ducts and a trauma surgeon with little elective experience in ductal surgery (i.e., choledocholithotomy or repair of stricture) should prompt immediate consultation with a specialist.

Ligation or Resection

It has been suggested that oversewing of a right or left hepatic duct might be preferable to a complex repair with its risks of biliary leakage, fistula, and abscess [60]. Such an approach has not been used in any of the large published series [1, 2, 6, 7, 11, 19], but would presumably result in atrophy of the involved lobe over time.

Hepatic resection is indicated only in the presence of a combination of injuries to the liver and a hepatic duct or the common hepatic duct.

Resection is performed in only 3 or 4 % of patients with hepatic injuries and continues to carry a mortality rate of 10–15 % [61].

The Whipple procedure is reserved for the rare injury to the distal bile duct associated with a macerated, devascularized, or actively bleeding pancreatoduodenal complex [62]. Even an extensive injury, such an avulsion of the ampulla of Vater, may be treated with a lesser procedure, such as anastomosis to a Roux-en-Y limb or reimplantation into the duodenum [19, 63].

Management of Complications After Repair of Extrahepatic Biliary Ducts

The morbidity of a biliary fistula after repair or reconstruction of an injured bile duct will depend on the volume of the output and the site of the leak. A low-output fistula (<200 mL/day) may be well tolerated if there is adequate external drainage, and observation alone can be considered. A moderate-output (200–500 mL/day) or high-output (>500 mL/day) fistula may cause dehydration, may cause electrolyte abnormalities, and may lead to fistulas from adjacent pancreatic or gastrointestinal repairs.

With fistulas of any volume, it is appropriate to rehydrate the patient, correct any electrolyte deficiencies, cease oral intake, and consider the injection of subcutaneous somatostatin analogue at a dose of 100–150 mcg three times a day. A moderate- or high-output fistula that persists is treated with biliary sphincterotomy and insertion of a #7 Fr or #10 Fr biliary stent at the site of the sphincterotomy or at the site of the fistula [64, 65]. The stent is removed when the fistula closes.

One of the sequelae of a significant breakdown of a primary biliary repair or bilioenteric anastomosis is that a stricture usually results as part of secondary healing. In addition to hyperbilirubinemia and elevation of alkaline phosphatase levels, episodes of cholangitis occur. Options for therapy are the same as for strictures that occur following laparoscopic cholecystectomy or previous biliary reconstruction – namely, balloon dilatation, endoscopic stenting, or reoperation individually or in combination [65].

Chapter adapted from Feliciano DV. Biliary injuries as a result of blunt and penetrating trauma. Surg Clin N Am. 1994; 897–907.

References

1. Feliciano DV, Bitondo CG, Burch JM, Mattox KL, Beall Jr AC, Jordan Jr GL. Management of traumatic injuries to the extrahepatic biliary ducts. Am J Surg. 1985;150:705–9.
2. Ivatury RR, Rohman M, Nallathambi M, Rao PM, Gunduz Y, Stahl WM. The morbidity of injuries of the extra-hepatic biliary system. J Trauma. 1985;25:967–73.
3. Jurkovich GJ, Hoyt DB, Moore FA, Ney AL, Morris Jr JA, Scalea TM, et al. Portal triad injuries – a multi-center study. J Trauma. 1995;39:426–34.
4. Rodriguez-Mentes JA, Rojo E, Martin LG-S. Complications following repair of extrahepatic bile duct injuries after blunt abdominal trauma. World J Surg. 2001;25:1313–6.
5. Michelassi F, Ranson JHC. Bile duct disruption by blunt trauma. J Trauma. 1985;25:454–7.
6. Busuttil RW, Kitahama A, Cerise E, McFadden M, Lo R, Longmire Jr WP. Management of blunt and penetrating injuries to the porta hepatis. Ann Surg. 1980;191:641–8.
7. Kitahama A, Elliott LF, Overby JL, Webb WR. The extrahepatic biliary tract injury. Perspectives in diagnosis and treatment. Ann Surg. 1982;196:536–40.
8. Drysdale TM. Case of rupture of the common duct of the liver. Formation of a cyst containing bile. Death occurring on the fifty-third day. Autopsy. Am J Med Sci. 1861;12:399–404.
9. Feliciano DV. Biliary injuries as a result of blunt and penetrating trauma. Surg Clin North Am. 1994;74:897–907.
10. Battle NH. Traumatic rupture of the common bile duct. Trans Clin Soc Lond. 1894;27:144–8.
11. Zollinger Jr RM, Keller RT, Hubay CA. Traumatic rupture of the right and left hepatic ducts. J Trauma. 1972;12:563–9.
12. Fletcher WS, Mahnke DE, Dunphy JE. Complete division of the common bile duct due to blunt trauma. Report of a case and review of the literature. J Trauma. 1961;1:87–95.
13. Lee JG, Wherry DC. Traumatic rupture of the extra-hepatic biliary ducts from external trauma. J Trauma. 1961;1:105–14.
14. Maier WP, Lightfoot WP, Rosemond GP. Extrahepatic biliary ductal injury in closed trauma. Am J Surg. 1968;116:103–8.
15. Haynes CD, Given KS, Stone HH, Smith RB III. Nonsurgical trauma to the extrahepatic bile ducts. South Med J. 1969;62:1323–6.
16. Sheldon GF, Lim RC, Yee ES, Petersen SR. Management of injuries to the porta hepatis. Ann Surg. 1985;202:539–45.
17. Fletcher WS. Nonpenetrating trauma to the gallbladder and extrahepatic bile ducts. Surg Clin North Am. 1972;52:711–7.
18. Carmichael DH. Avulsion of the common bile duct by blunt trauma. South Med J. 1980;73:166–8.
19. Fish JC, Johnson GL. Rupture of duodenum following blunt trauma: report of a case with avulsion of papilla of Vater. Ann Surg. 1965;162:917–9.
20. Cohn Jr I, Cotlar AM, Atik M, Lumpkin WM, Hudson TL, Wernette GJ. Bile peritonitis. Ann Surg. 1960;152:827–35.
21. Mason LB, Sidbury JB, Guiang S. Rupture of the extrahepatic bile ducts from nonpenetrating trauma. Ann Surg. 1954;140:234–41.
22. Root HD, Keizer PJ, Perry Jr JF. Peritoneal trauma, experimental and clinical studies. Surgery. 1967;62:679–86.
23. Abou-Mourad NN, Rogers LS. Extrahepatic biliary steering-wheel trauma simulating pancreatic carcinoma – a dilemma in management. J Trauma. 1980;20:180–2.
24. Wangensteen OH. On the significance of the escape of sterile bile into the peritoneal cavity. Ann Surg. 1926;84:691–702.
25. Jones KB, Thomas E. Traumatic rupture of the hepatic duct demonstrated by endoscopic retrograde cholangiography. J Trauma. 1985;25:448–9.
26. Thomson SR, Bade PG. Penetrating bile duct trauma. Injury. 1989;20:215–6.
27. Borgman MA, Spinella PC, Perkins JG, Grathwohl KW, Repine T, Beekley AC, et al. The ratio of blood products transfused affects mortality in patients receiving massive transfusions at a combat support hospital. J Trauma. 2007;63:805–13.
28. Cotton BA, Gunter OL, Isbell J, Au BK, Robertson AM, Morris JA, et al. Damage control hematology: the impact of a trauma exsanguination protocol on survival and blood product utilization. J Trauma. 2008;64:1177–83.
29. Rotondo MF, Schwab CW, McGonigal MD, Phillips III GR, Fruchterman TM, Kauder DR, et al. "Damage control": an approach for improved survival in exsanguinating penetrating abdominal injury. J Trauma. 1993;35:375–82.
30. Sandblom P, Tabrizian M, Rigo M, Fluckiger A. Repair of common bile duct defects using the gallbladder or cystic duct as a pedicled graft. Surg Gynecol Obstet. 1975;140:425–32.
31. Rutledge RH. Methods of repair of noncircumferential bile duct defects. Surgery. 1983;93:333–42.
32. Lucas CE, Walt AJ. Analysis of randomized biliary drainage for liver trauma in 189 patients. J Trauma. 1972;12:925–30.

33. Northover JMA, Terblanche J. A new look at the arterial supply of the bile duct in man and its surgical implications. Br J Surg. 1979;66:379–84.
34. Donald JW, Donald JG. Complete severance of the common bile duct due to nonpenetrating trauma. Ann Surg. 1958;148:855–8.
35. Dobbie Jr RP, Stormo AC. Complete transection of the common bile duct: the sole sequela of blunt abdominal trauma. J Trauma. 1968;8:9–18.
36. Williams GR. Experiences with surgical reconstruction of the hepatic ducts. Ann Surg. 1974;179:540–8.
37. Diethrich EB, Beall Jr AC, Jordan Jr GL, DeBakey ME. Traumatic injuries to the extrahepatic biliary tract. Am J Surg. 1980;112:756–9.
38. Longmire Jr WP. Early management of injury to the extrahepatic biliary tract. JAMA. 1966;195:623–5.
39. Bengtsson HJ, Broomé AEA, Rimér V. Repair of bile duct defect with full-thickness vascularized jejunal patch. World J Surg. 1986;10:510–5.
40. Sanchez RM, Halsted GO, Trivelde RR. Common bile duct stricture repair with serosal onlay technic. Am J Surg. 1978;135:258–9.
41. Senning A. Correction of common bile duct stricture by onlay patch of duodenum. World J Surg. 1979;3:775–9.
42. Michie W, Gunn A. Bile duct injuries. A new suggestion for their repair. Br J Surg. 1964;51:96–100.
43. Monk Jr JS, Church JS, Agarwal N. Repair of a traumatic noncircumferential hepatic bile duct defect using a vein patch: case report. J Trauma. 1991;31:1555–7.
44. Belzer FO, Watts JR, Ross HB, Dunphy JE. Auto-reconstruction of the common bile duct after venous patch graft. Ann Surg. 1965;162:346–55.
45. Cushieri A, Baker PR, Anderson RJL, Holley MP. Total and subtotal replacement of the common bile duct: effect of transhepatic silicone tube stenting. Gut. 1982;24:756–60.
46. Hartung H, Kirchner R, Baba N, Waldmann D, Strecker EP. Histologic laboratory and x-ray findings after repair of the common bile duct with a Teflon graft. World J Surg. 1978;2:639–42.
47. Thomas JP, Metropol HJ, Myers RT. Teflon patch graft for reconstruction of the extrahepatic bile ducts. Ann Surg. 1964;160:967–70.
48. Rydell Jr WB. Complete transection of the common bile duct due to blunt abdominal trauma. Arch Surg. 1970;100:724–8.
49. Waddell WR, Grover FL. The gallbladder as a conduit between the liver and intestine. Surgery. 1973;74:524–9.
50. Sarr MG, Cameron JL. Surgical management of unresectable carcinoma of the pancreas. Surgery. 1982;91:123–33.
51. Posner MC, Moore EE. Extrahepatic biliary tract injury: operative management plan. J Trauma. 1985;25:833–7.
52. Voyles CR, Blumgart LH. A technique for the construction of high biliary-enteric anastomoses. Surg Gynecol Obstet. 1982;154:885–7.
53. Blumgart LH. Hilar and intrahepatic biliary enteric anastomosis. Surg Clin North Am. 1994;74:845–63.
54. Strasberg SM, Hertl M, Soper NJ. An analysis of the problem of biliary injury during laparoscopic cholecystectomy. J Am Coll Surg. 2005;180:101–25.
55. Smith R. Hepaticojejunostomy with transhepatic intubation. Br J Surg. 1964;51:186–94.
56. McFadden PM, Tanner G, Kitahama A. Traumatic hepatic duct injury. New approach to surgical management. Am J Surg. 1980;139:268–71.
57. Mercado MA, Dominguez I. Classification and management of bile duct injuries. World J Gastrointest Surg. 2011;3:43–8.
58. Wu YV, Linehan DC. Bile duct injuries in the era of laparoscopic cholecystectomies. Surg Clin North Am. 2010;90:787–802.
59. Perera MTPR, Silva MA, Hegab B, Muralidharan V, Bramhall SR, Mayer AD, et al. Specialist early and immediate repair of post-laparoscopic cholecystectomy bile duct injures is associated with an improved long-term outcome. Ann Surg. 2011;253:553–60.
60. Flint LM. Discussion of Ivatury RR, Rohman M, Nallathambi M, Rao PM, Gunduz Y, Stahl WM. The morbidity of injuries of the extra-hepatic biliary system. J Trauma. 1985;25:967–73.
61. Feliciano DV, Mattox KL, Jordan Jr GL, Burch JM, Bitondo CG, Cruse PA. Management of 1000 consecutive cases of hepatic trauma (1979–1984). Ann Surg. 1986;204:438–45.
62. Feliciano DV, Martin TD, Cruse PA, Graham JM, Burch JM, Mattox KL, et al. Management of combined pancreatoduodenal injuries. Ann Surg. 1987;250:673–80.
63. Parkinson SW, Wisniewski ZS. Avulsion of the ampulla of Vater: an isolated injury following blunt abdominal trauma. Aust N Z J Surg. 1978;48:562–4.
64. Navarrete C, Gobelet JM. Treatment of common bile duct injuries after surgery. Gastrointest Endosc Clin N Am. 2012;22:539–53.
65. Pitt HA, Sherman S, Johnson MS, Hollenbeck AN, Lee J, Daum MR, et al. Improved outcomes of bile duct injuries in the 21st century. Ann Surg. 2013;258:490–9.

Acquisition of Surgical Skills in Animal and Simulation Laboratories

Robert F. Buckman Jr. and Mark W. Bowyer

Introduction

Trauma is a leading cause of morbidity and mortality worldwide and rapid identification and control of hemorrhage is essential for survival. As such it is imperative that all surgical trainees be proficient in the management of traumatically injured patients to include operative exposure and control of bleeding. The success of nonoperative management of trauma [1–4] and implementation of duty-hour restrictions has led to an overall decline in operative experience for surgical residents [5–7]. A recent 20-year review of Accreditation Council for Graduate Medical Education (ACGME) case logs demonstrated that graduating chief residents performed half the number of mean total designated trauma operations (39.4) and operations for intra-abdominal trauma (16.8) compared to two decades ago (72.5 and 30.9, respectively) [7].

The liver remains the most frequently injured abdominal organ, despite its relatively protected location [8, 9]. The management of hepatic trauma has undergone a paradigm shift over the past several decades with significant improvement in outcomes, shifting from mandatory operation to selective nonoperative treatment and, presently, to nonoperative treatment with selective operation [10–12]. As such experience with operative management of complex liver injuries is extremely limited among current surgical trainees and recent graduates. This is borne out in the recent review of ACGME case logs showing the mean number of liver operations for trauma for graduating chief residents decreasing from 3.9 to 1.9 in the last 20 years [7]. In fact in the most recent year of reporting (2011–2012), the average number of repairs of hepatic injuries was listed at 1.4, and the average number of hepatic resections for injury was listed at 0.1 for graduating chief residents [13].

This limited experience is of great concern, as several investigators have identified experience as one factor in gaining competence [14–17]. An additional consequence of declining experience is a decrease in surgeons' confidence to manage injuries and the potential increase in morbidity and mortality [18]. Though it is difficult to judge proficiency and competence by numbers alone, it is clear that the experience of trainees is lacking and that we are graduating surgeons who when called upon to care for victims of hepatic trauma may or may not have the requisite skill set to ensure optimal outcomes. As such there is a critical need to improve the way we train and maintain the skills of the surgeon caring for trauma in the future. In a thoughtful review of this subject, Lucas and Ledgerwood [19] concluded that the decrease in therapeutic laparotomies for liver

R.F. Buckman Jr., MD, FACS (✉)
Operative Experience Inc.,
500 Principio Parkway, North East, MD 21901, USA
e-mail: rfbuckman@comcast.net

M.W. Bowyer, MD
The Norman M. Rich Department of Surgery,
Uniformed Services University,
4301 Jones Bridge Road, Bethesda, MD 20814, USA
e-mail: mark.bowyer@usush.edu

R.R. Ivatury (ed.), *Operative Techniques for Severe Liver Injury*,
DOI 10.1007/978-1-4939-1200-1_16, © Springer Science+Business Media New York 2015

injury has created a training vacuum for future trauma surgeons. They further concluded that residents will need to supplement their clinical experience with solid organ hemostasis by practice on appropriate animal models of injury and cadaver dissections [19].

Animal Laboratory (ATOM, DST, EWS Courses)

The Advanced Trauma Operative Management (ATOM) course developed at Hartford Hospital (Hartford, CT, USA) and currently administered by the American College of Surgeons Committee on Trauma was specifically designed to enhance surgeons' knowledge, confidence, and skill in repairing penetrating injuries [20]. The ATOM course uses an anesthetized pig model and the curriculum includes management of liver trauma as the terminal event of the course. The Definitive Surgical Skills Course (DSTC) administered by the International Association of Trauma and Surgical Intensive Care is designed to teach qualified surgeons and advanced surgical trainees strategic thinking and decision-making in the management of the severely injured patients and provide them with practical surgical skills to manage major organ injuries. Taught by experienced trauma-trained surgeons, it is an intensive 2-day course comprising lectures, interactive case discussions, and laboratory-based surgical skills training. The surgical skills lab is variably comprised of cadaver, animal (pig or goat), or both animal and cadaver models depending on the local availability and cultural sensitivities regarding use of such models [21]. The US military has used an animal (pig) model as part of the Emergency War Surgery Course for more than 20 years to prepare deploying surgeons [22].

The use of animals for training has several advantages, but also several distinct limitations. Animals provide an excellent representation of human physiology, with tissue that is very similar to that of humans and bleeds when cut and can be dissected and sutured using standard instruments and supplies, and there are potential consequences (death of the animal) if the procedure is not done correctly [23, 24]. The logistics of maintaining an animal lab are great, requiring veterinary support, animal care facilities, sterile operating room facilities, and the means to dispose of the animals in an accepted fashion. The use of animals is also a highly visible and emotionally charged issue decried by very active and vocal animal rights groups [22]. Additionally, the availability of the live animal model for training is highly variable across the world and in fact is prohibited in many areas. Though still available in the United States, there are multiple and repeated efforts being put forward to legislatively outlaw the use of live animals for trauma training, and there is likely to be a continuing onslaught of similar efforts and the surgical community must be proactive in searching for meaningful alternatives that can replace live tissue training though the development of physical or virtual reality-based models that can be validated in head to head comparison with existing animal models and incorporated into meaningful curricula.

Cadaver Course

Cadaver-based training has also been a longstanding mainstay of surgical training and is particularly useful for teaching vascular exposures in humans, a skill essential to the effective treatment of vascular injuries [23–26]. The availability and cost of cadavers are highly variable as is the cultural acceptability of using cadaveric material around the world. One of the authors (MWB) has helped develop and promulgate the Advanced Surgical Skills Exposures for Trauma (ASSET) course developed by the American College of Surgeons Committee on Trauma [18, 27]. This course uses human cadavers to teach vascular exposures for the management of vascular trauma, to include mobilization of and practice of the skills required to manage liver trauma. The ASSET course requires access to fresh or fresh frozen human cadavers, and the cost of obtaining cadavers is highly variable ranging from no cost to as high as $8000 depending upon which state in the United States one desires to conduct the course. Cultural and religious factors and practices make the use of cadavers impossible in many parts of the world. Even in areas where it is possible to obtain cadaveric material, the number of adequate specimens is not sufficient to meet the needs.

Though cadavers are an excellent representation of human anatomy, the anatomy is specific to that particular cadaver. As there is great variability in human anatomy, this represents a potential limitation of using the human cadaver. The way in which a cadaver is preserved also affects the utility of the cadaver model. Cadavers preserved in formalin have much different characteristics than found in a fresh or fresh frozen cadaver. The other limitation of cadaver training for vascular surgery or hemorrhage control in particular is the absence of flow within vessels and the lack of bleeding and hematoma encountered in the living. Attempts to improve the fidelity of cadaveric specimens have been made by cannulating the vessels of very fresh cadavers and perfusing them with artificial blood in a pulsatile fashion [28, 29]. Initially developed for neurosurgical training [28], this perfused cadaver model has been modified as a potential tool for training trauma surgical procedures [29]. Pulsatile flow was obtained using a modified intra-aortic balloon pump system and injuries were created in the right atrium and ventricle, as well as to the lung, liver, and inferior vena cava allowing for repair in a "bleeding human model" [29]. Though this technique improves the fidelity of the cadaveric model, it requires significant preprocessing and equipment as well as very fresh cadaveric material making it currently impractical for widespread use and adoption.

Surgical Simulation

In response to the aforementioned limitations of traditional methods of training, there has been significant interest in new ways to impart surgical training. Led by the US military, there has been an explosion in the application of emerging simulation technologies to surgical and trauma skills training [22, 30]. There has been widespread adoption of simulation in surgical training [31–37] and nearly all academic centers have invested in creating simulation-based skills labs. In the field of minimally invasive surgery, both physical and computer-based simulators have been shown to predict and improve actual performance in the operating room [38, 39]. This is achievable by using simulation solutions that provide feedback to trainees through carefully structured performance metrics and by requiring training on these simulators until some objectively assessed level of performance is achieved. While simulation for the skills required to manage the trauma patient is more challenging than for minimally invasive surgery, the potential benefit is great. The training of surgeons in the techniques of operation is different from almost any other form of technical training that might be taught using simulation. In particular, the number of variables that must be considered, the anatomic relationships, and the actual tactics and techniques required are much more extensive in major surgical operations than in most other technical fields. There are several efforts underway to improve simulation technologies to teach trauma and there have been some initial success with limited procedures [22, 40–42].

The remainder of this chapter will focus on advances in simulated physical models that have the potential to revolutionize the way in which vital trauma operative skills are taught. The goal is to display the potential value of novel high-fidelity, surgical simulators, linked to an appropriate curriculum, to teach the elements of surgical anatomy and operative tactics and techniques that are most important in the management of severe liver trauma. It is essential to recognize that simulation itself does not constitute education or training. It is merely a tool to be used to transmit, by demonstration and practice, technical curriculum content. The value of simulation-based methods for teaching major surgical operations is, at present, largely unproven. The present chapter will display the use of a prototype simulator to demonstrate selected maneuvers that might be taught and practiced using such a system. The specific and detailed techniques of operation for massive hepatic trauma have been discussed elsewhere in the text by surgeons of wide experience. Therefore, the focus will be on the potential value of the model with specific applications guided by the authors' combined 60 plus year experience with the management of hepatic trauma.

The essence of major, open operations for trauma generally includes the sudden presentation of a patient with an unusual, life-threatening emergency, associated with hemodynamic compromise. The patterns of anatomic injury associated with these emergencies are highly variable. Often the surgeon has not encountered the injury pattern that he or she is facing at present. Operative maneuvers rarely required in daily surgical practice must be now executed promptly and expertly. It is possible that, in the future, the preparation of the surgeon to manage such emergencies will be enhanced because he or she would have practiced the treatment of similar injuries in a simulation laboratory. Although simulation has been used to train surgeons for many generations, the advent of high anatomical fidelity simulators for major, open, emergency operations is a recent development. Such simulators permit the demonstration of surgical techniques using three-dimensional representations of traumatic injuries or other pathologies and allow the practice of techniques using real surgical instruments within an environment of accurate regional anatomy.

The principal limitation of the artificial, major operation simulators available thus far has been the inability to precisely duplicate the properties of biologic tissues. This is not a disabling limitation so long as the trainee has already mastered basic tissue handling skills prior to training in major operations. In this connection, it may be observed that the anatomy of experimental animals and the tissues of cadavers also present constraints in the training of complex technical procedures as previously discussed.

The prototype simulators displayed in the present chapter have non-water-based, viscoelastic tissues. The simulators can be used to display a nearly limitless number of injury patterns and can be subjected to operation with standard instruments. Demonstration of technique on a three-dimensional model permits high-quality photography and videotaping with almost unlimited camera angles and a clearer view of the operation than can be achieved with actual intraoperative photography in clinical situations. The images thus obtained constitute a valuable heuristic tool by themselves, constituting a new form of publication, and one that can be reviewed at any time using a handheld device such as a smartphone or tablet.

Simulation-based training is particularly well suited to the convenient teaching and practice of uncommon, high-stakes emergency operations. Systematic, curriculum-driven training offers the opportunity to teach approved solutions to difficult technical problems, based on the consensus opinion of experts. In this role, it may potentially transmit the understanding, born of operative experience of senior surgeons, to trainees in a manner that is more efficient than catch-as-catch-can clinical experience. Recognition of various injury patterns, and the immediate and orderly execution of approved tactics and techniques to correct the problems, can be demonstrated. Moreover, repetitive, orderly, systematic, mentored, step-by-step practice in the management of complex injuries becomes practical when simulators rather than unstable trauma patients constitute the test-bed for such practice.

Ideal simulation-based training would be part of a standardized surgical curriculum and would transmit all of the cognitive and psychomotor information necessary for a person of ordinary skills to perform all subtasks of specified operations, according to standard metrics. It is a further ideal that the trainees should prove cognitive and psychomotor proficiency in the operations, by objective testing at the completion of training. Methods and systems to achieve these ideals are currently under development and will require validation, refinement, and cost-effectiveness studies.

Massive hepatic trauma, accompanied by uncontained hemorrhage, is uncommon enough and its patterns are so variable that, with rare exceptions, the personal, operative experience of a single surgeon, even over a period of many years, will not be extensive. Recommendations concerning the ideal conduct of operations to control hepatic hemorrhage, offered by any particular expert, must be viewed in this light. Very little, if any, firm scientific foundation undergirds operative recommendations. The basis of most operative practices in hepatic trauma is the published experience of surgeons with large experience and/or high interest in this topic. Doctrines have evolved, particularly over the last 20 years, in favor of nonoperative therapies and "damage control" operations [8–12], although the teaching of some techniques that have a dismal clinical record and that should be of historical interest only, such as atriocaval shunting, continues [20].

The basic techniques for the control of hepatic hemorrhage demonstrated hereafter are based on observations that appear to have the strongest experiential foundations. The first of these evidence-based observations and one that has been repeatedly confirmed since the advent of CT scanning is that hepatic injuries, even those involving extensive destruction of the hepatic parenchyma and laceration of intrahepatic blood vessels, have a favorable prognosis, even without operation, if there has been spontaneous containment of hemorrhage by the capsule and/or ligaments of the liver [43–49]. Containment or tamponade of hemorrhage is all that is necessary to prevent death or severe morbidity. Although angiography and embolization of persistent intraparenchymal hepatic artery bleeding is sometimes necessary, the loss of containment more than 24 h after injury with hemorrhage requiring operative intervention is uncommon [50]. The corollary of this observation is that, when surgical intervention is required because of active bleeding, operative containment or tamponade of the hemorrhage by the simplest measures possible, without any necessity for definitive repair of the parenchyma or vessels, is a sufficient treatment.

A second, well-founded observation of high practical value is that the effective control of uncontained hemorrhage by gauze packing, performed early in the operation carries a lower mortality risk than attempts at definitive repair followed by desperation packing when repair fails [44, 45, 51–53].

A third and related observation, based on a collective review of reported experience, is that

attempts at direct repair of the juxtahepatic vena cava and hepatic veins, although sometimes successful, have a higher overall mortality risk than control of such injuries by packing or other measures to contain the hemorrhage [50]. Our belief in the soundness of these basic observations and personal experience with the consequences of departing from them informs the following demonstrations of techniques that we believe are most valuable. However, as previously indicated, our purpose here is to demonstrate the potential value of simulation to demonstrate techniques for operative control of major hepatic hemorrhage rather than to advocate for or against particular techniques or beliefs.

The techniques demonstrated in the images of this chapter are some of those that have been described elsewhere in this volume for the operative management of the most dangerous forms of hepatic injury, those involving hemorrhage that has escaped containment and tamponade by the hepatic parenchyma, capsule, and ligaments.

A stepwise approach to the patient with massive bleeding from hepatic trauma is paramount. Coincident with preparing to take the unstable patient to the operating room, massive transfusion protocol to include large volume infusions of red blood cells, plasma, and platelet packs in an approximate ratio of 1:1:1 should be initiated and continued until control of hemorrhage is achieved. The first expedient in operations for massive trauma is to gain immediate, if sometimes temporary, control of the bleeding. This control is usually achieved by manual pressure or gauze packing accompanied by a Pringle maneuver. Initial control allows further resuscitation of the patient and allows for the surgeon to plan subsequent steps in a more controlled fashion.

One of the authors (RFB) has pioneered the development of novel hyperrealistic physical models with characteristics of human tissue that can be operated on using real surgical instruments. This novel technology has enabled the creation of realistic appearing and bleeding models with true representations of human anatomy and the surgical planes encountered by surgeons. The liver and adjacent structures have been successfully modeled and can be used to replicate

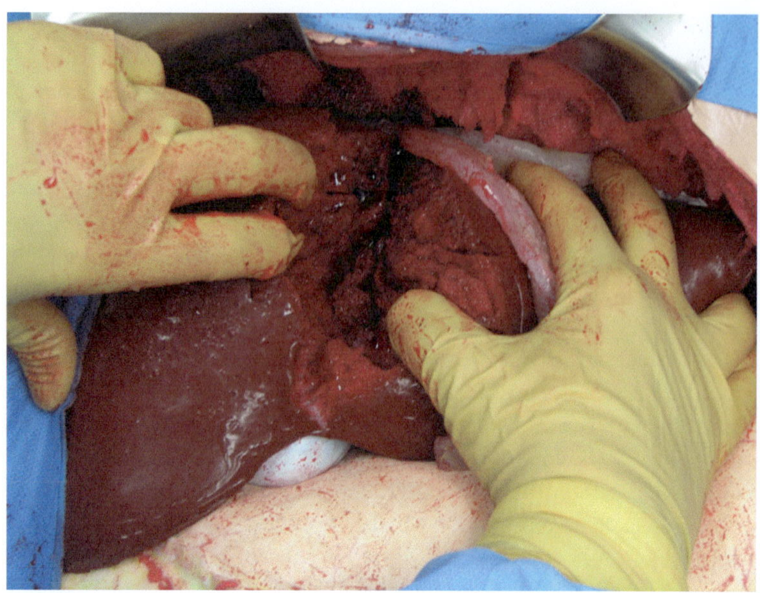

Fig. 16.1 This figure shows a complex, stellate hepatic fracture within the interlobar plane between the gallbladder bed and inferior vena cava in a high-fidelity surgical simulator. Hepatic venous bleeding is evident from the depths of the fracture. Modern technology makes it possible to create not only this wound but a wide variety of hepatic injury patterns within artificial tissues (Image courtesy of Operative Experience Inc.)

traumatic injuries that can be incorporated into curricula to teach the operative management of hepatic trauma. Figure 16.1 demonstrates the degree of fidelity that can be achieved with such models, showing a simulated liver with a deep, stellate, parenchymal fracture extending along the interlobar plane between the gallbladder bed and the vena cava. This type of injury frequently involves a laceration of the middle hepatic vein. The model displays simulated bleeding from the depths of the hepatic fracture. The injury pattern also includes injury to branches of the hepatic artery and portal vein often concealed within the many overhangs, crags, and fissures of the complex wound zone.

Because of the massive disruption of the hepatic parenchyma and capsule, spontaneous containment of hemorrhage is impossible in the type of wound depicted in Fig. 16.1. Patients with this pattern of injury often present in hemorrhagic shock. A positive FAST exam or peritoneal tap results in rapid transport of the patient to the operating room for exploratory laparotomy and continued resuscitation.

We propose that a comprehensive curriculum, based on this high-fidelity physical model/surgical simulator, could be developed to teach the operative management of severe hepatic trauma. Such a curriculum might include training in maneuvers such as manual compression of the liver; mobilization of the liver; perihepatic packing; Pringle maneuver; control of accessible, intrahepatic artery branches using clips or ligatures; mobilization of the omentum; omental packing of the liver; and placement of deep liver sutures. These maneuvers which are rarely performed in clinical practice are fundamental to the management of a complex liver injury. The simulator permits not only the demonstration but also the repeated and systematic practice of all these maneuvers, using standard surgical instruments. Additionally, the standardized nature of the model would allow for rigorous assessment of trainees to ensure correct performance.

The physical model takes into account the fact that the liver has a somewhat pyramidal shape that makes manual compression of the very thick, deep central zone difficult. By constructing the simulated liver in a three-dimensional anatomically correct fashion, it is possible to fold down the left lateral segment, as shown in Fig. 16.2. This allows the liver to assume a more globular shape that facilitates manual compression of the deep portions of the liver where the largest segments of the intraparenchymal hepatic veins reside. Compression of this deep posterior central zone of the liver is essential to immediate hemorrhage control because hepatic vein bleeding is

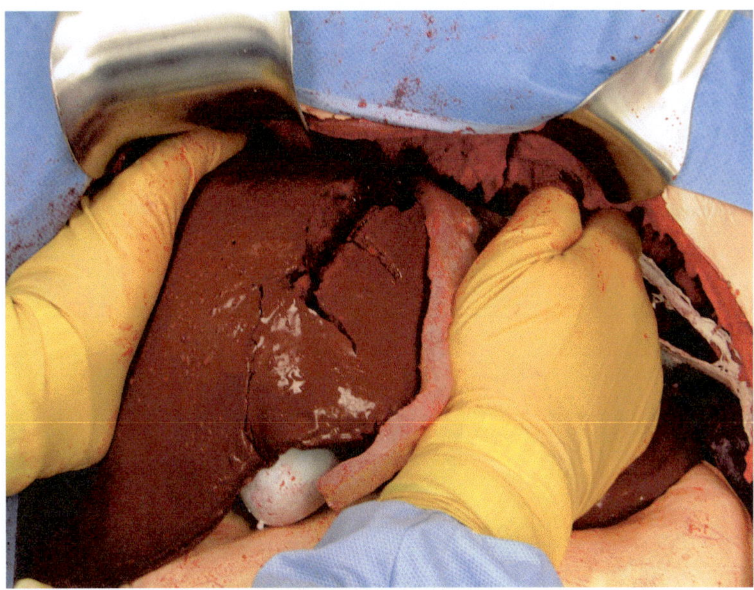

Fig. 16.2 A demonstration of manual compression of the liver after mobilization of the left triangular and falciform ligaments. The anterior body wall of the simulator has been removed to facilitate photography (Image courtesy of Operative Experience Inc.)

not controlled by a Pringle maneuver. Mobilization of the left lateral segment can then be achieved by taking down the left triangular ligament in a way that does not involve a major entry into the bare area of the liver.

The photograph of Fig. 16.2 shows the cut left triangular and falciform ligaments. The falciform ligament has been divided all the way back to the vena cava within the areolar tissue of the bare area. This is potentially a tactical error, leading to bad outcomes. The injury pattern shown on the simulator carries a risk of associated injury to the retrohepatic vena cava or the extraparenchymal hepatic veins. In such a case, hepatic mobilization that destroys the suspensory ligaments of the liver, exposing the bare area, is extremely dangerous because it may release uncontrollable hemorrhage from injured retrohepatic, major veins.

Wide hepatic mobilization has long been recommended by most experts as an early, and almost automatic, step in the management of liver injuries. In most cases, it facilitates exposure and is safe. However, an exception to this rule exists in patterns of injury that might be associated with retrohepatic venous injuries. Mobilization of the liver should be a rational rather than an automatic decision. In our opinion, mobilization should be limited to the left triangular ligament and the falciform ligament anterior to the coronary ligaments, if there is a possibility that a spontaneously contained retrohepatic venous injury may exist.

Taking down the hepatic ligaments is easy to do but impossible to undo. Destruction of the spontaneous containment of a retrohepatic venous injury by surgical division of the coronary and triangular ligaments may leave the operator with no choice but to attempt a direct repair of the venous injury, using an atriocaval shunt, venovenous bypass, or some other heroic and high-risk approach. This potential catastrophe is largely avoidable if the operator is circumspect about hepatic mobilization in cases in which a contained retrohepatic/bare area hemorrhage may exist. In such cases, if the hepatic suspensory ligaments are damaged with leakage of blood or if injudicious hepatic mobilization has already begun when the blood is encountered, the suspensory ligaments should be repaired or reinforced to restore bare area containment.

Hepatic inflow occlusion by the Pringle maneuver is, together with manual compression and packing, one of the key initial maneuvers for hepatic hemorrhage control. Although almost any type of vascular clamp or a Rumel tourniquet could be used, we have found that a highly angled vascular clamp such as that shown in Fig. 16.3 is

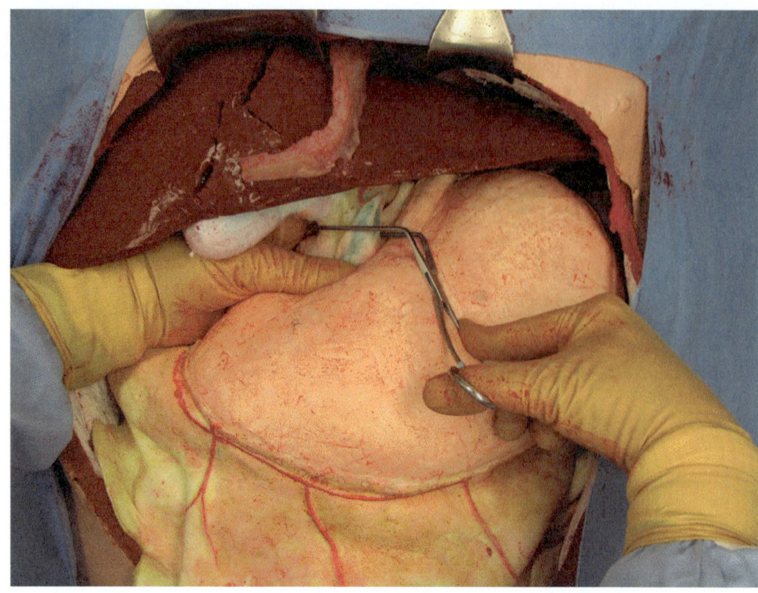

Fig. 16.3 A demonstration of the Pringle maneuver: with a finger in the foramen of Winslow, an angled vascular clamp is placed across the hepatic inflow vessels (Image courtesy of Operative Experience Inc.)

ideal. The clamp may be rapidly placed if the operator places the index finger of the left hand through the foramen of Winslow, loops the finger around the portal structures, and passes the clamp from a medial to lateral direction against the finger through the lesser omentum as shown in Fig. 16.3. With this direction of clamping, the handle of the clamp lies on the anterior stomach and remains out of the way during the rest of the operation.

Effective hepatic inflow occlusion abolishes arterial and portal perfusion of the liver, except in the case of an aberrant left hepatic artery. The persistence of dark bleeding through or around the liver after hepatic inflow occlusion indicates hepatic venous injury. Bleeding through the fractured liver indicates an injury of the intraparenchymal portion of the hepatic veins. Dark blood issuing through the suspensory ligaments of the liver indicates potential extraparenchymal hepatic venous or retrohepatic vena cava injury.

Figure 16.4 shows the appearance of a rolled gauze pack. Over the years, one of the authors (RFB) has found multiple uses for gauze packs made in this way, particularly as an adjunct to manual pressure on bleeding sites, including injuries of the inferior vena cava. They also work well as rapidly placed tampons in large soft tissue wounds of the abdominal and flank muscles

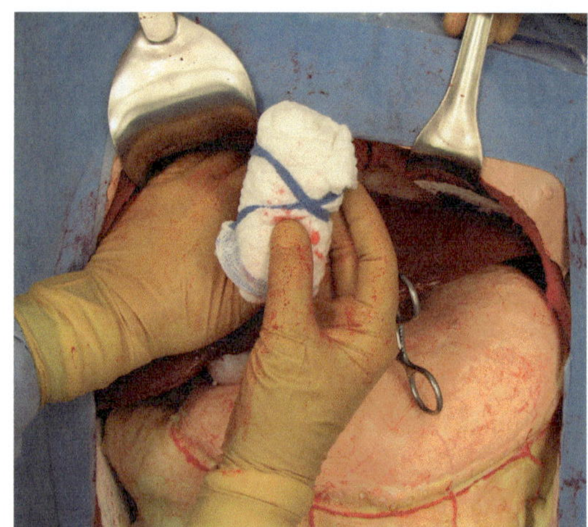

Fig. 16.4 The use of rolled gauze packs allows the application of focal pressure at selected points on the liver. The packs are created by folding standard laparotomy pads in thirds and rolling them into tight cylinders with the ribbon maintaining the shape. They are often used in combination with loose gauze packing (Image courtesy of Operative Experience Inc.)

while attention is directed to more pressing injuries. In liver trauma, they are useful for perihepatic and subhepatic packing because they maintain their structure and can be placed and stacked in precise locations, for example, along the dome of the liver or against the hepatic suspensory ligaments.

As is true for many things in operative surgery, there has been no trial comparing the efficacy of packs made in this way to standard, loose gauze packing with regard to the control of bleeding. If the packs are premade and stored in sterile bags, dozens of them can be made available at the beginning of a case, which allows for extremely rapid abdominal packing, including the use of stacked rolls at actively bleeding sites.

High-energy transfer injuries of the liver, whether due to blunt bursting fractures or high-energy gunshot wounds, create extremely complex wounding patterns within the parenchyma. The area of destruction often contains, in addition to the primary laceration, multiple secondary and tertiary crevices, crags, and overhangs. Tissue within the wounded parenchyma is extremely friable. In the absence of major hemorrhage from hepatic vein injury, an effective Pringle maneuver permits entry into the injury site where accessible arterial and portal vein branches may be directly controlled with hemostatic surgical clips. This approach is illustrated in Fig. 16.5. High-pressure bleeding from arteries is the real target. The lesser branches of the portal vein and intraparenchymal hepatic veins which are low pressure vessels can be controlled by omental packing, deep hepatic sutures, and perihepatic gauze packing.

It is extremely difficult if not impossible to completely control all bleeding sites within complex burst fractures of the liver using direct measures such as surgical clips. Intraparenchymal packing with gauze is not widely used although the long-standing prejudice against this practice, based on clinical experiences, does not appear to have a strong scientific foundation. The best expedient for packing within the substance of the liver is the omental pack based on the right gastroepiploic artery.

In severe hepatic fractures, that is, those in which intraparenchymal hemostatic packing may be contemplated, the structural integrity of the omentum should be preserved during initial exploration of the lesser sac. Rather than clamping across the omentum to gain access to the lesser sac, the slightly more time-consuming expedient of mobilizing the omentum from the

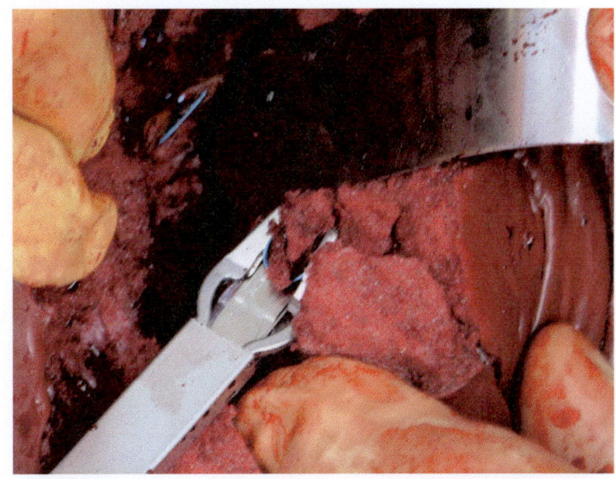

Fig. 16.5 After an effective Pringle maneuver, surgical clips can be used to control accessible bleeding vessels and bile ducts within the hepatic injury zone. Because the disrupted tissue is very friable, the use of suture ligatures is slower and generally less satisfactory than the use of the clips. Even the clips are not absolutely secure. One should be careful not to displace them during subsequent omental packing of the liver (Image courtesy of Operative Experience Inc.)

transverse colon in the avascular plane preserves the entire omentum for later use. The thickness of the omentum varies widely from individual to individual; in obese individuals it may be very substantial, whereas in lean young males, it may have relatively little fat.

The ability to demonstrate on the model the procedure for mobilizing the omentum on the right gastroepiploic artery and using it to pack a major liver defect is shown in Figs. 16.6, 16.7, 16.8, 16.9, 16.10, and 16.11. In nearly all patients no matter how obese, there is a thin area of the greater omentum below the left inferior aspect of the greater curvature of the stomach. This area is easily penetrated with finger dissection, which is the first step in mobilization. It is desirable to start the mobilization of the omentum in this location, just inferior to the short gastric arteries, because it makes virtually the entire omentum available for later use (Fig. 16.6).

The dissection of the omentum is carried down to the greater curvature. The gastric branches of the gastroepiploic artery are now divided between clamps, along the wall of the stomach (Fig. 16.7). This process is repeated all along the greater curvature until a sufficient

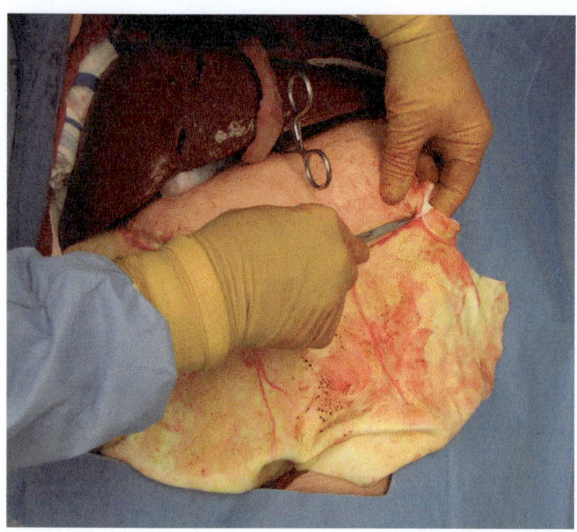

Fig. 16.6 Beginning mobilization of the greater omentum along the curvature of the stomach. Finger dissection has opened a rent in the thinnest portion of the omentum. The gastric branches of the gastroepiploic artery are isolated and divided between clamps (Image courtesy of Operative Experience Inc.)

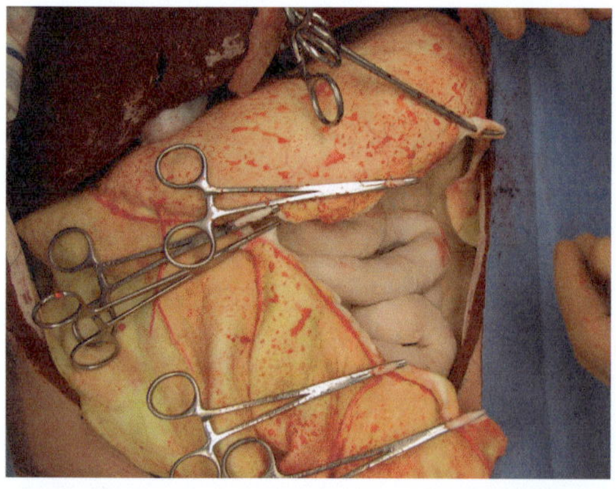

Fig. 16.7 Continued mobilization of the momentum from the greater curvature (Image courtesy of Operative Experience Inc.)

amount of omentum has been mobilized for the desired use.

The arteries on both the stomach side and the arterial side must be securely ligated (Fig. 16.8). The branches of the gastroepiploic artery that are going to be packed into the liver with the omentum must be tied carefully to avoid the displacement of the ligature during hepatic packing as this would create a source of arterial bleeding from the hemostatic pack itself.

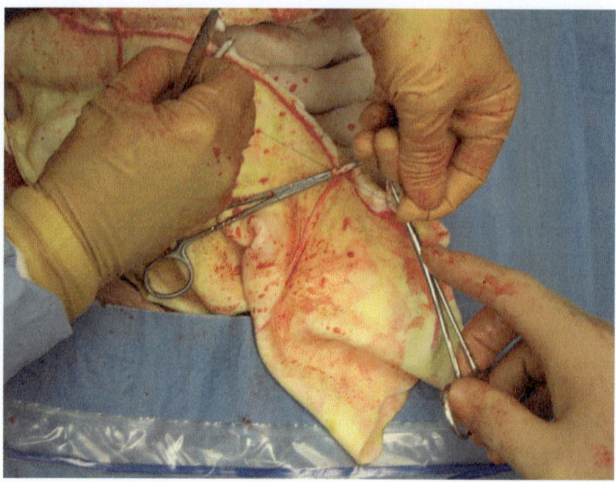

Fig. 16.8 Secure ligation of the branches of the gastroepiploic artery that will be packed into the liver is absolutely essential. The use of hemostatic clips is not recommended for this maneuver because the clips will be susceptible to displacement as the omentum is packed into the liver wound (Image courtesy of Operative Experience Inc.)

After full mobilization and with care to avoid a 360° twist of the gastroepiploic artery pedicle, the omentum is inserted into the hepatic fracture (Fig. 16.9). This maneuver must be done with delicacy to avoid lacerating vessels in the omentum, pushing clips off the vessels in the liver parenchyma, or displacing ties on the gastroepiploic artery. With finger pressure on the omentum within the crevice in the liver, a series of large liver sutures of # 1 Chromic on a blunt-tipped needle are used to bridge the defect and secure the omental pack in place (Fig. 16.10). Bolsters are generally not required although a delicate touch is necessary while tying the sutures to avoid having them cut through the liver. The main role of these sutures is to hold the pack in place while exerting some compression of the liver against the pack. However, perihepatic packing, often using rolled gauze packs, is almost invariably required to further compress the liver against the omental pack (Fig. 16.11).

Summary

Educating surgical trainees to proficiently and competently manage victims of trauma has become ever more challenging in this era of

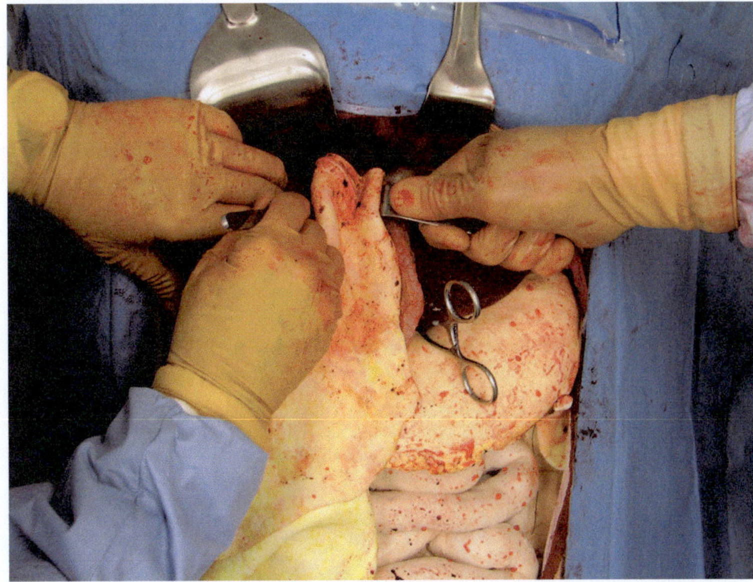

Fig. 16.9 The mobilized omentum is packed into liver injury with care to avoid a 360° twist of the pedicle or injury to the arteries within the omental pack (Image courtesy of Operative Experience Inc.)

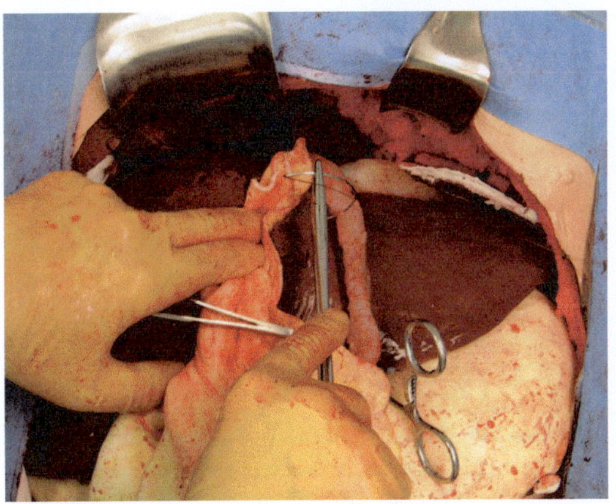

Fig. 16.10 The omental pack is secured within the liver with large sutures of number 1 Chromic on a blunt-tipped liver needle (Image courtesy of Operative Experience Inc.)

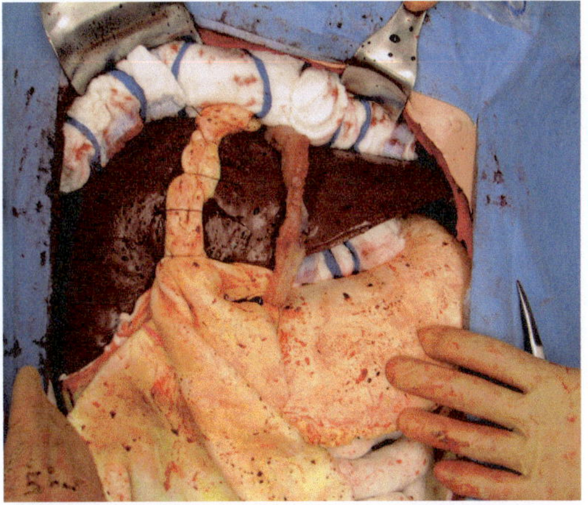

Fig. 16.11 Perihepatic packing using rolled gauze packs complements the hemostatic compression of the liver. The anterior body wall of the simulator has been removed to facilitate visualization. In clinical practice, packs would be inserted between the anterior surface of the liver and the diaphragm (Image courtesy of Operative Experience Inc.)

nonoperative management of trauma and mandated work-hour restrictions. We will likely not be able to train longer; thus, we need to develop ways to train smarter. We believe that the use of simulation technology and validated, consensus-driven curricula based upon hyperrealistic physical models such as the liver model presented in this chapter can revolutionize surgical education. Using this template, we have the ability to create models for virtually any pathology and operative technique desired for train-

ing. Such models have the potential of augmenting and perhaps replacing currently used animal and cadaver models. We envision a day when surgical residents will be able to perform all of the essential and uncommon operations on a hyperrealistic physical model guided by a rigidly standardized consensus-driven curriculum. This standardized curricular approach will allow for rigorous assessment of skill and the ability to produce surgeons who can confidently "perform as advertised" with resultant improvements in outcomes.

Disclaimer/Disclosure The views expressed herein are those of the authors and are not to be construed as official or reflecting the views of the Department of Defense. The lead author (RFB) is the founder and chief executive officer of Operative Experience Inc. (North East Maryland) which develops, manufactures, and distributes high-fidelity surgical simulation systems. There are no other disclosures.

References

1. Hawkins ML, Wynn JJ, Schmacht DC, Medeiros RS, Gadacz TR. Nonoperative management of liver and/or splenic injuries: effect on resident surgical experience. Am Surg. 1998;64:552–6.
2. Lukan JK, Carillo EH, Franklin GA, Spain DA, Miller FB, Richardson JD. Impact of recent trends for noninvasive trauma evaluation and nonoperative management in surgical resident education. J Trauma. 2001;50:1015–9.
3. Bulinski P, Bachulis B, Naylor DF, Kam D, Carey M, Dean RE. The changing face of trauma management and its impact on surgical resident training. J Trauma. 2003;54:161–3.
4. Bittner 4th JG, Hawkins ML, Medeioros RS, Beatty JS, Atteberry LR, Ferdinand CH, Mellinger JD. Nonoperative management of solid organ injury diminishes surgical resident operative experience: is it time for simulation training? J Surg Res. 2010;163:179–85.
5. Sadababa JR, Urso S. Does the introduction of duty-hour restrictions in the United States negatively affect the operative volume of surgical trainees? Interact Cardiovasc Thorac Surg. 2011;13:316–9.
6. Damadi A, Davis AT, Saxe A, Apelgren K. ACME duty-hour restrictions decrease resident operative volume: a 5-year comparison at an ACGME-accredited university general surgery residency. J Surg Educ. 2007;64:256–9.
7. Drake FT, Van Eaton EG, Huntington CR, Jurkovich GJ, Aarabi S, Gow KG. ACGME case logs: surgery resident experience in operative trauma for two decades. J Trauma Acute Care Surg. 2012;73:1500–6.
8. Ochiai T, Igari K, Yagi M, Ito H, Kumagai Y, Iida M, et al. Treatment strategy for blunt hepatic trauma: analysis of 183 consecutive cases. Hepatogastroenterology. 2011;58:1312–5.
9. Morrison JJ, Bramley KE, Rizzo AG. Liver trauma—operative management. J R Army Med Corps. 2011;157(2):136–44.
10. Kozar RA, Feliciano DV, Moore EE, Moore FA, Cocanour CS, West MA, et al. Western Trauma Association/critical decisions in trauma: operative management of adult blunt hepatic trauma. J Trauma. 2011;71:1–5.
11. Jiang H, Wang J. Emergency strategies and trends in the management of liver trauma. Front Med. 2012;6:225–33.
12. Stein DM, Scalea TM. Nonoperative management of spleen and liver injuries. J Intensive Care Med. 2006;21:296–304.
13. Accreditation Council for Graduate Medical Education online- http://www.acgme.org/acgmeweb/Portals/0/GSNatData1112.pdf. Accessed Jan 6 2013.
14. Bell R. Why Johnny cannot operate. Surgery. 2009;146:533–42.
15. Compeau C, Tryhitt J, Shargall Y, Rotstein L. A retrospective review of general surgery training outcomes at the University of Toronto. Can J Surg. 2009;52:E131–6.
16. Suwanabol PA, McDonald R, Foley E, Weber SM. Is surgical resident comfort level associated with experience? J Surg Res. 2009;156:240–4.
17. Fonza JS, Prystowsky JP, Darosa D, Fryer JP. Surgical residents' perception of confidence and relevance of the clinical curriculum to future practice. J Surg Educ. 2012;69:792–7.
18. Kuhls DA, Risucci DA, Bowyer MW, Luchette FA. Advanced surgical skills for exposure in trauma: a new surgical cadaver course for residents and fellows. J Trauma Acute Care Surg. 2013;74(2):664–70.
19. Lucas CE, Ledgerwood AM. The academic challenge of teaching psychomotor skills for hemostasis of solid organ injury. J Trauma. 2009;66:636–40.
20. Jacobs LM, Burns KJ, Kaban JM, Gross RI, Cortes V, Brautigam RT, et al. Development and evaluation of the advanced trauma operative management course. J Trauma. 2003;5:471–9.
21. Ryan JM, Roberts P. Definitive surgical trauma skills: a new skills course for specialist registrars and consultants in general surgery in the United Kingdom. Trauma. 2002;4:184–8.
22. Ritter EM, Bowyer MW. Simulation for trauma and combat casualty care. Min Invas Ther Allied Technol. 2005;14:224–34.
23. Reeds MG. Trauma training using the live tissue model. J Trauma. 2010;69:999–1000.
24. Sohn VY, Miller JP, Koeller CA, Gibson SO, Azarow KS, Myers JB, et al. From the combat medic to the forward surgical team: they Madigan model for improving trauma readiness of brigade combat teams fighting the Global War on Terror. J Surg Res. 2007;138:25–31.
25. Gambhir RPS, Agrawal A. Training in trauma management. Med J Armed Forces India. 2010;66:354–6.
26. Gunst M, O'Keeffe T, Hollett L, Hamill M, Gentilello LM, Frankel H, et al. Trauma operative skills in the era of nonoperative management: the trauma exposure course. J Trauma. 2009;67:1091–6.

27. Kuhls DA, Risucci DA, Bowyer MW, Luchette FA. ASSET: an effective educational experience for practicing surgeons. Bull Am Coll Surg. 2012;97:31–5.
28. Aboud E, Al-Mefty O, Yasargil MG. New laboratory model for neurosurgical training that simulates live surgery. J Neurosurg. 2002;97:1367–72.
29. Aboud ET, Krisht AF, O'Keefe T, Nader R, Hassan M, Stevens CM, et al. Novel simulation training for trauma surgeons. J Trauma. 2011;71:1484–90.
30. Kaufmann C, Lui A. Trauma training: virtual reality applications. Stud Health Technol Inform. 2001;81:236–41.
31. Evgeniou E, Loizou P. Simulation-based surgical education. ANZ J Surg. 2012;82:1445–2197.
32. De Visser H, Watson MO, Salvado O, Passenger JD. Progress in virtual reality simulators for surgical training and certification. Med J Aust. 2011;194:S38–40.
33. Fried GM. Lessons from the surgical experience with simulators: incorporation into training and utilization in determining competency. Gastrointest Endosc Clin N Am. 2006;16:425–34.
34. Kneebone R. Simulation in surgical training: educational issues and practical implications. Med Educ. 2003;37:267–77.
35. Windsor JA. Role of simulation in surgical education and training. ANZ J Surg. 2009;79:127–32.
36. Tan SS, Sarker SK. Simulation in surgery: a review. Scott Med J. 2011;56:104–9.
37. Cherry RA, Ali J. Current concepts in simulation-based trauma education. J Trauma. 2008;65:1186–93.
38. Seymour N, Gallagher A, Roman S, O'Brien MK, Bansal VK, Andersen DK, et al. Virtual reality training improves operating room performance: results of a randomized. Double-blinded study. Ann Surg. 2002;236:458–64.
39. Grantcharov T, Kristianson V, Bendix J, Bardram L, Rosnenburg J, Funch-Jensen P. Randomized clinical trial of virtual reality simulation for laparoscopic skills training. Br J Surg. 2004;91:146–50.
40. Knudson MM, Khaw L, Bullard MK, Dicker R, Cohen MJ, Staudenmayer K, et al. Trauma training in simulation: translating skills from SIM time to real time. J Trauma. 2008;64:255–63.
41. Bowyer MW, Manahal M, Acosta E, Stutzmen J, Lui A. Far forward feasibility: testing a cricothyroid simulator in Iraq. Stud Health Technol Inform. 2008;132:37–41.
42. Acosta E, Lui A, Armonda R, Fiorill M, Haluck R, Lake C, et al. Burrhole simulation for an intracranial hematoma simulator. Stud Health Technol Inform. 2007;125:1–6.
43. Moore EE. Critical decisions in the management of hepatic trauma. Am J Surg. 1984;148:712–6.
44. Carmona RH, Peck DZ, Lim RC. The role of packing and planned reoperation in severe hepatic trauma. J Trauma. 1984;24:779–84.
45. Sheridan R, Driscoll D, Felsen R. Packing and temporary closure in a liver injury. Injury. 1997;28:711–2.
46. Carillo EH, Wohltmann C, Richardson JD, Polk Jr HC. Evolution in the treatment of complex blunt liver injuries. Curr Probl Surg. 2001;38:1–60.
47. Christmas AB, Wilson AK, Manning B, Franklin GA, Miller FB, Richardson JD, et al. Selective management of blunt hepatic injuries including nonoperative management is a safe and effective strategy. Surgery. 2005;138:606–11.
48. Liu PP, Chen CL, Cheng YF, Hsieh PM, Tan BL, Jawan B, et al. Use of a refined operative strategy in Combination with the multidisciplinary approach to manage blunt juxtahepatic venous injuries. J Trauma. 2005;59:940–5.
49. Kozar RA, McNutt MK. Management of adult blunt hepatic trauma. Curr Opin Crit Care. 2010;16:596–601.
50. Buckman RF, Miraliakbari R, Badellino MM. Juxtahepatic venous injuries: a critical review of reported management strategies. J Trauma. 2000;48:978–84.
51. Feliciano DV, Mattox KL, Jordan Jr GL. Intra-abdominal packing for control of hepatic hemorrhage: a reappraisal. J Trauma. 1981;21:285–90.
52. Feliciano DV, Mattox KL, Burch JM, et al. Packing for control of hepatic hemorrhage. J Trauma. 1986;26:738–43.
53. Beal S. Fatal hepatic hemorrhage: an unresolved problem in the management of complex liver injuries. J Trauma. 1990;30(2):163–9.

Acquisition of Surgical Skills by Hepatobiliary Rotation

Brian G. Harbrecht and J. David Richardson

Introduction

The changes that have occurred over the last several decades regarding the management of liver injuries have been described in several recent publications [1–3]. The number of liver injuries being identified has increased over time associated with improvements in techniques for diagnosis and the widespread use of computed tomography (CT) in injured patients [1, 2]. However, the incidence of major, high-grade hepatic injuries has remained largely unchanged in 12–15 % of all liver injuries [1–4]. Most liver injuries in patients with satisfactory hemodynamics are now managed nonoperatively [3, 5, 6]. While some have reported that this shift in management has not changed resident operative experience [5], others have noted a significant decline in the resident operative experience in the management of liver trauma [6, 7]. Lucas reported that recent graduating chief surgical residents performed a mean of 1.2 operations for hemostasis with liver injuries with most having no experience with complex techniques of liver injury management such as tractotomy or hepatic resection [7]. Given the preponderance of nonoperative management, it may take years for a surgeon to accrue substantial personal experience in the operative management of patients with complex, high-grade liver injuries. Currently, patients with liver injuries undergoing operative treatment are frequently the subset of patients with the most severe liver injuries, unstable hemodynamics, and the most severe physiologic derangements. The relatively infrequent presentation of patients with complex liver injuries requiring operative treatment combined with their typically unstable hemodynamics has created a challenging scenario for the training of future trauma surgeons. What is the best way to train surgeons to manage an injury that occurs infrequently in even the busiest trauma centers but when present, requires rapid decision making, challenging surgical exposure of the site of bleeding, and potentially complex operative techniques for hemostasis?

The pitfalls of dealing with complex liver injuries are different compared than those of severe injuries of the spleen and kidney even though these injuries are often combined into outcome studies on "solid organ injuries." For the spleen and kidney, mobilization and excision are often an expeditious way to deal with the actively bleeding and extensively damaged organ. However with the liver, especially when major venous injuries are present, mobilization for exposure can increase hemorrhage and potentially complicate operative management [8]. Perihepatic packing can help achieve hemostasis with selected severe liver injuries even when major venous injuries are present as long as the retroperitoneal tissues have not been significantly violated and can be used to

B.G. Harbrecht, MD • J.D. Richardson, MD (✉)
Department of Surgery,
University of Louisville Hospital,
550 South Jackson Street,
Louisville, KY 40292, USA
e-mail: jdrich01@louisville.edu

R.R. Ivatury (ed.), *Operative Techniques for Severe Liver Injury*,
DOI 10.1007/978-1-4939-1200-1_17, © Springer Science+Business Media New York 2015

help tamponade bleeding [3, 8, 9]. Unfortunately, some injuries will not respond to perihepatic packing, will continue to bleed even when packed, and require direct repair. Deciding when to abandon packing and proceed with direct repair requires experience, judgment, and then familiarity with techniques to expose and repair this challenging injury.

In order to optimize outcome from major hepatic injuries, the surgeon needs to be fully prepared to rapidly execute several operative steps and have a variety of techniques in their armamentarium. The maneuvers and techniques that can be applied are discussed in recent publications [3, 10] and in previous chapters of this work. How to become facile in these techniques when the injury is uncommon is an ongoing challenge since residency, fellowship, and even years of practice may expose the surgeon to few severe hepatic injuries. A combination, though, of structured training and self-directed learning can familiarize the surgeon or trainee with the relevant anatomy and techniques for surgical exposure that prove useful in managing these injuries.

Cadaver Dissection

Use of cadavers for medical education to study anatomy has been practiced for centuries. More recently, cadavers have been used to develop or practice techniques in laparoscopic and vascular surgery, help compensate for decreased trainee exposure to operative procedures imposed by work hour restrictions, and disseminate new techniques [11–13]. The use of "lightly" or "softly" embalmed cadavers has helped avoid decomposition problems associated with the use of fresh cadavers while preserving anatomic planes, tissue feel, and the appearance of fresh tissue that helps the surgeon prepare for dissection in a living patient [13]. The development of a fresh tissue or "lightly embalmed" tissue dissection program for surgical training requires extensive institutional support and commitment, multidisciplinary involvement to optimize utilization, and a supply of donor cadavers from the community to name a few of the obstacles.

While an objective educational benefit to trainees with the use of cadaver dissections has been difficult to prove, prior experience with a procedure in a controlled, nonbleeding environment with cadavers improves trainee confidence and subjectively enhances their education [11, 12]. Our institution has had an active multidisciplinary tissue dissection laboratory for several decades. It has formed the basis for a number of important investigations in the fields of anatomy, orthopedic surgery, plastic and microsurgery, and general surgery [14]. In addition to its use in formal anatomic research, it is a valuable educational tool for our general surgery residents to practice and become facile with several operative exposures for injured patients including mobilization of the liver, exposure of the hepatic veins, dissection of the supra- and infrahepatic vena cava, and isolation of the portal triad structures. While the number of patients with complex liver injuries that any individual resident or fellow manages may be limited, the number of fresh tissue dissections and exposures can be extensive.

Organ Procurement Rotation

Preparation of abdominal organs for procurement for subsequent transplantation involves exposure and control of major vascular structures, isolation and control of the vena cava, and dissection of the hepatic hilar vessels in a manner that emphasizes avoidance of injury to the organ to be transplanted. Experience in these maneuvers will be performed in a similar manner for patients with liver injuries. A rotation on an organ procurement team has been shown to improve resident knowledge of anatomy and technical skill in vascular control relevant to the patient with complex liver injuries [15].

The value of an organ procurement rotation will be directly proportional to the volume of the procurement/transplant service and the effectiveness of the local Organ Procurement Organization (OPO) in achieving donations. At our institution, residents cover the organ procurement service as senior-level residents and gain valuable experience in the exposure and control of major vascular structures, retroperitoneal anatomy, and dissection of the portal triad in heart-beating subjects. Incorporating this experience while on clinical services that are less busy provides a valuable experience within work hour constraints.

Hepatobiliary Rotation

Experience performing an operation under elective conditions should improve the ability to perform an operation under emergency conditions. Rotation on a busy liver transplant, hepatobiliary (HPB), or hepatic resection service is an excellent way for the trainee to become familiar with several aspects of hepatic surgery that may prove useful when managing complex hepatic injuries. These include an improved knowledge of anatomy for vascular isolation and control, mobilization of the liver and exposure of key structures, hilar anatomy, techniques for parenchymal transaction, techniques and new technologies for hemostasis, and methods for the prevention/management of postoperative bile leaks [16].

While extensive experience in elective liver surgery may be the most productive way to gain experience for emergency liver surgery, there are significant obstacles that must be overcome. Despite national increases in the number of hepatic resections being performed [17], graduating general surgery residents completing training report relatively few major hepatic resections during training [18, 19]. This finding may be due to progressive regionalization of elective liver resection to high-volume surgeons in high-volume centers [20]. If this trend continues, rotations on HPB services may be limited to training programs in larger medical centers which may or may not coincide with programs that train most surgeons who will go on to practice trauma care. In addition, some estimates of the increasing number of HPB fellowship-trained surgeons entering the workforce suggest that an oversupply of HPB surgeons may exist in the near future [17]. How this disparity would affect distribution of cases, hospital volumes, and the operative experience of general surgery residents who will manage injured patients in their career remains to be determined. If an HBP rotation is used to secure this type of training, it is imperative that the trainee be actively involved in important technical aspects of the case. Often such experience is reserved for an HBP trainee who may unfortunately have little interest in or involvement with the management of hepatic injuries.

Future Considerations

The discussion of how to train trauma surgeons to deal with an infrequent yet technically challenging injury has focused primarily on the period of general surgery residency and trauma/critical care fellowship. It cannot be stressed too strongly however that a career in trauma, as with other areas of surgery, requires a strong commitment to lifelong learning and self-education. In order to best serve our patients, it also demands that each surgeon objectively assess his or her own skills and knowledge base so that additional time and effort can be devoted to specific ongoing education in those areas where individual experience has not been extensive. We endorse the concept, as pointed out by Peitzman and Marsh [10], that when dealing with complex liver injuries, the most useful step even for experienced surgeons may be to enlist the assistance of the most experienced set of hands available to assist in these complex cases. The trauma surgeon should not hesitate to rapidly take full advantage of all resources available at their hospital to stop bleeding with these complex injuries before coagulopathy and hypothermia develop. It is equally imperative that maneuvers (such as stapling techniques) utilized in elective hepatic operations should be considered in the treatment of complex liver injuries.

References

1. Richardson JD, Franklin GA, Lukan JK, Carrillo EH, Spain DA, Miller FB, Wilson MA, Polk Jr HC, Flint LM. Evolution in the management of hepatic trauma: a 25 year perspective. Ann Surg. 2000;232:324–30.
2. Richardson JD. Changes in the management of injuries to the liver and spleen. J Am Coll Surg. 2005;200:648–69.

3. Pachter HL. Prometheus bound: evolution in the management of hepatic trauma-from myth to reality. J Trauma. 2012;72:321–9.
4. Tinkoff G, Esposito TJ, Reed J, Kilgo P, Fildes J, Pasquale M, Meredith JW. American Association for the surgery of trauma organ injury scale I: spleen, liver and kidney validation based on the national trauma data bank. J Am Coll Surg. 2008;207:646–55.
5. Jennings GR, Poole GV, Yates NL, Johnson RK, Brock M. Has nonoperative management of solid visceral injuries adversely affected resident operative experience? Am Surg. 2001;67:597–600.
6. Hawkins ML, Wynn JJ, Schmacht DC, Medeiros RS, Gadacz TR. Nonoperative management of liver and/ or splenic injuries: effect on resident surgical experience. Am Surg. 1998;64:552–7.
7. Lucas CE, Ledgerwood AM. The academic challenge of teaching psychomotor skills for hemostasis of solid organ injury. J Trauma. 2009;66:636–40.
8. Buckman Jr RF, Miraliakbari R, Badellino MM. Juxtahepatic venous injuries: a critical review of reported management strategies. J Trauma. 2000;48:978–84.
9. Cogbill TH, Moore EE, Jurkovich GJ, Feliciano DV, Morris JA, Mucha P. Severe hepatic trauma: a multicenter experience with 1,335 liver injuries. J Trauma. 1988;28:1433–8.
10. Peitzman AB, Marsh JW. Advanced operative techniques in the management of complex liver injuries. J Trauma Acute Care Surg. 2012;73:765–70.
11. Gilbody J, Prasthofer AW, Costa ML. The use and effectiveness of cadaver workshops in higher surgical training: a systematic review. Ann R Coll Surg Engl. 2011;93:347–52.
12. Reed AB, Crafton C, Giglia JS, Hutto JD. Back to basics: use of fresh cadavers in vascular surgery training. Surgery. 2009;146:757–63.
13. Juang R, Cook P, Blyth P. A comparison of embalming fluids for use in surgical workshops. Clin Anat. 2011;24:155–61.
14. Acland RD. The inguinal ligament and its lateral attachments: correcting an anatomical error. Clin Anat. 2008;21:55–61.
15. Ahmed N, Chung R. Multiple organ procurement: a tool for teaching operative technique of major vascular control. J Trauma. 2008;65:1093–4.
16. Gonzalez RJ, Barnett Jr CC. A technique for safely teaching major hepatectomy to surgical residents. Am J Surg. 2008;195:521–5.
17. Scarborough JE, Pietrobon R, Bennett KM, Clary BM, Kuo PC, Tyler DS, Pappas TN. Workforce projections for hepato-pancreato-biliary surgery. J Am Coll Surg. 2008;206:678–84.
18. Cofer JB, Adams RB. Fundamentals of liver surgery for the practicing surgeon. Am Surg. 2010;76:461–9.
19. Stain SC, Biester TW, Hanks JB, Ashley SW, Valentine RJ, Bass BL, Buyske J. Early tracking would improve the operative experience of general surgery residents. Ann Surg. 2010;252:445–51.
20. Scarborough JE, Pietrobon R, Clary BM, Marroquin CE, Bennett KM, Kuo PC, Pappas TN. Regionalization of hepatic resections is associated with increasing disparities among some patient populations in use of high-volume providers. J Am Coll Surg. 2008;207:831–8.